Epidemiologic Methods in Physical Activity Studies

Epidemiologic Methods in Physical Activity Studies

Edited by

I-Min Lee
Associate Professor of Medicine
Harvard Medical School
Boston, Massachusetts

SECTION EDITORS

Steven N. Blair
Professor of Exercise Science
Arnold School of Public Health
University of South Carolina
Columbia, South Carolina

JoAnn E. Manson
Professor of Medicine and
the Elizabeth Fay Brigham
Professor of Women's Health
Harvard Medical School
Boston, Massachusetts

Ralph S. Paffenbarger, Jr.
Professor of Epidemiology, Emeritus
Stanford University School of Medicine
Stanford, California

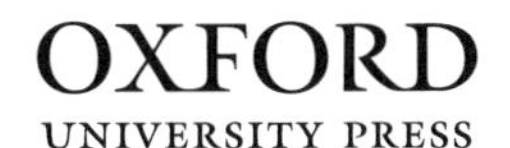

2009

OXFORD
UNIVERSITY PRESS

Oxford University Press, Inc., publishes works that further
Oxford University's objective of excellence
in research, scholarship, and education.

Oxford New York
Auckland Cape Town Dar es Salaam Hong Kong Karachi
Kuala Lumpur Madrid Melbourne Mexico City Nairobi
New Delhi Shanghai Taipei Toronto

With offices in
Argentina Austria Brazil Chile Czech Republic France Greece
Guatemala Hungary Italy Japan Poland Portugal Singapore
South Korea Switzerland Thailand Turkey Ukraine Vietnam

Published by Oxford University Press, Inc.
198 Madison Avenue, New York, New York 10016
www.oup.com

Library of Congress Cataloging-in-Publication Data

Epidemiologic methods in physical activity studies / [edited by] I-Min Lee ... [et al.].
p. ; cm. Includes bibliographical references.
ISBN 978-0-19-518300-9 (cloth)
1. Physical fitness--Health aspects. 2. Epidemiology. I. Lee, I-Min. [DNLM: 1. Physical Fitness.
2. Epidemiologic Methods. 3. Health Status. 4. Motor Activity. QT 255 E64 2008]
RA781.E62 2008 613.7--dc22
2008000397

9 8 7 6 5 4 3 2 1

Printed in the United States of America
on acid-free paper

To the memory of Paff, and to GBK

Preface

The idea that physical activity can be beneficial to health is not new. Ancient texts from China and India dating back as far as 3000 BC refer to exercises developed for health promotion. Hippocrates and Galen, some 2500 years later, also advised that a lack of physical exercise was detrimental to health, further adding that overexertion was unwise (prescient, given recent data on the transient risks of sudden death associated with vigorous exercise, particularly among those habitually sedentary, discussed in Chapter 13). Belief in the health benefits of physical activity apparently continued through the eighteenth century, with the English physician William Heberden describing a patient with angina who "set himself a task of sawing wood for half an hour every day, and was nearly cured." The arrival of the Industrial Revolution with its attendant technological advances and increased productivity, however, allowed mankind to increasingly eschew physical labor for a sedentary way of life. Physical activity no longer seemed favored in the early twentieth century: Henry Ford, father of the modern assembly line, reputedly remarked, "Exercise is bunk; if you are healthy, you don't need it; if you are sick, you shouldn't take it."

As labor-saving developments continued during the twentieth century, chronic diseases—such as coronary heart disease—gained ascendancy. Public health researchers sought reasons for this increase, and there emerged a hypothesis that lack of physical activity may be partly responsible. Following the pioneer investigations of Professor Jerry Morris in Britain (*see* Chapter 1) and Professor Ralph Paffenbarger in the United States (*see* Chapter 6) on coronary heart disease, there has since accumulated a large body of evidence documenting myriad health benefits associated with physical activity. Today, physical activity may be as close to a "magic bullet" that we have for health, decreasing the risks of many chronic diseases and increasing longevity (*see* Chapters 8–12). And so we have come full circle in belief regarding physical activity and health.

Much of the data on the health benefits of physical activity derive from epidemiologic studies. As such research continues, it has become apparent that although standard epidemiologic methods can be used to study the relation between physical activity and health, there are methodologic issues specific to the study of physical activity. Professors Morris and Paffenbarger had already begun to adopt and to adapt standard epidemiologic methods for the study of physical activity more than a half-century ago; over the past one to two decades, refinements of these methods have increased in pace. Previously, a primary question would have been: Does physical activity reduce the risk of this health outcome? Today, with clear evidence that physical activity does, indeed, reduce the risk of many poor health outcomes, research questions now focus on details relevant to public health: what kinds of activity (e.g., moderate- or vigorous-intensity activity? Aerobic or strength-training activity?)

are needed? How much activity—30 or 60 minutes/day? What patterns of activity (e.g., single long bout or multiple short bouts)? Is there a dose–response; if so, what is the shape of the dose–response curve? What genetic influences are there in an individual's response to physical activity? Also, with some urgency, how can we promote physical activity, even as activities of daily living require less and less physical effort? And, how do we monitor trends in physical activity behavior of populations; what activities "count" toward these trends?

The need to document and clarify methodologic issues that arise in epidemiologic studies addressing research questions such as these has been the impetus for this book. The book is intended primarily for researchers investigating physical activity and health—whether those new to epidemiology, or established epidemiologists merely new to the study of physical activity. Additionally, other researchers and professionals using physical activity data—including exercise physiologists, public health researchers and professionals, and health economists—can benefit from understanding how physical activity data are collected, analyzed, and used. Finally, those interested in physical activity and health—including physicians and journalists—who want to understand and appropriately interpret the results from studies of physical activity may find this book useful.

The book is divided into four sections. Chapter 1 provides a historical perspective: it represents the personal observations of Professor Jerry Morris, describing the circumstances and reasoning behind initial investigations of a link between physical activity and risk of coronary heart disease. The second section, encompassing Chapters 2 through 7, covers methodologic issues relevant to epidemiologic studies of physical activity and health. In particular, this section discusses issues to be considered when measuring physical activity and inactivity (Chapter 2) and assessing the reliability and validity of such measurements (Chapter 3); issues relevant to examining dose–response (Chapter 4) and the role of genetics in studies of physical activity and health (Chapter 5); topics to be addressed when designing, conducting, and analyzing data from cohort studies investigating physical activity (Chapter 6); and points to be considered in surveys of physical activity and inactivity (Chapter 7). The third section, encompassing Chapters 8 through 14, provides data on the relationship between physical activity and health outcomes, both beneficial and adverse. Substantive knowledge in this area is rapidly evolving and so these chapters are not intended to provide an exhaustive review of the relationships between physical activity and health. Rather, their aim is to provide current data, at the time of publication, on the association of physical activity with several important health outcomes and to use these data as a springboard to illustrate pertinent methodologic issues that arise. The last section, covering Chapters 15 and 16, describes how physical activity recommendations have evolved over time and the implications (Chapter 15) as well as the methodological concerns to be considered in designing and evaluating interventions to increase physical activity at a population level (Chapter 16).

Finally, I and the section editors, Steven N. Blair, JoAnn E. Manson, and Ralph S. Paffenbarger, Jr., are deeply indebted to the contributors, experts in the field, who have generously shared their expertise and experience in the various chapters. Although much has been learned regarding physical activity and health—both methods of study, as well as knowledge regarding the associations—over the past half-century, it is also patent from the chapters that much remains to be discovered. We thus hope this book will stimulate interest in and continued research on physical activity.

I-Min Lee
Boston, MA
December 2007

Contents

Contributors

BARBARA E. AINSWORTH Department of Exercise and Wellness, Arizona State University, Mesa, Arizona, USA

DAVID R. BASSETT, JR. Department of Exercise, Sport, and Leisure Studies, The University of Tennessee, Knoxville, Tennessee, USA

SHARI S. BASSUK Division of Preventive Medicine, Brigham and Women's Hospital, Harvard Medical School, Boston, Massachusetts, USA

ADRIAN BAUMAN Center for Physical Activity and Health, School of Public Health, University of Sydney, Sydney, Australia

STEVEN N. BLAIR Department of Exercise Science, Arnold School of Public Health, University of South Carolina, Columbia, South Carolina, USA

CLAUDE BOUCHARD Human Genomics Laboratory, Pennington Biomedical Research Center, Baton Rouge, Louisiana, USA

KELLIANN DAVIS Physical Activity and Weight Management Research Center, Department of Health and Physical Activity, University of Pittsburgh, Pittsburgh, Pennsylvania, USA

EUGENE C. FITZHUGH Department of Exercise, Sport, and Leisure Studies, The University of Tennessee, Knoxville, Tennessee, USA

WILLIAM L. HASKELL Stanford Prevention Research Center, Stanford University School of Medicine, Stanford, California, USA

JENNIFER M. HOOTMAN Division of Adult and Community Health, National Center for Chronic Disease Prevention and Health Promotion, Centers for Disease Control and Prevention, Atlanta, Georgia, USA

GANG HU Department of Public Health, University of Helsinki, Department of Health Promotion and Chronic Diseases Prevention, National Public Health Institute, Helsinki, Finland

JOHN M. JAKICIC Physical Activity and Weight Management Research Center, Department of Health and Physical Activity, University of Pittsburgh, Pittsburgh, Pennsylvania, USA

C. DEXTER KIMSEY JR. Division of Nutrition, Physical Activity, and Obesity, National Center for Chronic Disease Prevention and Health Promotion, Centers for Disease Control and Prevention, Atlanta, Georgia, USA

HAROLD W. KOHL III Division of Epidemiology and Department of Kinesiology and Health Education, University of Texas School of Public Health and University of Texas, Austin, Texas, USA

ANDREA M. KRISKA Department of Epidemiology, Graduate School of Public Health, University of Pittsburgh, Pittsburgh, Pennsylvania, USA

TIMO A. LAKKA Department of Physiology, Institute of Biomedicine, University of Kuopio, Kuopio Research Institute of Exercise Medicine, Kuopio, Finland, USA

MICHAEL J. LAMONTE Department of Social and Preventive Medicine, University at Buffalo, The State University of New York, Buffalo, New York, USA

I-MIN LEE Division of Preventive Medicine, Brigham and Women's Hospital, Harvard Medical School, Boston, Massachusetts, USA

JOANN E. MANSON Division of Preventive Medicine, Brigham and Women's Hospital, Harvard Medical School, Boston, Massachusetts, USA

JERRY MORRIS Public & Environmental Health Research Unit, Department of Public Health and Policy, London School of Hygiene and Tropical Medicine, London, United Kingdom

AMY D. OTTO Physical Activity and Weight Management Research Center, Department of Health and Physical Activity, University of Pittsburgh, Pittsburgh, Pennsylvania, USA

RALPH S. PAFFENBARGER, JR. (1922–2007) Division of Epidemiology, Department of Health Research and Policy, Stanford University School of Medicine, Stanford, California, USA

KELLEY K. PETTEE Department of Exercise and Wellness, Arizona State University, Mesa, Arizona, USA

PHILAYRATH PHONGSAVAN Center for Physical Activity and Health, School of Public Health, University of Sydney, Sydney, Australia

KRISTEN POLZIEN Physical Activity and Weight Management Research Center, Department of Health and Physical Activity, University of Pittsburgh, Pittsburgh, Pennsylvania, USA

KENNETH E. POWELL Epidemiology and Public Health Consultant, Atlanta, Georgia, USA

TUOMO RANKINEN Human Genomics Laboratory, Pennington Biomedical Research Center, Baton Rouge, Louisiana, USA

JACOB SATTELMAIR Department of Epidemiology, Harvard School of Public Health, Boston, Massachusetts, USA

BARBARA STERNFELD Division of Research, Kaiser Permanente, Oakland, California, USA

KRISTI L. STORTI Department of Epidemiology, Graduate School of Public Health, University of Pittsburgh, Pittsburgh, Pennsylvania, USA

JAAKKO TUOMILEHTO Department of Public Health, University of Helsinki, Department of Health Promotion and Chronic Diseases Prevention, National Public Health Institute, Helsinki, Finland

Epidemiologic Methods in Physical Activity Studies

1

Physical Activity Versus Heart Attack: a Modern Epidemic

Personal Observations

Jerry Morris

Returning eagerly to civil life after the long years of World War II, health researchers found an unusually favorable situation. Notably, we were presented with a major Public Health challenge: heart attack/myocardial infarction (MI), a serious, often fatal condition, newly common during the century and evidently increasing, that had been quite little investigated! Little was known of its etiology, nothing that could be applied in prevention.

Such was the situation as Keys and colleagues in Minneapolis, the Framingham initiative in Boston, we in Britain, and several others, embarked on *population* studies—we evidently were dealing with *mass* situations—from our various perspectives. In my case it was *social epidemiology* cum *clinical medicine*; I had been a privileged personal student of the great Thomas Lewis.

The first investigation by the Medical Research Council's Social Medicine Unit in this field was historical. I examined the basis of it all: the condition of the coronary arteries and myocardium, in middle and early old age, as this was *routinely* recorded in *every* (NB "every") *post mortem* examination from 1907 to 1949 at the London Hospital, that famed academic center serving its large East End population. It was this mode of recording instituted by Professor Turnbull that I felt permitted some extrapolation to the general population, and 1907 to 1949 were the years that saw the emergence of heart attack to national and international eminence. After interminable hours with the *post mortem* folios, the main findings were a steep rise over those years of reports of *fresh coronary thrombosis* and of *acute MI* associated with this or with evidence of *previous thrombosis* in men; this finding was rather less in women and was from very low bases in both. Unexpectedly, and despite intensive search, I could find no indication of increase during the period in the underlying coronary atherosclerosis that was prevalent throughout (Morris, 1951; Meade, 2001).[1]

The multiple indications in clinical experience, vital statistics, medical examiners' reports, and such pathology, of a new and serious *population* hazard, the rise of coronary thrombosis and myocardial infarction (MI), was of course particularly challenging for us in *social* medicine "for causes may be discoverable in changing ways of living, in people who

[1] I tried to repeat this study elsewhere but failed to locate another hospital/pathology department with the crucial *routine post mortem* recording of coronary arteries and myocardium at every *post mortem* in Britain, and failing also at the Massachusetts General Hospital and Johns Hopkins.

are changing in a changing environment" (Morris, 1951). It appeared that this ancient disease had been mutating from relative obscurity into the "modern epidemic" of heart attack … And half-a-century later it is plausible to attribute some of this transformation to mass decline in physical activity in work, getting about, recreation, and the home—technological/social/behavioral shifts of the twentieth century—and to the biologic maladjustments in response.

Mapping Population Incidence

In 1948 we set about assessing for the first time morbidity of coronary heart disease (CHD) across the population for the first time—"bliss was it in that time to be alive"! We aimed to provide some basic Public Health data to complement the national mortality statistics. Choice of sentinel indicator of CHD was critical. Three were on offer: incidence, attack rate, and prevalence. Which was likeliest to be revealing also on possible causes? Unqualified prevalence surely least. But Bradford Hills' text (1942), our bible that I knew inside out, did not distinguish "incidence"—the *first*—from *other* attack, thus producing an overall "attack rate". Our previous *clinical* experience decided us in favor of *incidence* because the diagnosis of CHD could itself lead to changes in ways of living, possibly losing any such *prior* associations with occurrence of the disease. Hopefully, that this was 1947/1948 will excuse such simplicities. Incidence was defined as *any first clinical manifestation (episode) of CHD.*

At the time, we had a "hunch" that CHD, and its main presentation MI, might be related to occupation: the condition manifestly was more common in men than women and in middle age than younger men, there was Osler on angina, and there were hints in the Registrar General's national death rates.

So we began to explore CHD incidence in men across a wide range of occupations: two professions, medical practitioners and schoolteachers; a large group of factory workers; a variety of grades in London Transport; the nation's postmen; and miscellaneous office workers in several departments across government—large organizations with developed Occupational Health Services that were keen to participate in our studies. All possibly relevant sickness data, reporting from the new universal National Health Service (General primary care Practitioners and hospital specialist Consultants) and through Occupational Health, were assembled by our Unit with multiple clinical and statistical checks, and all death certificates, including those *via* the Coroner (Medical Examiner) and his pathologist.

"Natural Experiment"?

During 1949, the first year of these studies, a pattern emerged in the first comprehensive data-set to be established—that for the two men doing different jobs on London Transport's double-decker buses: the *driver* self-evidently sedentary and the *conductor* unavoidably active. The main feature was fewer first clinical manifestations of CHD in the conductors and, in particular, fewer "sudden deaths" without preceding sickness absence. Some months later, an astonishingly similar pattern emerged through government medical services in the national populations of *postmen* vs. three grades of *office staff* in the postal service and across Departments; there were of course also multiple social differences within these. It may be recalled that those were difficult days for everyone (Kynaston, 2007).

The illustration in Table 1.1 extends to the first 4 years' data of this most serious (dysrhythmic?) of acute coronary syndromes, *sudden death as first clinical manifestation.*

Table 1.1 Fatal Incidence of CHD 1949–52

	Age-Standardized Rates per 1000/year	
	"Sudden death" in first clinical episode[1]	*Deaths later, within first 3 months of first episode*
Men ages 35–64		
Conductors	0.5	0.3
Drivers	1.1	0.5
Men ages 35–59		
Postmen	0.4	0.3
Telephonists	0.8	0.6

[1] Technically defined as deaths without preceding sickness absence. Many were medical examiner's (Coroner's) cases. There will of course also be deaths after 3 months.
Subjects were London busmen, British postmen, and male Government telephonists, mainly in Security and Foreign Office.

(Data from Morris et al., 1953.)

It proved to be the main occupational difference and was greater in early than later middle age. Overall, non-fatal as well as fatal incidence figures showed a similar trend, although it was not as strong.

The contrast in *physical activity* in these occupational groupings straightaway appealed a likelier explanation to us than more nebulous psychological "stress" or social variation that indeed had previously stumped us in our first occupational observation: higher CHD incidence in General Practitioners than in hospital Consultants and other doctors (Morris et al., 1952). After often heated debate among ourselves and discussions with busmen, their managers and Union officials, a sample of postmen, and Treasury (Government) Medical Service personnel, and in face of much collegial skepticism (except among the physiologists), we chose to focus on physical activity and to reorganize accordingly. With regret, I have to record that unlike the United States, British cardiology was quite uninterested in what we were doing. For example, when we published, Paul White telephoned for a long and searching discussion, and Jim Watt, Head of the National Heart Institute of Health, flew over... We became personal and family friends with both.[2]

Follow-up of Physical Activity

How do we now proceed? Clinically, we knew that *hypertension* and *diabetes* affected CHD, and the notion of *selection* was also familiar from experience of the effects of illness on mode of life, including occupation ("reverse causality"/"survival bias"?), as previously recalled. But surely, we felt, there must be more to this *newly* widespread affliction, and the possibility of some protection against it by physical activity, than such ancient lore?

More pressing, we had arrived, unexpectedly and unprepared, at the classic issue: how to test a causal hypothesis by *observation* and without planned *experiment*—"dealing," as we put it at the time, "with material impossible to control." NB this was 1950, 1951.

[2] It may be worth mentioning that 1949/1950 preceded the mass immigration from the Caribbean, and a spot-check showed that virtually all the busmen, drivers, and conductors smoked, although I can't now recall why we looked at this.

We had little epidemiology to guide us, no formulation yet of the pitfalls of "confounding", "life course", "risk factors", "randomized trials". The several innovative cardiovascular population studies indeed were a major contributor to the focused chronic disease epidemiology that was emerging (e.g., Morris, 1957, 1964, 1975). The only strategy available was to exploit the potential of *observation* as best we could by making as many, and as different, approaches as possible, "depending on the power of simultaneous attack... from different directions... using independent bodies of material... testing the provisional hypothesis by observing the capacity to predict in a variety of situations..." (Morris et al., 1953).

Too many opportunities were on offer... Clinical survey of CHD from ruptured heart at one extreme to unnoticed angina at the other... pathological survey... comprehensive statistics in young and old... and, of course, physical activity of occupation vs. exercise in leisure time. There is no mention in the records of observing the disease in women. That indeed today is an incomprehensible "blank" in our studies.

Our first published report, not until the end of 1953 (to much media speculation on a possible "cause" that I had no idea how to handle) and including a precautionary repeat of the original observations, also detailed two different approaches, both of which extended as well as tested the main initial finding. In one, independent experts in Occupational Health classified all the men in several years of national mortality statistics by the physical activity entailed in the occupation on the death certificate, and we analyzed "blind" the rates certified to CHD—which of course also included deaths in a later, rather than the first, clinical episode. The other test postulated that physically active workers do not merely suffer less CHD but, as suggested in the experience of conductors and postmen, *less severe* disease, age for age, presenting more often as angina. Both tests yielded favorable results (i.e., as "predicted").

Evidence in Men's Hearts

We next sought to combine two of our previous approaches in a sample survey across Britain, after much consultation (that was highly educational) of *pathology* of coronary disease by physical activity of occupation. Virtually the entire national specialist Pathology–Morbid Anatomy community participated; they were much intrigued by our approach (unlike the clinicians previously – why?). The issue raised was whether it was possible to identify signs in the hearts of men of the kind of work they had done, particularly the physical activity that had been entailed. There were problems again regarding the validity of the occupation on death certificate as an indicator of mode of life: ill health as said before can lead to change of occupation. However, examination of the occupational histories of Doll and Bradford Hill's grand representative series (which they kindly made available in 1954) revealed unexpectedly little such change. Moreover, changes most likely to affect our hypothesis—a move from heavy to lighter work—would *attenuate* any protection against CHD by active occupation and thus were not so worrying.

Table 1.2 provides the main findings in those simple pre-angiography days. They focus on the necropsies we regarded as likely to provide the most valid account of the general population—the "non-coronary", "non-vascular", deaths ascribed to injuries, infections, cancers. There were two interesting trends. What the morbid-anatomists recognized as *ischemic myocardial fibrosis* was more common in the lighter occupations, particularly the occasional scars of large healed (possibly silent) infarcts. So, too, was complete or near-complete *occlusion of a main coronary artery*, but not the *overall prevalence* of plaques (Morris and Crawford, 1958).

Table 1.2 National Sample of Coronary Artery and Myocardial Disease at *Post Mortem* in Men, Ages 45–70 Years, Britain 1956

	Rates (Percent)		
Physical Activity of Occupation at Death			
	Heavy	*Moderate*	*Light*
Coronary atherosclerosis	82	82	85
Much coronary atherosclerosis as defined	14.6	15	15.7
Complete, or near-complete occlusion of main coronary artery	2.5	3.0	3.7
Ischemic myocardial fibrosis	4.8	6.3	9.2

Based on 2697 "non-coronary," "non-vascular" deaths, those certified to injuries, infections, cancers, etc.
The age distribution in the three occupation groups was similar.

(Data in Morris and Crawford, 1958.)

Body Mass, Uniforms: Selection?

During the 1950s and 1960s, we made sample surveys with the busmen, our friends by now, regarding physique, lipids, blood pressure, lifestyles, including aspects of diet (confirming higher kcal/kg body mass in the conductors [Morris et al., 1977]); and assorted attitudes. Disappointingly, practical technology for population study of thrombogenesis (i.e., not requiring admission to hospital) wasn't available, despite much interest among laboratory experts.

CHD was being related to obesity, and drivers manifestly were fatter, from their entry to the job. Study of *uniform sizes* in the two occupations—for example, the trouser waistband (validated clinically)—illustrated this. But slim, average, or portly (the tailors' *patois*) conductors suffered fewer CHD "sudden deaths" than comparable drivers—the main occupational advantage previously found (Heady et al., 1961). Concern in those days, long before formulation of the "metabolic syndrome" (e.g., Reaven, 1995), was already with waist circumference and the emerging significance of central adiposity (e.g., the apples and pears).

Culture—Biology

The next step was to assemble a small representative cohort of busmen from 1956 to 1960 and to follow this up for incidence of CHD from 1960 to 1965. The importance of levels of casual systolic blood pressure and, crucially, plasma cholesterol (supplemented later with β-lipoprotein low-density lipoprotein cholesterol and low-density Sf fractions) emerged in the two occupations. Both factors, age-for-age, were higher in drivers, and they accounted statistically for much of their higher CHD attack rate (Morris et al., 1966). This was an effort at deliberate joint study of the main current approaches to etiology of CHD—in counterpoint of the social/behavioral and the biologic—i.e., lifestyles such as physical activity together with the physiologic, metabolic "risk factors" that were being identified in clinical cases by the Framingham and other studies.

Recreational Exercise Versus Coronary Heart Disease

Such was the pace of technologic change—so evident in men's work—that by the early 1960s it was becoming clear that any material contribution of physical activity to Public Health would have to be through *exercise in leisure time*. The historic studies of Paffenbarger et al. (Paffenbarger et al., 1970; Paffenbarger and Hale, 1975) and others supported an occupational activity hypothesis (e.g., Karvonen, 1981). Methods of assessing *non-occupational* exercise are becoming more objective and accurate (Brage et al., 2005), and cf. the present volume. Our own main effort that we believed valid enough, reproducible, and acceptable was laborious and too expensive (Yasin et al., 1967). Nevertheless, in 1968, we mounted a prospective incidence study of 18,000 middle-age men in a lower management grade of government service nationwide. The by now familiar army of clerks was mobilized and trained... those halcyon pre-computer days!

Our hypothesis, derived from the occupational and pathology studies, stated that high totals of activity would provide some protection against CHD. But there was no evidence of this in 8.5 years of follow-up. Instead, and essentially, men engaging in vigorous (as defined) "sports" experienced fewer attacks than the rest. Other men age 50–65 years who reported heavy recreational "work" also showed some benefit, but not those initially 40–49 years (Morris et al., 1980).

This was disappointing indeed, especially the unwelcome intimation that in formulating our hypothesis we hadn't paid due heed to signals in the *nature* as well as the *quantity* of the hypothetical protective activity of bus conductors and postmen—forever *climbing stairs*, the hours and hours of *walking*.

How do we respond? Do we accept the new and unexpected observation as a possible step forward for Public Health or directly *test* it in a new *ad hoc* survey? The opportunity costs of any such survey would be formidable indeed for our modest Research Unit. There was no hope of salvation in experiment.

After seemingly endless deliberation, we decided to proceed with a fresh survey to directly test the new hypothesis using a different method to gather far more information on both nature and amount and accompaniments of the physical activity being reported. Whatever this found, it would hopefully be a clearer message for the science to Public Health and to the public. Table 1.3 reports the main results. Two messages were clear in intensive study of the new data.

First, *current and ongoing dynamic aerobic exercise*, likely to reach *7.5 kcal/min* (6 METS) alone consistently showed some protection against heart attack. We were unable to identify any benefit in CHD incidence from any and all other activity, including the vast amount of recreational "work", even heavy work, reported.

Second, this observation withstood everything that we were able to throw at it over the years. In large and small studies, singly or in combination, we explored possible confounding in family history, smoking, Body Mass Index, aspects of diet, personal history of exercise from childhood, other physical activity, total energy expenditure, medical history and multiple disease associations, total mortality, attitudes to exercise, to health, to life! As indicated, we couldn't study thrombogenesis (Morris et al., 1990; Morris, 1996).

Exercise, Training, and Fitness?

The 7.5 kcal/min of dynamic aerobic exercise, much discussed with physiologist friends, would be likely to yield a "training" effect in such a population of healthy and, it may be postulated, average-sized 70-kg middle-aged, sedentary workers. The 7.5 kcal/min ≡ 6 METS ≡ 21.6 ml Kg^{-1} min^{-1} O_2. To be sustainable, it may further be suggested that such

Table 1.3 Total Incidence of Coronary Heart Disease in 9376 men, Ages 45–64 Years, Followed An Average of 9.3 Years, 1976–1986, Britain

<table>
<tr><th></th><th colspan="3">Age-Standardized Rates per 1000 Man-Years</th></tr>
<tr><th>Times*</th><th>Reporting vigorous sports[1]</th><th>Non-vigorous sports[2]</th><th>Heavy work[3]</th></tr>
<tr><td>0</td><td>5.8</td><td>5.4</td><td>5.5</td></tr>
<tr><td>1–3</td><td>4.5</td><td>5.9</td><td>5.6</td></tr>
<tr><td>4–7</td><td>4.1</td><td>5.9</td><td>5.5</td></tr>
<tr><td>8–11</td><td rowspan="2">2.1</td><td>3.5</td><td>4.2</td></tr>
<tr><td>≥12</td><td>6.9</td><td>5.5</td></tr>
<tr><td></td><td>$p < 0.005$</td><td>NS</td><td>NS</td></tr>
</table>

*Spells of sports, hours of heavy work, in past 4 weeks.
Subjects were executive grade civil servants with no history or record of CHD. Nationwide sample.
[1]Liable to reach peaks of energy expenditure of 7.5 kcal/minute (6 METS).
For example, swimming, racket games, jogging, football and hockey (mainly coaching, refereeing), hill-climbing. Also fast walking (over 6.4 km/hour) and defined much cycling.
[2]For example, golf, ballroom dancing, table tennis, and specified long walks, less cycling.
[3]The heaviest jobs about the house, garden, and on the car. For example, moving furniture, concreting, shifting earth, heavy digging, rusty repairs.
Our second cohort study (1976 et seq).

(Data in Morris et al., 1990.)

exercise would have to be no more than about half of individual VO_2 max. Therefore, that could be proposed as in the low 40ies of mL/kg/min—that is, in the upper reaches of national sample figures averaging about 39 mL/kg/min—that later became available in our National Fitness Survey (and Canadian figures were similar).

The absence of any indication of benefit from the "heavy work" of Table 1.3 and numerous other analyses also focused attention on *dynamic aerobic* activity against the typically more *static resistance* effort entailed in such "work".

This raises the further issue of whether it is the apparently beneficial exercise that is effective or, plausibly, the training and resultant *physical fitness* (Williams, 2001). We could not take this crucial question further.

Hoist With Our Own Petard?

Another concern surfaced: Was our intensively studied civil service population, so narrowly homogenous, so selected to exclude "noise" of income, locality, education, class, that any generalization from it must be suspect? They were also a "healthy worker" cohort, and our experience of Government personnel medical service indicated this was no formality. Less expected by other than U.K. readers: 91% of our men were gardeners, typical of this stratum of the middle class. "It's what keeps us sane", they repeatedly told us. And the gardening often was altogether more serious than the common U.S. "yard work", and so forth. (Paffenbarger et al., numerous communications over the years). Multiple standardizing for the amount, nature, and effort of this manual "work" didn't tell us anything. But the effect so much miscellaneous recreational activity had on our total picture—creating a population not basically sedentary—and therefore demanding the additional high 7.5 kcal/min level for specific CHD benefit (Haskell, 2005). This might also account for the discrepancy between our experience and the common finding elsewhere that *moderate* and *total activity* levels also can be protective (Lee, 2004). We were unable to identify an analogous population study for comparison. (An independent proposal by the leading University Department of Exercise Science for physiologic study of middle-aged men, including busmen, postmen, and office staff couldn't be funded.) But again, confluence on the main issue of so many and so various worldwide studies, each with its own unwelcome selection bias, hopefully provides some reassurance against critical negative confounding (Powell et al., 1987).

Observation and Experiment

It seems worth venturing, perhaps as prompt for a seminar, that the three principal lifestyle etiologies of CHD—diet, smoking, and physical activity—all originated and remain dependent on *observation*, explicated and reinforced now in a wealth of *experiment* (e.g., the present volume; Orma, 1957).

National Fitness

During the second half of the 1980s, I devoted half my working time in this field to the analyses of the civil servants' study and half to the English National Fitness Survey (previously mentioned) that was executed in 1990. Inspired by the pioneer Canadian experience, the English scientific community determined to do even better, and I hope that our reports are in your library (Main Report, 1992; Technical Report, 1994). They are a model production, I feel entitled to claim, designed to appeal also to our political lords and masters. Alas, they were familiarly uninterested, an experience of rejection it is scant consolation by no means unique to the U.K. Table 1.4 illustrates how we have also sought to express the laboratory physiologic data in everyday terms that all could appreciate (Morris and Hardman, 1997).

Table 1.4 Proportions in 1990 of an English National Population Sample (n = 2699), By Age and Sex, Who Can *Comfortably Sustain Walking for 1.6 km* at 4.8 km/hour on the Level (*a "Basic" Fitness Level*), and on a Slope of 1 in 20 (*a "Desirable" Fitness Target*).*

Age (y)	*Men (%)*	*Women (%)*
Walking comfortably at 4.8 km/hour on the level		
25–34	98	88
35–44	92	81
45–54	91	62
55–64	70	51
Walking comfortably at 4.8 km/hour on a slope of 1 in 20, or at 6.4 km/hour on the level		
25–34	89	51
35–44	77	32
45–54	57	19
55–64	30	9

*"Comfortably"—that is, without exceeding 70% of maximal heart rate.

(Data of English National Fitness Survey; Morris and Hardman, 1997.)

This work was done before the current increase of interest in "fitness" among the *clinical* community—in direct translation from the physiology and epidemiology. Such are its diagnostic and predictive possibilities that regular inclusion of fitness-testing by treadmill or cycle into clinical practice is beginning to be realistic (e.g., Kraus and Douglas, 2005). In England, on the other hand, we have been piloting a relatively simple step-test, suitable also for routine local Public Health practice. Hopefully, usable results can be provided in 2008.

Personal Perspective

Anti-Aging?

The health community may, at last, be onto a winner. After decades of scant success in persuading people to be more active, response to the global alarm on obesity is gloomily awaited (the possible contribution also vs. climate change may help). I wonder if the *anti-aging* potentials of exercise could now be some *personal* answer, regardless of the commonly discouraging *environment?* Gains in *older age* from exercise are plain, the fruit of epochal physiologic research: in cardiovascular and overall fitness, muscle mass and strength, joint-stability and balance; and there are encouraging hints on the brain. We can thereby be more optimistic about the ubiquitous "deconditioning", "physical decay" of older age—greater personal mobility, weight control, the limiting of disability, in social participation, better sleep possibly, and thus about "well-being," autonomy, and even the fashionable "happiness"! Apparently, improvement in quality of living can realistically be achieved even from exercise *started in* old age (Young and Dinan, 2000). As older people experience longer life, "extra time" (life expectancy in United States at 65 years in 1970 = 15.2 years, in 2003 = 18.4 years), older people themselves surely have specific contributions to make: first is *self-care* in the multiple prevalent chronic disabilities (some related to previous physical *in*activity), and second we now can also, in some measure, *counter the actual processes* of aging—reduce them and retrieve. When Roth the master mourns (2006) that old age is not a battle but a massacre, is he not plain wrong? But what an uphill task for us, the health community.

And another hopefully familiar thought.

Evolution?

We in the West are the first generations in human history in which the mass of the population has to deliberately exercise to be healthy. How can society's *collective* adaptations match? And again, what are our responsibilities in the health community?

ACKNOWLEDGMENT My respects and gratitude to fellow workers across the world and to my colleagues and comrades over so many years. The principal investigators in the studies of the MRC Social Medicine Unit are listed as the authors of publications below.

References

Bradford Hill A. *Principles of Medical Statistics.* 3rd Ed. London: The Lancet Ltd. 1942.

Brage S, Brage N, Franks PW, Ekelund V, Wareham NJ. 2005. Reliability and validity of the combined heart and movement sensor Actiheart. *Eur J Clin Nutr* 59:561–70.

Haskell WL. Addition to Chapter 19. In M Marmot & P Elliot (Eds.), *Coronary heart disease epidemiology: from aetiology to public health.* 2nd ed. Oxford: Oxford University Press, 2005.

Heady JA, Morris JN, Kagan A, Raffle PAB. 1961. Coronary heart disease in London busmen: a progress report with particular reference to physique. *Br J Prev Soc Med* 15: 143–53.

Karvonen MJ. 1981. Occupation, daily activities and leisure as sources of fitness and health. *Hermes (Leuven)* 15: 303–23.

Kraus WE, Douglas PS. 2005. Where does fitness fit in? *N Engl J Med* 353: 517–9.

Kynaston D. Austerity Britain: 1945–51. London: Bloomsbury, 2007.

Lee I-M. 2004. No pain, no gain? Thoughts on the Caerphilly Study. *Br J Sports Med* 38: 4–5.

Meade TW. 2001. Cardiovascular disease—linking pathology and epidemiology. *Int J Epidemiol* 30: 1179–83.

Morris JN. 1951. Recent history of coronary disease. *Lancet* I: 1–7, 69–73.

Morris JN, Heady JA, Barley RG. 1952. Coronary heart disease in medical practitioners. *BMJ* I: 503–20.

Morris JN, Heady JA, Raffle PAB, Roberts CG, Parks JW. 1953. Coronary heart disease and physical activity of work. *Lancet* II: 1053–7, 111–20.

Morris JN. *Uses of Epidemiology*. 1st Ed. 1957, 2nd Ed. 1964, 3rd Ed. 1975. Edinburgh & London: Churchill, Livingstone.

Morris JN, Crawford MD. 1958. Coronary heart disease and physical activity of work: evidence of a national necropsy survey. *BMJ* II: 1485–96.

Morris JN, Pattison DC, Gardner MJ, Raffle PAB. 1966. Incidence and prediction of ischaemic heart disease in London busmen. *Lancet* II: 553–9.

Morris JN, Marr JW, Clayton DG. 1977. Diet and Heart: a postscript. *BMJ* II: 1307–14.

Morris JN, Everitt MG, Pulland R, Chave SP, Semmence AM. 1980. Vigorous exercise in leisure time: protection against coronary heart disease. *Lancet* II: 1207–10.

Morris JN, Clayton DG, Everitt MG, Semmence AM, Burgess EH. 1990. Exercise in leisure-time: coronary attack and death rate. *Br Heart J* 63: 325–34.

Morris JN. 1996. Exercise versus heart attack: questioning the consensus. *Research Quart Exercise Sport* 67: 216–20.

Morris JN, Hardman AE. 1997. Walking to health. *Sports Med* 23: 306–332; 24: 96.

National Fitness Survey: Main Findings. Morris JN, Hoinville G, Fentem P. London: Sports Council and Health Education Authority, 1992.

National Fitness Survey: Technical Report. Fentem P, Collins M, Tuxworth W, Walker A. London: Sports Council and Health Education Authority, 1994.

Orma EJ. 1957. Effect of physical activity on athero-genesis: an experimental study in cockerels. *Acta Physiol Scand* 41 (Suppl): 142.

Paffenbarger RS, Laughlin ME, Gima AS, Black RA. 1970. Work activity of longshoremen as related to death from coronary heart disease and stroke. *N Engl J Med* 282: 1109–14.

Paffenbarger RS, Hale WE. 1975. Work activity and coronary heart mortality. *N Engl J Med* 292: 545–50.

Powell KE, Thompson PD, Caspersen CJ, Kendrick JS. 1987. Physical activity and the incidence of coronary heart disease. *Ann Rev Public Health* 8: 253–87.

Reaven GM. 1995. Characteristics of metabolic syndrome X. *Endocrinol Metabol* 2 (Suppl B): 37–42.

Roth P, Everyman. Boston: Houghton Mifflin, 2006.

Williams PT. 2001. Physical fitness and activity as separate heart disease risk factors: a meta-analysis. *Med Sci Sports Exerc* 33: 754–61.

Yasin S, Alderson MR, Marr JW, Pattison DC, Morris JN. 1967. Assessment of habitual physical activity apart from occupation. *Br J Prev Soc Med* 21: 163–9.

Young A, Dinan S. Active in later life. In G McLatchie, M Harries, C Williams, & J King (Eds.), ABC of Sport Medicine. 2nd ed. London: BMJ Books, 2000.

I

Epidemiologic Methods

2 Measurement of Physical Activity and Inactivity in Epidemiologic Studies

Kelley K. Pettee, Kristi L. Storti,
Barbara E. Ainsworth, and
Andrea M. Kriska

Due to the physiological links between physical activity/inactivity and many chronic diseases, past and present public health researchers have been incorporating physical activity into the methodological design of many research efforts (USDHHS, 1996). Physical activity is often measured to determine the association between activity and the development of a particular disease. Physical activity can also be assessed as part of an intervention strategy to eliminate or improve the burden of disease at both the individual and population level. As more investigators incorporate physical activity assessment and/or intervention in their public health efforts, a tremendous need arises for a better understanding of how to assess physical activity accurately across a variety of settings and populations.

Physical activity is a complex behavior, and selecting the proper assessment tool(s) is challenging, particularly among free-living populations. The lack of a reasonable gold standard measure and inconsistent use of physical activity terminology have contributed to the confusion in this field. Measurement is further complicated by the fact that there are several health-related dimensions of physical activity (Caspersen, 1989), which may require the use of different assessment tools. The qualitative difference among the various dimensions of physical activity contributes to the diversity in the biological mechanisms underlying the relationship of physical activity with specific diseases and, therefore, influences how physical activity should be assessed. When examining the relationship between physical activity and a disease or condition, it is important to focus on the dimension(s) of physical activity that is most likely to be associated with the specific outcome of interest (for additional discussion, *see* Chapter 4).

Definition and Terms

Energy expenditure is defined as the exchange of energy required to perform biological work. Components of total energy expenditure include basal metabolic rate (which typically encompasses 50%–70% of total energy), the thermic effect of food (TEF, which accounts for another 7%–10%), and physical activity (Ravussin, 1992). Physical activity is the most variable component of total energy expenditure and includes structured (sports, leisure, transportation, and occupational activity) and non-structured activities (housework, childcare, and activities of daily living). Physical activity as a variable component of the total energy expenditure is greater for active individuals compared to their sedentary counterparts.

Although similar, the terms physical activity and exercise have different meanings. Physical activity is defined as any bodily movement produced by skeletal muscles that result in increased energy expenditure (Caspersen, 1985). Therefore, activities such as housework, gardening, occupational, and recreational activity may all be considered types of physical activity. On the other hand, exercise is defined as planned, structured, and repetitive bodily movements done to improve or maintain one or more components of physical fitness and is usually associated with sport or conditioning activities (Caspersen, 1985). When differentiating between the two, exercise is a type of physical activity, but not all physical activity is considered exercise (Table 2.1).

Table 2.1 Definitions of Terms Related to the Assessment of Physical Activity

Term	Definition
Basal metabolic rate	The number of kilocalories your body needs to properly function while at rest (Ravussin, 1992).
Duration	The dimension of physical activity referring to the amount of time (e.g., minutes, hours, days) an activity is performed.
Energy expenditure	The total exchange of energy required to perform a specific type of biological work. Often used to express the *volume of physical activity* performed during a defined time frame. (Ravussin, 1992)
Exercise	Planned, structured, and repetitive bodily movement done to improve or maintain one or more components of physical fitness. Exercise is a specific subcategory of physical activity (Caspersen, 1985)
Frequency	The dimension of physical activity referring to how often an activity is performed. Frequency is often expressed over a defined time frame (e.g., how many times per week).
Intensity	The dimension of physical activity referring to the level of effort or physiological demand required to perform the activity (e.g., how hard is the activity).
Kilocalories (kcal)	Used to express the energy expended during physical activity. Physical activity can be expressed as the amount of kilocalories expended over a given period of time, such as per week (kcals/week).
Metabolic equivalent (MET)	A unit used to estimate the metabolic cost (oxygen consumption) of physical activity. One MET equals the resting metabolic rate of approximately 3.5 mL of $O_2 \cdot kg^{-1} minute^{-1}$, or 1 kcal $\cdot kg^{-1} hour^{-1}$. Often expressed as METs per minute (MET-minutes) or METs per hour (MET-hours).
Mode	The dimension of physical activity that identifies the specific type of activity (e.g., walking, weight lifting, gardening, housework) being performed.
Physical activity	Any bodily movement produced by skeletal muscles that results in energy expenditure (Caspersen, 1985)
Physical fitness	A set of attributes (e.g., muscle fitness [strength and endurance], cardiorespiratory fitness, flexibility, body composition) that people have or achieve that relate to the ability to perform physical activity (Caspersen, 1985).
Thermic effect of food	The number of kilocalories your body uses digesting food (Ravussin, 1992).
Total energy expenditure	Components of total energy expenditure include basal metabolic rate, which typically encompasses 50–70% of total energy, and the thermic effect of food, which accounts for another 7–10% (Ravussin, 1992).

Physical activity is often quantified in terms of the frequency, duration, intensity, and type of activity performed. Frequency is often defined as the number of sessions or days per week or month an activity is performed. The duration usually refers to the time (in minutes or hours) spent in one bout of a specific activity. Intensity refers to the level of effort required to perform a specific activity and is often expressed in terms of metabolic equivalents (METs), which are defined as the ratio of the energy cost of an activity divided by the energy cost of the resting metabolic rate (RMR; 1 MET). One MET is roughly equivalent to 1 kilocalorie per kilogram body weight per hour (1 kcal/kg/hour) (Taylor, 1978). Physical activity is often expressed as time per week or can be weighted by an estimate of intensity and expressed as MET-time/week (MET-hours/week or MET-minutes/week). This summary variable is created by multiplying the appropriate weighted MET value for each activity (Ainsworth, 2000b) by the amount of time spent performing that specific activity during a given week (Table 2.1).

Objective Measures of Energy Expenditure

Energy expenditure due to physical activity comprises a complex series of biochemical processes that result in the transfer of metabolic energy to drive skeletal muscle contraction (Brooks, 1996). A large amount of heat energy is produced during the coupling of energy transfer and skeletal muscle contraction and is directly proportional to the net activity-related energy expenditure. Energy expenditure can be directly quantified by measuring body heat at rest or during exercise (Jequier, 1987; Montoye, 1996). The oxidation of food substrates is a primary source of energy production at rest, during activity, and following physical activity. Based on some assumptions about the energy cost of the specific substrate oxidized, activity-related energy expenditure can be indirectly estimated by measuring the fractional concentrations of expired carbon dioxide and oxygen at rest or during physical activity (Brooks, 1996; Jequier, 1987; Montoye, 1996). Laboratory and field methods exist for these direct (e.g., room calorimetry) and indirect measures of energy expenditure (e.g. ventilatory gas exchange detected by indirect calorimetry).

Direct Measures of Energy Expenditure

Direct Calorimetry

The measurement of body heat production is known as direct calorimetry and is the most precise measure of energy expenditure (Brooks, 1996; Jequier, 1987; Horton, 1983; Montoye, 1996). Calorimetry is typically performed under laboratory conditions with the individual in an airtight chamber. Measurements are typically made over a 24-hour period and follow a 10- to 12-hour fast so that RMR can be accurately assessed. Room calorimeters are typically small and confined; therefore, they are not practical for assessing activity-related energy expenditure for a variety of free-living activity patterns. Cost and technical limitations make direct calorimetry generally impractical for assessing activity-related energy expenditure in large epidemiological studies. Although it provides highly precise measures of energy expenditure, a number of limitations should be noted. For one, laboratory methods generally restrict the type and pattern of physical activity that can be studied. In addition, these techniques are often conducted over short periods of time. However, these measures are often used to validate more feasible field measures of energy expenditure (*see* Chapter 3 for additional discussion on assessing validity of field measures of energy expenditure, including examples of studies).

Indirect Measures of Energy Expenditure

Rather than measure body heat production, activity-related energy expenditure can be estimated by measuring the rate of oxygen uptake and carbon dioxide production associated with the energy transfer of substrate oxidation (Ferrannini, 1988; Jequier, 1987). Oxygen and carbon dioxide measurements can be based on expired ventilatory gas analysis (CO_2O_2 and flow), stable isotope enrichments (deuterium and ^{18}oxygen) obtained from serial urine samples (doubly labeled water [DLW]) or isotope-labeled bicarbonate.

Indirect Calorimetry

Whole Room Calorimeter. The heat energy released from substrate oxidation during physical activity can be estimated from measured $\dot{V}O_2$, or oxygen uptake. Energy expenditure estimates are based on assumed relationships between VO_2 and the caloric cost of substrate oxidation (Ferrannini, 1988; Jequier, 1987; Ravussin, 1986). Individuals are confined to a metabolic chamber for the duration of the assessment. Similarly to the room calorimeter (*see* Direct Calorimetry), the respiratory chamber is an air-tight, insulated, and temperature- and humidity-controlled room (Brooks, 1996; Jequier, 1983; Jequier, 1987; Montoye, 1996). Room air with measured concentrations of O_2 and CO_2 are introduced to the respiratory chamber at a controlled rate of airflow. Fractional concentrations of O_2 and CO_2 are measured as the air leaves the system. Based on the gas concentrations and flow rate of expired air, $\dot{V}O_2$ and $\dot{V}CO_2$ can be determined. This technique can be used for validation of other measures of physical activity in both children (Ventham, 1999) and adults (Strath, 2003; Starling, 1999). However, due to the restrictions of the chamber, this technique does not give accurate measures of free living energy expenditure (Seale, 1997).

Metabolic Carts and Portable Indirect Calorimetry. Methods for performing oxygen uptake-based indirect calorimetry outside the chamber have been developed. These techniques utilize an integrated measurement system comprised of an O_2 and CO_2 analyzer, a ventilation flow-volume meter, and a microcomputer to process expired air collected through a fitted hood, face mask, or mouthpiece (Davis, 1996). Typically, these techniques are used to assess task specific activities such as treadmill walking/running, cycling, housework, yardwork, and occupational activity (Strath, 2002).

Doubly Labeled Water

DLW is a technique that estimates total energy expenditure through the use of biological markers that reflect the rate of metabolism in the body. Combined with measured RMR and TEF (or an assumed percentage, e.g. 10%), activity related energy expenditure can be calculated. DLW utilizes water labeled with stable isotopes (^2H_2O and $H_2{}^{18}O$) dosed according to total body water. Urinary isotope elimination is generally followed over 7 to 21 days using an isotope-ratio mass spectrometer. Labeled hydrogen (^2H_2O) is excreted as water, whereas labeled oxygen is lost as water ($H_2{}^{18}O$) and CO_2 ($C^{18}O_2$) produced by the carbonic anhydrase system. The difference in the isotope turnover rates provides a measure of metabolic $\dot{V}CO_2$. Oxygen uptake and total body energy expenditure is extrapolated from $\dot{V}CO_2$ and an estimate of the respiratory quotient (RQ) is obtained from published equations (Black, 1986). Under steady-state conditions, RQ reflects the relative percentage of carbohydrate and fat oxidation and is calculated as $\dot{V}CO_2 / \dot{V}O_2$. Inherent error will exist in DLW energy expenditure measures when RQ is estimated and when measurements are made under non-steady-state conditions such as with weight loss, unless one accounts for body energy stores used during the period (DeLany, 1989; de Jonge, 2007).

Although DLW provides precise estimates of free-living energy expenditure over prolonged periods (e.g., a week), a major shortcoming of this technique is that, when combined with measures of RMR, it only provides total activity related energy expenditure. As such, DLW is unable to provide information pertaining to the duration, frequency, or intensity of activity-related energy expenditure. Therefore, physical activity patterns or dose–response issues must be measured using other assessment techniques. Unfortunately, DLW is not often feasible for use in large population studies because of high cost, availability of the isotopes (has certainly been an issue in the past), and technical difficulties associated with the isotope analyses.

Isotope Labeled Bicarbonate

The labeled bicarbonate (radioactive $NaH^{14}CO_3$) method is very similar to DLW and has been used to measure free-living total daily energy expenditure over shorter observation periods (e.g., days) than in studies of DLW (Elia, 1992). More recent research suggests the possibility of using a stable isotope labeled bicarbonate ($NaH^{13}CO_3$) as well (Fuller, 2000; Raj, 2006). A specific amount of isotope is infused at a constant rate and eventually diluted by the body's CO_2 pool. Labeled carbons are recovered from expired air, blood, urine, or saliva. Metabolic $\dot{V}CO_2$, is determined from an isotope dilution curve. Total energy expenditure is estimated from $\dot{V}CO_2$ and assumptions made about RQ. Limitations of this method are similar to those discussed for DLW, but can be used to measure energy expenditure over shorter periods of time than DLW.

Objective Measures of Physical Activity

As mentioned previously, physical activity is the most variable component of total energy expenditure and includes structured and non-structured activities of a range of intensities. Because RMR and the thermic effect of food are relatively stable, it is participation in physical activity that is directly modifiable and is the focus of disease prevention and treatment efforts. Objective assessment tools have the ability to capture components of physical activity that subjective measures often cannot including unstructured activities and those activities of lower intensity.

Direct Observation Techniques

Direct observation techniques have been used to study human behavior in natural settings and often provide information during specific windows of time. The reader is referred to McKenzie (2002) for a detailed description of the various methods available. Direct observation systems are often developed for target populations in specific settings and include the following characteristics: a well defined observation strategy to sample activities per unit of time, a list of activity categories to code movement types, a list of associated variables that may influence behavior (e.g., context, teacher behavior, environmental settings), supplemental methods to record concurrent levels of energy expenditure, data entry procedures (e.g., pencil and paper, computer, palm pilot), and detailed scoring schemes used to summarize the data. Direct observation is predominantly conducted in children because of their limited ability to accurately recall physical activity or properly complete records, logs, and questionnaires and typically takes place in the school or home setting. Direct observation is often not a viable assessment technique for large epidemiological studies because of the time and expense required for data collection. Also, it provides information on activity performed only during the assessment period and not activity performed at other times.

Movement Monitors

Accelerometers

Accelerometers are small battery-operated devices worn on the waist, arm, or ankle that measure the rate and magnitude of truncal or body limb movement. These monitors are non-invasive and are useful in laboratory or field settings. Movement is measured in single or multiple planes. Microcomputer technology integrates and sums the absolute value and frequency of acceleration forces over a defined observation period (e.g., every minute). Physical activity data is output as an activity "count." Regression equations have been developed from controlled laboratory experiments to allow for the estimation of activity-related energy expenditure from the activity counts (Freedson, 1998; Melanson, 1995).

Accelerometers have been shown to be valid and reliable in a number of populations, including children (Trost, 2002; Eston, 1998; Rodriguez, 2002), adults (LeMasurier, 2003; Leenders, 2000; Campbell, 2002), and older adults (Koschersberger, 1996; Leemer, 2001). Accelerometers have also been used to validate physical activity questionnaires (Matthews, 2005; Strath, 2003; Matthews, 1995) and quantify associations between physical activity behaviors and health outcomes (Matthews, 2000).

Accelerometers provide information about the frequency, duration, intensity, and patterns of physical activity and have the capability to record and store information over long periods of time. Unfortunately, information regarding the specific type of physical activity (i.e., gardening *vs.* walking) is not captured. Accelerometers tend to underestimate lifestyle activity-related energy expenditure and do not account for energy expenditure owed to upper body involvement, water activities, or uphill walking (Ainsworth, 2000a). It is likely that many of these limitations reflect the accuracy of the regression equations used to predict activity-related energy expenditure rather than imprecision of motion detection by the accelerometer. Subject compliance issues, potentially altered physical activity patterns, and the cost of the more sophisticated instruments are additional limitations to the practicality of accelerometers as measures of activity-related energy expenditure among free-living populations (*see* Chapter 3 for additional discussion, including examples of studies).

Pedometers

Pedometers have gained widespread popularity in research and practice settings to quantify ambulation in terms of accumulated steps in free-living settings. Pedometers are small, inexpensive, battery-operated devices worn at the waist that have the ability to measure ambulatory activity in terms of steps taken (and distance walked if stride length is available; Bassett, 1996). The vertical forces of foot-strike cause movement of a spring-suspended lever arm to open and close an electrical circuit, which registers a "step." In theory, step registration should reflect only the vertical forces of foot-strike and, hence, ambulatory activity. However, any vertical force through the hip area (e.g., sitting down hard on a chair, riding on a bike or in a car over rough terrain) can also trigger the device.

Pedometers have demonstrated reasonable precision for use in research and clinical settings where walking is the primary type of activity. Moreover, their ease of administration makes them a practical assessment tool for individuals, encompassing nearly all age groups (Scruggs, 2003; Bassett, 2000; Coleman, 1999; Macko, 2002). Finally, pedometers have the ability to promote behavior change and have been increasingly used in intervention settings as an intervention tool.

Pedometers do not provide information relating to activity type, duration, or intensity. Therefore, accurate quantification of activity-related energy expenditure, time spent in type- or intensity-specific activities, and patterns of activity (e.g., short vs. continuous bouts) cannot be assessed using the pedometer. Similarly to other movement monitors, pedometers do not have the capability to quantify upper body movements (Tudor-Locke, 2001) and have difficulty accurately assessing activity levels in individuals at slower gait speeds (Storti, 2008; Bassett, 1996) (*see* Chapter 3 for additional discussion, including examples of studies).

Objective Measures of Physical Fitness

Physical fitness is a set of attributes, such as cardiorespiratory fitness, that people have or can achieve that relate to the ability to perform physical activity participation (Caspersen, 1985) and, therefore, has been used as a surrogate measure or marker for recent physical activity. The measurement of physical fitness is common practice in both preventive and rehabilitative exercise programs. The purposes of fitness testing include: educating individuals about current fitness status relative to population norms, collecting baseline and follow-up data to measure progress in an exercise program, motivation of exercise participants, and risk stratification for chronic disease development (ACSM, 2000).

Maximum Oxygen Uptake

Maximal oxygen uptake, or VO_{2max}, is the most accurate measure of cardiovascular (aerobic) fitness, one of the five components of physical fitness. Cardiovascular fitness relates to how well the cardiorespiratory system works to transport and utilize oxygen in the body. VO_{2max} can be defined as the highest level of oxygen consumption that is utilized by the body during peak physical exertion (ACSM, 2000).

VO_{2max} protocols may not be possible in large epidemiological studies where there are a large number of participants due to cost and the necessity of wearing instruments that likely alters usual patterns of physical activity. In addition, when examining population studies, there is only a moderate relationship between physical activity and physical fitness (Siconolfi, 1985; Jacobs, 1993). This lack of a strong relationship could result from the fact that there are other factors besides activity, such as genetics (Bouchard, 1988), gender, age, and relative weight (Leon, 1981), that influence physical activity.

In instances where VO_{2max} testing is not practical, such as with large epidemiological studies, cardiovascular fitness can be measured indirectly using submaximal VO_2 and field-test protocols. Submaximal VO_2 tests use heart rate (HR) to predict the oxygen consumption that would have occurred during maximal workloads (VO_{2max}). Submaximal VO_2 tests are able to predict VO_{2max} because of the linear relationship that exists between HR and exercise workload/intensity (as workland/intensity increases, HR increases; ACSM, 2000). Examples of submaximal VO_2 tests include the YMCA Cycle Ergometer Test and McArdle Step Test. Similarly, field tests use either the distance that is covered or the amount of time it took to cover a particular distance to estimate VO_{2max} using established prediction equations (ACSM, 2000). Examples of field tests include the Rockport Walking Test and 1.5-mile run test.

Heart Rate Monitoring

Heart rate has been used to estimate activity-related energy expenditure based on the assumption of a linear relationship between HR and $\dot{V}O_2$ (Wilmore, 1971). The administrative and technical issues associated with measuring activity-related energy expenditure by indirect calorimetry in the field are difficult; therefore, HR is often used as a measure of physical fitness. Because the HR–VO_2 relationship is somewhat attenuated during low and very high-intensity activities (Acheson, 1980), and because of considerable between-person and day-to-day HR-VO_2 variability (Li, 1993; McCroy, 1997), individual HR–VO_2 calibration curves (Haskell, 1993) are necessary for estimation of activity-related energy expenditure. This technique is easy and quick to administer and can be utilized in either a laboratory or free-living setting. It is relatively accurate in the assessment of physical activity intensity and has been utilized in both children (Beghin, 2002) and adults (Strath, 2002; Kashiwazaki, 1986). However, measuring HR may become cumbersome over longer assessment periods and with a large sample size.

Body temperature, size of the active muscle mass (e.g., upper vs. lower body), type of exercise (static vs. dynamic), stress, and medication all influence HR without having substantial effects on oxygen uptake (Acheson, 1980; Montoye, 1996). This may result in an imprecise estimation of activity-related energy expenditure. Day-to-day HR variability also reduces the reliability of estimated energy expenditure (Washburn, 1986). Recent advancements in technology may overcome previous limitations by combining HR and motion monitoring into one instrument (for additional discussion, *see* Chapter 3). Instrumentation costs and the development of individual calibrations make this method less suitable for routine use in free-living settings.

Subjective Measures of Physical Activity

Physical Activity Questionnaires

Self-reporting questionnaires are the most frequently used method of assessing physical activity levels among free-living individuals. Questionnaires vary in their complexity, time frame, and type of activity that is assessed. Each of these considerations will be outlined in more detail in the following sections. (Additionally, Chapter 3 provides discussion on assessing reliability and validity of physical activity questionnaires, and Chapter 6 provides selected examples of questionnaires used by ongoing epidemiologic studies of physical activity.)

Complexity

Physical activity questionnaires vary in their complexity, from global, single-item questionnaires to more complex quantitative history questionnaires estimating physical activity over a lifetime. Global activity questionnaires are typically short surveys that can be self-administered (Siscovick, 1988; Sternfeld, 2000) or given as a phone interview (Macera, 2001) to obtain a general index of physical activity. Single-item questionnaires may ask individuals whether they are more active than others of their age and sex (National Center for Health Statistics, 1988) or whether the person exercises long enough to break a sweat (Paffenbarger, 1978; Washburn, 1990). Global questionnaires provide crude detail on specific types and patterns of physical activity and generally provide simple classifications of activity status (e.g., active vs. inactive). Such simple single-item questions are often used to adjust for the confounding influence of physical activity when exploring associations among other variables (Caspersen, 1989). Although the precision and reproducibility of global activity questionnaires have been satisfactory (Ainsworth, 1993; Jacobs, 1993), misclassification on activity status can often occur (Macera, 2001), and lack of detail precludes comprehensive investigations of physical activity dimensions and patterns.

More complex questionnaires, such as recall questionnaires, attempt to survey a wide range of popular activities over a defined time frame. Recall questionnaires detail the frequency, duration, and types of activities performed during a defined recall period (e.g., past day, week, month, or year). These instruments can be interview-based (Ainsworth, 2000a; Kriska, 1997; Blair, 1985; Jacobs, 1989) or self-administered (Baecke, 1982; Paffenbarger, 1986; Wolf, 1994).

Quantitative histories record the frequency and duration of occupational, leisure, and other physical activities over the past year (Kriska, 1997; Montoye, 1971; Taylor, 1978) or lifetime (Chasan-Taber, 2002; Friedenreich, 1998; Kriska, 1988). These surveys may be interview-based (Friedenreich, 1998; Kriska, 1997; Taylor, 1978) or self-administered (Chasan-Taber, 2002; Montoye, 1971). Quantitative activity histories are useful for investigators and practitioners who are interested in physical activity patterns over long periods of time because of the presumed influence on chronic disease with a long developmental phase (Chasan-Taber, 2002; Friedenreich, 1998; Kriska, 1988). Chronic diseases such as osteoporosis or cancer have a latent, long-term development period; therefore, chronic exposure to physical inactivity can accelerate disease development. The intensive administrative burden and recall effort limits the feasibility and practicality of these instruments in many settings.

Time Frame

The activity questionnaire can either ask about usual activity or inquire about activity done within the past day, week, month, year, or even over a lifetime. Participants may be asked to use diaries and logs to record activities over 1 day, 3 days, or the past week. Questionnaires focusing on a long time frame, such as 1 year, are more likely to reflect usual activity patterns and have been used extensively in epidemiologic studies. Questionnaires with short time frames have two advantages over those with longer time frames: the estimates are less vulnerable to imprecise recall and are more practical to validate with objective tools. However, assessment over a short time period is less likely to reflect "usual" behavior, as activity levels may vary with seasons or as a result of illness or time constraints (Kriska, 1997). To obtain the best estimate of physical activity levels, some questionnaires include assessments over both a short and long time period.

Activity Type

Physical activity comprises several different domains, including transportation, sports/leisure, school/occupation, and housework/child or elderly care. Early studies in physical activity epidemiology estimated physical activity performed at work (Morris, 1953; Paffenbarger, 1975) and typically did no more than inquire about job titles. In contrast, more recent occupational physical activity questionnaires query the frequency, duration, and intensity of activities performed by individual workers on the job (Ainsworth, 1999; Kriska, 1990; Montoye, 1971; Yore, 2005). However, because physical activity levels at work have continued to decline in most industrialized countries (Powell, 1987), assessment of leisure-time physical activity is often assumed to be the best representation of physical activity in a population. For this reason, most contemporary physical activity surveys only assess leisure-time activities that require energy expenditure above that of daily living. Some questionnaires include both leisure and occupational activity components to be used in situations where the contribution of these components are either unknown or cannot be assumed (Kriska, 1992; Sallis, 1985).

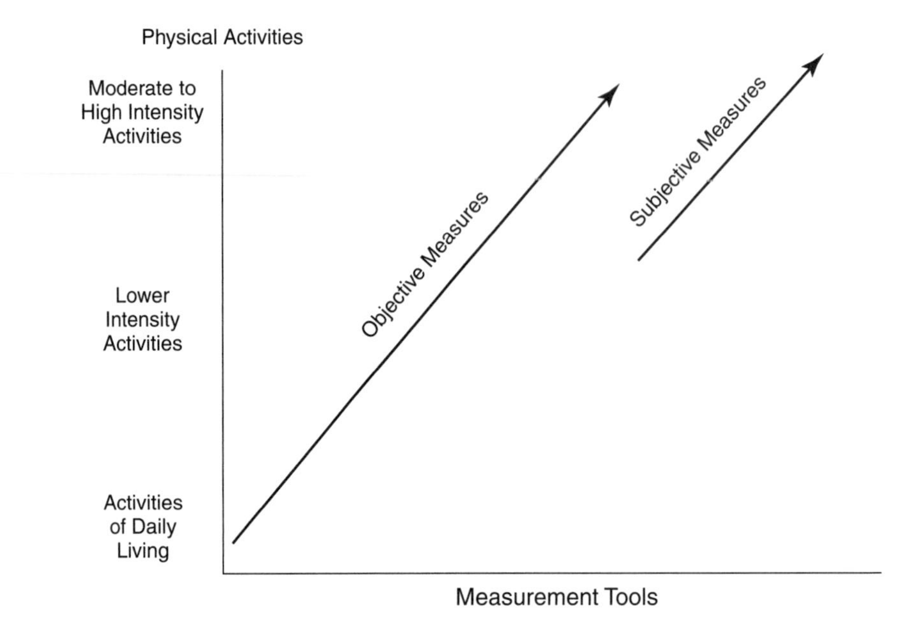

Figure 2.1 Spectrum of Physical Activity Assessment. (Adapted from Kriska, 2000.)

Although subjective measures accurately assess moderate to higher intensity activity, focusing solely on leisure (in particular sport) and/or occupational activity may only be valid for younger and healthier populations. It is well-established that certain subgroups of the population (older adults and women) acquire most of their physical activity in lower intensity activities, which subjective measures tend to do a poor job assessing (Kriska, 1997; Jacobs, 1993). Therefore, the supplemental use of objective measures may be required for a more accurate assessment of physical activity participation in these populations. This is particularly important when lower intensity and/or unstructured activities comprise the bulk of energy expenditure (Kriska, 2000; Fig. 2.1).

Activity information obtained by self-reporting measures is subject to response bias (e.g., imprecise recall, social desirability) that may influence the precision in measures of physical activity and related energy expenditure (Coughlin, 1990; Durante, 1996). Bias appears to be highest for low-intensity physical activities that are habitual behaviors (e.g., walking, housework) compared to higher intensity structured activities such as sport and conditioning activities, which are planned and intentional behaviors (Durante, 1996).

Measures of Physical Inactivity

Physical inactivity is defined as a state in which body movement is minimal (Dietz, 1996). Inactivity can be categorized into behaviors that are modifiable, such as television viewing and recreational computer use, vs. necessary sedentary behaviors such as sleeping, sitting while engaging in homework (children) or occupational activities. Although the U.S. Surgeon General has determined that physical inactivity is a major health risk factor for various chronic diseases, the quantification of physical inactivity has received far less attention than physical activity. Furthermore, there is limited published evidence in current literature regarding the reliability and validity of measures that can be used to accurately assess sedentary behavior (Gordon-Larsen, 2000).

Researchers often focus on modifiable sedentary activities when quantifying physical inactivity. In both children and adults, researchers typically examine the average amount of time spent viewing television or videos and playing computer/video games and sometimes even include reading and/or napping. (Fitzgerald, 1997; Andersen, 1998; Vaz de Almeida, 1999; Fung, 2000; Gordon-Larsen, 2000; 2002; Hu, 2001; Manson, 2002; Feldman, 2003; Jakes, 2003; Utter, 2003; Evenson, 2005).

Recently, a number of intervention efforts specifically targeting modifiable sedentary behaviors have been developed to decrease the occurrence of inactivity and promote activity participation. Earlier attempts in inactivity intervention included the use of daily activity logs in which participants recorded the time spent in modifiable sedentary behaviors (Epstein, 2002; Ford, 2002). More recent and innovative measures have included objective electronic television time managers and event loggers that assist in budgeting the amount of time spent watching television, watching videotapes (DVDs), and playing video games (Robinson, 1999; Epstein, 2002; Ford, 2002). Recently, novel approaches have been developed in which a modifiable sedentary behavior is contingent upon activity participation. More specifically, in interventions targeting children, television viewing was contingent upon pedaling a stationary/electronically braked cycle ergometer to decrease inactivity and increase activity participation (Faith, 2001).

There has also been considerable interest in assessing physical inactivity through the use of objective monitoring, such as accelerometers (Matthews, 2005). As mentioned previously, accelerometers have the capability to provide information relating to patterns of physical activity. Data are output as counts per minute, which is an expression of change in acceleration during a 1-minute time period. Therefore, a count of zero may indicate time spent in sedentary activity, especially if zero counts are accumulated over longer periods of time. For example, zero counts accumulated over a 30-minute span may indicate that the individual was inactive during that time period. However, because a zero count may also be reflective of removal of the monitor, this information should be used with caution. The use of a supplemental activity diary indicating wear-time may allow the investigator to better differentiate between monitor removal and inactivity.

Issues in Assessing Physical Activity

Reliability and Validity Measures

Reliability and validity studies help ensure the accuracy and quality of physical activity assessment. A reliable questionnaire consistently provides the same results under the same circumstances. Reliability studies typically use test–retest reliability coefficients or intraclass correlation coefficients. Validity studies assess how well the questionnaire measures what it was designed to measure. Reliability does not equal validity; therefore, an assessment tool should be both reliable and valid to accurately assess physical activity levels (Kriska, 1997; *see* Chapter 3 for additional discussion on establishing reliability and validity of physical activity assessment tools).

Early studies in the field of physical activity epidemiology often published significant results on the relationship between physical activity and decreased risk of chronic diseases, with the assumption that such results automatically implied that the instrument was reliable and valid. Unfortunately, such studies ran the risk of finding a spurious result and may have been published under the influence of positive publication bias. Today, evidence of instrument reliability and validity is becoming a scientific norm (Kriska, 1997).

Reliability and validity are affected by cognitive factors, such as a person's ability to store and retrieve information (Durante, 1996; Baranowski, 1988). Reliability and validity of the data collected can also be influenced by interviewer or respondent bias, the day of the week being probed, and the sequence of administration of the physical activity questions within the battery of other measures collected. Future methodological research examining the reliability and validity of physical activity questionnaires should focus on these issues as well as on socio-demographic and cultural issues (Craig, 2003; Kriska, 1997; Warnecke, 1997; LaPorte, 1985).

Seasonality

Environmental changes in temperature, precipitation, and number of daylight hours are believed to also provoke seasonal changes in physical activity levels (Matthews, 2001; Kriska, 1997). Therefore, in parts of the United States where weather patterns fluctuate with the changing seasons, it is highly probable that activity levels may also vary by season. For example, in the southwestern United States, physical activity levels may drop during the summer months because of the hot and dry climate. In contrast, in the northeast, physical activities may decline during the cold, snowy winter months. A number of previous investigations set in geographical areas with four distinct seasons reported peak physical activity levels during months in which weather patterns were more conducive to being physically active (Uitenbroek, 1993; Matthews, 2001; Tudor-Locke, 2004).

Considerations for Selecting an Appropriate Assessment Tool

When selecting the appropriate physical activity assessment tool, several methodological issues should be considered, such as study and population characteristics (Fig. 2.2). In brief, study characteristics include geographic location, budget, sample size, and study outcome. Population characteristics such as age, health status, level of cognition, race/ethnicity/culture, socioeconomic status, and gender should also be considered when selecting the appropriate assessment tool(s).

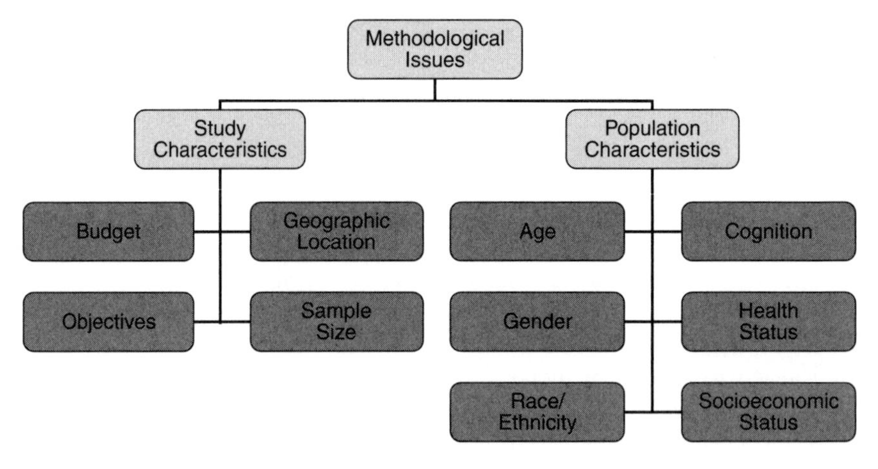

Figure 2.2 Factors that need to be considered when selecting an appropriate physical activity assessment tool.

Study Characteristics

There are many methodological issues that need to considered when deciding on an appropriate physical activity assessment tool. The assessment tool should be specific to the proposed study objectives. Furthermore, it should adequately measure the type of activity that is most related to the outcome of interest. For example, when examining the relationship between obesity and physical activity, a tool that measures total physical activity may be more appropriate than one that solely assesses higher intensity activities. The type of study design and number of associated assessment time-points will aid in the decision-making process. Study budget, cohort size, and available staffing are also important issues to consider when selecting an appropriate assessment tool. Large epidemiological studies with limited funding and staffing may opt for the less expensive questionnaire rather than the more expensive activity monitors. Geographic location, including climate/weather, is also an important concern when selecting an appropriate physical activity assessment tool. For example, a study in Boston, Massachusetts, may need to consider issues of seasonality, which may not be as relevant for study populations in Honolulu, Hawaii.

Population Characteristics

The characteristics inherent to the study population will also help assist in the selection process for the appropriate assessment tool. The measurement tool should have the ability to accurately assess physical activities that are specific to the population of interest. For example, when measuring physical activity in an older cohort, an assessment tool that primarily captures time spent solely in higher intensity structured exercise may be inappropriate, as many older adults tend to participate in lower intensity, unstructured activities. Demographic factors such as age, gender, race/ethnicity, and socioeconomic status are all important considerations when selecting the appropriate technique. The study investigator should also evaluate both the physical and cognitive status of the study participants. For example, a study cohort of individuals with Parkinson's disease should not rely solely on measures that assess ambulatory movement because of the associated symptoms/side effects (tremors). Furthermore, individuals with dementia will most likely have problems accurately recalling physical activity using a survey approach; therefore, objective measures of physical activity may be more suitable for this group. Finally, native language and level of educational attainment are important considerations when developing and/or translating an activity questionnaire and/or movement monitor instructions. Furthermore, the questionnaire or instructions should not only be translated into the native language but also pilot-tested in a representative sample.

To obtain a true estimate of participation in physical activity, investigators need to closely examine both the characteristics of the study, as well as the specific details of the individuals who comprise the study population. By doing so, the investigator will be able to establish the most appropriate method or methods needed to assess physical activity levels in the selected study population.

Personal Perspective

For over 40 years, physical activity researchers have been assessing physical activity levels in public health research to determine both the association between activity and health status and to identify individuals in need of physical activity intervention. The specific components of physical activity that we have focused on, as well as our definition of inactivity, have changed over these years; the challenge has been to modify the assessment tools to reflect these changes. Initial interest in the field focused on higher intensity, well-defined sports and recreational activities and/or occupational activities. The assessment of physical activity at that point in time was determined primarily with questionnaires, which were found to be relatively accurate for assessment of those higher intensity activities. However, more recently, our focus has evolved to that of total activity and overall movement. Technological advances such as cars, elevators, and remote controls have decreased the amount of movement necessary to get us through a day, causing us to redefine what it means to be "inactive." It is no longer the absence of a significant amount of intense activity in an occupation or in leisure time that is considered "inactive" but more the lack of substantial movement during the course of a day or week. To measure this latter level of physical activity, which would encompass both low- and high-intensity activities, we need to include objective measures of physical activity in our repertoire of tools. {Andrea Kriska}

The growth in technology has increased the precision of physical activity assessment, where it is now possible to simultaneously measure limb movement, the physiological responses to physical activity, and spatial characteristics of human movement. In addition, it is possible to electronically collect data about physical activity patterns using computer, Internet, and wireless technology. The challenge in this new era of physical activity assessment is in understanding how to integrate multiple modes of data and to identify the most important types of data that characterize physical activity patterns related to health status.

It remains difficult to capture all types of physical activity with physical activity monitors. In the future, it is likely that electronic instruments will continue to be developed, refined, and used to assess physical activity; however, because of their expense, questionnaires will still be used as a primary method to assess physical activity in epidemiological studies. Instead of developing new questionnaires to assess physical activity, we should evaluate previously evaluated questionnaires for their reliability and validity in various population groups, such as ethnic and racial minorities, disabled persons, and individuals of all ages and socioeconomic status. Also, when possible, we should continue to combine objective and subjective measures to assess physical activity, thus obtaining a broad pattern of physical activity performed in desired settings. {Barb Ainsworth}

ACKNOWLEDGMENTS We thank Vanisha L. Brown, Jonathan A. Wyno, and Dr. James DeLany for their contribution to this chapter.

References

Acheson KJ, Campbell IT, Edholm OG, Miller DS, Stock MJ. 1980. The measurement of daily energy expenditure—an evaluation of some techniques. *Am J Clin Nutr* 33: 1155–64.

Ainsworth BE, Bassett DR, Strath SJ, et al. 2000a. Comparison of three methods for measuring the time spent in physical activity. *Med Sci Sports Exerc.* 32(9 Suppl): S457–64.

Ainsworth BE, Haskell WL, Whitt MC, et al. 2000b. Compendium of physical activities: an update of activity codes and MET intensities. *Med Sci Sports Exerc.* 32(9 Suppl): S498–504.

Ainsworth BE, Richardson MT, Jacobs DR, Leon AS, Sternfeld B. 1999. Evaluation of occupational activity surveys. *J Clin Epidemiol.* 52: 219–27.

Ainsworth BE, Jacobs DR Jr., Leon AS. 1993. Validity and reliability of self-reported physical activity status: The Lipid Research Clinics Questionnaire. *Med Sci Sports Exerc.* 25: 92–8.

American College of Sports Medicine. 2000. ACSM's guidelines for exercise testing and prescription (6th ed.). Baltimore, MD: Lippincott Williams & Wilkins.

Andersen RE, Crespo CJ, Bartlett SJ, Cheskin LJ, Pratt M. 1998. Relationship of physical activity and television watching with body weight and level of fatness among children: results from the Third National Health and Nutrition Examination Survey. *JAMA* 279: 938–42.

Baecke JAH, Burema J, Frijters JER. 1982. A short questionnaire for the measurement of habitual physical activity in epidemiological studies. *Am J Clin Nutr* 36: 936–42.

Baranowski T. 1988. Validity and reliability of self report measures of physical activity. An information-processing perspective. *Res. Quarter Exerc Sport*. 59: 314–27.

Bassett DR, Ainsworth BE, Swartz AM, Strath SJ, O'Brien WL, King GA. 2000. Validity of four motion sensors in measuring moderate intensity physical activity. *Med Sci Sports Exerc*. 32(9 Suppl): S471–80.

Bassett DR, Ainsworth BE, Leggett SR, et al. 1996. Accuracy of five electronic pedometers for measuring distance walked. *Med Sci Sports Exerc*. 28: 1071–77.

Beghin L, Michaud L, Guimber D, et al. 2002. Assessing sleeping energy expenditure in children using heart-rate monitoring calibrated against open circuit indirect calorimetry: a pilot study. *Br J Nutr*. 88: 533–543.

Black AE, Prentice AM, Coward WA. 1986. Use of food quotients to predice respiratory quotients for the doubly labeled water technique. *Human Nutr: Clin Nutr* 40C: 381–91.

Blair SN, Haskell WL, Ho P, et al. 1985. Assessment of habitual physical activity by a seven-day recall in a community survey and controlled experiments. *Am J Epidemiol* 122: 794–804.

Bouchard C, Boulay MR, Simoneau JA, Lortie G, Perusse L. 1988. Heredity and trainability of aerobic and anaerobic performance: an update. *Sports Med*. 5: 69–73.

Brooks GA, Fahey TD, White TP. 1996. Exercise physiology. *Human bioenergetics and its applications* (2nd ed.), Mountain View, CA: Mayfield.

Campbell KL, Crocker PRE, McKenzie DC. 2002. Field Evaluation of energy expenditure in women using Tritrac accelerometers. *Med Sci Sports Exerc*. 34: 1667–74.

Caspersen, CJ. 1989. Physical activity epidemiology: Concepts, methods and applications to exercise science. *Exerc Sport Sci Rev* 17: 423–73.

Caspersen CJ, Powell KE, Christenson GM. 1985. Physical activity, exercise, and physical fitness: definitions and distinctions for health-related research. *Public Health Reports* 100(2): 126–31.

Chasan-Taber L, Erickson JB, Nasca PC, Chasan-Taber S, Freedson PS. 2002. Validity and reproducibility of a physical activity questionnaire in women. *Med Sci Sports Exerc*. 34: 987–92.

Coleman KL, Smith DG, Boone DA, Joseph AW, del Aguila MA. 1999. Step activity monitor: Long-term, continuous recoding of ambulatory function. *J Rehab Res Dev*. 36: 8–18.

Coughlin SS. 1990. Recall bias in epidemiologic studies. *J Clin Epidemiol* 43: 87–91.

Craig CL, Marshall AL, Sjöström M, et al. 2003. The International Physical Activity Questionnaire (IPAQ): a comprehensive reliability and validity study in twelve countries. *Med Sci Sports Exerc*. 35: 1381–95.

Davis JA. 1996. Direct determination of aerobic power. In PJ Maud & C Foster (Eds.), *Physiological assessment of human fitness*, Champaign, IL: Human Kinetics, pp. 9–17.

de Jonge L, DeLany JP, Nguyen T, et al. 2007. Validation study of energy expenditure and intake during calorie restriction using doubly labeled water and changes in body composition. *Am J Clin Nutr*. 85:73-9.

DeLany JP, Schoeller DA, Hoyt RW, Askew EW, Sharp MA. 1989. Field use of D2180 to measure energy expenditure of soldiers at different energy intakes. *J Appl Physiol*. 67:1922-29.

Dietz WH. 1996. The role of lifestyle in health: the epidemiology and consequences of inactivity. *Proc Nutr Soc* 55: 829–40.

Durante R and Ainsworth BE. 1996. The recall of physical activity: using a cognitive model of the question-answering process. *Med Sci Sports Exerc* 28: 1282–1291.

Elia M, Fuller NJ, Murgatroyd PR. 1992. Measurement of bicarbonate turnover in humans: applicability to estimation of energy expenditure. *Am J Physiol* 263: E676-87.

Epstein LH, Paluch RA, Consalvi A., et al. 2002. Effects of manipulating sedentary behavior on physical activity and food intake. *J Pediatr* 140: 334–9.

Eston RG, Rowlands AV, Ingledew DK. 1998. Validity of heart rate, pedometry, and accelerometry for predicting the energy cost of children's activities. *J Appl Physiol*. 84: 362–71.

Evenson KR, McGinn AP. 2005. Test-retest reliability of adult surveillance measures for physical activity and inactivity. *Am J Prev Med* 28: 470–8.

Faith MS, Berman N, Heo M, et al. 2001. Effects of contingent television on physical activity and television viewing in obese children. *Pediatrics* 107: 1043–8.

Feldman DE, Barnett T, Shrier I, Rossignol M, Abenhaim L. 2003. Is physical activity differentially associated with different types of sedentary pursuits? *Arch Pediatr Adolesc Med* 157: 797–802.

Ferrannini E. 1988. The theoretical bases of indirect calorimetry. *Metabolism* 37: 287–301.

FitzGerald S, Kriska AM, Pereira MA, de Courten M. 1997. Associations among physical activity, television watching, and obesity in adult Pima Indians. *Med Sci Sports Exerc.* 29: 910–15.

Ford BS, McDonald TE, Owens AS, Robinson, TN. 2002. Primary care interventions to reduce television viewing in African-American children. *Am J Prev Med* 22: 106–9.

Freedson PS, Melanson E, Sirard J. 1998. Calibration of the Computer Science and Applications, Inc. accelerometer. *Med Sci Sports Exerc.* 30: 772–81.

Friedenreich CM, Courneya KS, Bryant HE. 1998. The lifetime total physical activity questionnaire: development and reliability. *Med Sci Sports Exerc.* 30: 266–74.

Fuller NJ, Harding M, McDevitt R, Jennings G, Coward WA, Elia M. 2000 Comparison of recoveries in breath carbon dioxide of H13CO-3 and H14CO-3 administered simultaneously by single 6 h constant unprimed intraveneous infusion. *Br J Nutr.* 84:269-74.

Fung TT, Hu FB, Yu J, et al. 2000. Leisure-time physical activity, television watching, and plasma biomarkers of obesity and cardiovascular disease risk. *Am J Epidemiol* 152: 1171–8.

Gordon-Larsen P, Adair LS, Popkin BM. 2002. Ethnic differences in physical activity and inactivity patterns and overweight status. *Obes Res* 10: 141–9.

Gordon-Larsen P, McMurray RG, Popkin BM. 2000. Determinants of adolescent physical activity and inactivity patterns. *Pediatrics* 105: E83.

Haskell WL, Yee MC, Evans A, Irby PJ. 1993. Simultaneous measurement of heart rate and body motion to quantitate physical activity. *Med Sci Sports Exerc.* 25: 109–15.

Horton ES. 1983. An overview of the assessment and regulation of energy balance in humans, *Am J Clin Nutr* 38: 972–7.

Hu FB, Li TY, Colditz GA, Willett WC, Manson JE. 2003. Television watching and other sedentary behaviors in relation to risk of obesity and type 2 diabetes mellitus in women. *JAMA* 289: 1785–91.

Jacobs DR Jr., Ainsworth BE, Hartman T, Leon AS. 1993. A simultaneous evaluation of 10 commonly used physical activity questionnaires. *Med Sci Sports Exerc.* 25: 81–91.

Jacobs DR, Hahn LP, Haskell WL, Pirie P, Sidney S. 1989. Reliability and validity of a short physical activity history: CARDIA and the Minnesota Heart Health Program. *J Cardiopulm Rehab* 9: 448–59.

Jakes RW, Day NE, Khaw KT, et al. 2003. Television viewing and low participation in vigorous recreation are independently associated with obesity and markers of cardiovascular disease risk: EPIC-Norfolk population-based study. *Eur J Clin Nutr* 57: 1089–96.

Jequier E, Acheson K, Schutz Y. 1987. Assessment of energy expenditure and fuel utilization in man. *Ann Rev Nutr* 7: 187–208.

Jequier E and Schutz Y. 1983. Long-term measurements of energy expenditure in humans using a respiratory chamber. *Am J Clin Nutr* 38: 989–98.

Kashiwazaki H, Inaoka T, Suzuki T, Kondo Y. 1986. Correlations of pedometer readings with energy expenditure in workers during free-living daily activities. *Eur J Appl Physiol.* 54: 585–90.

Kochersberger GA, McConnell E, Kuchibhatla MN, Pieper C. 1996. The reliability, validity, and stability of a measure of physical activity in the elderly. *Arch Phys Med Rehabil.* 77: 793–5.

Kriska AM. 2000. Ethnic and cultural issues in assessing physical activity. Part of the "Measurement of Physical Activity: Reliability, Validity, and Methodological Issues Conference." *Res. Quarter Exerc Sport* 71: 47–53.

Kriska AM and Caspersen CJ. 1997. Introduction to the Collection of Physical Activity Questionnaires in A Collection of Physical Activity Questionnaires for Health-Related Research. Kriska and Caspersen editors. Centers for Disease Control and Prevention. *Med Sci Sports Exerc.* 29 (Suppl): S5–9.

Kriska AM and Bennett PH. 1992. An epidemiological perspective of the relationship between physical activity and NIDDM: From activity assessment to intervention. *Diabetes/Metabolism Rev* 8: 355–72.

Kriska AM, Knowler WC, LaPorte RE, et al. 1990. Development of questionnaire to examine the relationship of physical activity and diabetes in Pima Indians. *Diabetes Care* 13: 401–11.

Kriska AM, Sandler RB, Cauley JA, LaPorte RE, Hom DL, Pambianco G. 1988. The assessment of historical physical activity and its relation to adult bone parameters. *Am J. Epidemiol.* 127: 1053–63.

LaPorte RE, Montoye HJ, Caspersen CJ. 1985. Assessment of physical activity in epidemiologic research: problems and prospects. *Public Health Reports* 100(2): 131–46.

Le Masurier GC and Tudor-Locke C. 2003. Comparison of pedometer and accelerometer accuracy under controlled conditions. *Med Sci Sports Exerc*. 35: 867–71.

Leenders NYJM, Sherman WM, Nagaraja HN. 2000. Comparisons of four methods of estimating physical activity in adult women. *Med Sci Sports Exerc*. 32: 1320–26.

Lemmer JT, Ivey JM, Ryan AS, et al. 2001. Effect of strength training on resting metabolic rate and physical activity: age and gender comparisons. *Med Sci Sports Exer*. 33: 532–41.

Leon AS, Jacobs DR, DeBacker G, Taylor HL. 1981. Relationship of physical characteristics and life habits to treadmill exercise capacity. *Am J Epidemiol*. 113: 653–60.

Li R, Deurenberg P, Hautvast JGAJ. 1993. A critical evaluation of heart rate monitoring to assess energy expenditure in individuals. *Am J Clin Nutr*. 58: 602–7.

Macera CA, Ham SA, Jones DA, Kimsey CD, Ainsworth BE, Neff LJ. 2001. Limitations on the use of a single screening question to measure sedentary behavior. *Am J Pub Health* 91: 2010–2.

Macko RF, Haeuber E, Shaughnessy M, et al. 2002. Microprocessor-based ambulatory activity monitoring in stroke patients. *Med Sci Sports Exerc*. 34: 394–9.

Manson JE, Greenland P, LaCroix AZ, et al. 2002. Walking compared with vigorous exercise for the prevention of cardiovascular events in women. *N Engl J Med*. 347: 716–25.

Matthews CE, Ainsworth BE, Hanby C, et al. 2005. Development and testing of a short physical activity recall questionnaire. *Med Sci Sports Exerc*. 37: 986–94.

Matthews CE, Freedson PS, Hebert JR, et al. 2001. Seasonal variation in household, occupational, and leisure time physical activity: longitudinal analyses from the seasonal variation of blood cholesterol study. *Am. J. Epidemiol*. 153: 172–83.

Matthews CE, Freedson PS, Hebert JR, Stanek EJ, Merriam PA, Ockene IS. 2000. Comparing physical activity assessment methods in the Seasonal Variation of Blood Cholesterol Study. *Med Sci Sports Exerc*. 32, 976–84.

Matthews CE. Freedson PS. 1995. Field trial of a three-dimensional activity monitor: comparison with self report. *Med Sci Sports Exerc*. 27: 1071–8.

McCroy MA, Mole PA, Nommsen-Rivers LA, Dewey KG. 1997. Between-day and within-day variability in the relation between heart rate and oxygen consumption: effect on the estimation of energy expenditure by heart rate monitoring. *Am J Clin Nutr* 66: 18–25.

McKenzie TL. 2002. Use of direct observation to assess physical activity. In GJ Welk (Ed.), *Physical Activity Assessments for Health-Related Research*, Champaign, IL: Human Kinetics, pp. 179–196.

Melanson EL, Freedson PS. 1995. Validity of Computer Science and Applications, Inc. (CSA) activity monitor. *Med Sci Sports Exerc*. 27: 934–40.

Montoye HJ, Kemper HCG, Saris WHM, Washburn RA. 1996. *Measuring physical activity and energy expenditure*. Champaign, IL: Human Kinetics.

Montoye HJ. 1971. Estimation of habitual physical activity by questionnaire and interview, *Am J Clin Nutr*. 24: 1113–8.

Morris JN, Heady JA, Raffle PAB, Roberts CG, Parks JW. 1953. Coronary heart disease and physical activity of work. *Lancet*, 265: 1053–57, 1111–20.

National Center for Health Statistics. 1988. Health promotion and disease prevention. United States, 1985. Vital Health Stat 10 (163): 1985. Washington, DC.; U.S. Government Printing Office.

Paffenbarger RS, Hyde RT, Wing AL, Hsieh CC. 1986. Physical activity, all-cause mortality, and longevity of college alumni. *N Engl J Med*. 314: 605–13.

Paffenbarger RS, Wing AL, Hyde RT. 1978. Physical activity as an index of heart attack risk in college alumni. *Am J Epidemiol* 108: 161–75.

Paffenbarger RS Jr. and Hale WE. 1975. Work activity and coronary heart disease mortality. *N Engl J Med*. 292: 545–50.

Powell KE, Thompson PD, Caspersen CJ, Kendrick JS. 1987.Physical activity and the incidence of coronary heart disease. *Ann Rev Public Health*. 8: 253–87.

Raj T, D'Souza G, Elia M, Kurpad AV. 2006. Measurement of 24 h energy expenditure in male tuberculosis patients. *Indian J Med Res*. 124:665–76.

Ravussin E and Bogardus C. 1992. A brief overview of human energy metabolism and its relationship to essential obesity. *Am J Clin Nutr.* 55(suppl): 242S–45S.

Ravussin E, Lillioja S, Anderson TE, Christin L, Bogardus C. 1986. Determinants of 24-hour energy expenditure in man. *J Clin Invest.* 78: 1568–78.

Robinson TN. 1999. Reducing children's television viewing to prevent obesity: a randomized controlled trial. *JAMA* 282: 1561–7.

Rodriguez G, Beghin L, Michaud L, et al. 2002. Comparison of the TriTrac-R3D accelerometer and a self report activity diary with heart-rate monitoring for the assessment of energy expenditure in children. *Br J Nutr* 87: 623–31.

Sallis JF, Haskell W, Wood P, et al. 1985. Physical activity assessment methodology and the Five-City Project. *Am J Epidemiol.* 121: 91–106.

Scruggs PW, Beveridge SK, Eisenman PA, Watson DL, Shultz BB, Ransdell LB. 2003. Quantifying physical activity via pedometry in elementary physical education. *Med Sci Sports Exerc.* 35: 1065–71.

Seale JL & Rumpler WV. 1997. Comparison of energy expenditure measurements by diet records, energy intake balance, doubly labeled water and room calorimetry. *Eur J Clin Nutr.* 51: 856–863.

Siconolfi SF, Lasater TM, Snow RCK, Carleton RA. 1985. Self-reported physical activity compared with maximal oxygen uptake. *Am J Epidemiol* 122: 101–5.

Siscovick DS, Ekelund LG, Hyde JS, Johnson JL, Gordon DJ, LaRosa JC. 1988. Physical activity and coronary heart disease among asymptomatic hypercholesterolemic men. *Am J Public Health* 78: 1428–31.

Starling RD, Mathews DE, Ades PA, Poehlman ET. 1999. Assessment of physical activity in older individuals: A doubly labeled water study. *J Appl Phys.* 86: 2090–6.

Sternfeld B, Cauley J, Harlow S, Liu G, Lee M. 2000. Assessment of physical activity with a single global question in a large, multiethnic sample of midlife women. *AmJ Epidemiol* 152: 678–87.

Storti KL, Pettee KK, Brach JS, Talkowski JB, Richardson CR, Kriska AM. 2008. Gait Speed and Step-Count Monitor Accuracy in Community-Dwelling Older Adults. *Med Sci Sports Exerc.* 40: 59–64.

Strath SJ, Bassett DR, Swartz AM. 2003. Comparison of MTI accelerometer cut-points for predicting time spent in physical activity. *Int J Sports Med.* 24: 298–303.

Strath SJ, Bassett DR, Thompson DL, Swartz AM. 2002. Validity of the simultaneous heart rate-motion sensor technique for measuring energy expenditure. *Med Sci Sports Exerc* 34: 888–94.

Taylor HL, Jacobs DR Jr., Schucker B, Knudsen J, Leon AS, De Backer G. 1978. A questionnaire for the assessment of leisure time physical activities. *J Chronic Dis.* 31: 741–44.

Trost SG, Pate RR, Sallis JF, et al. 2002. Age and gender differences in objectively measured physical activity in youth. *Med Sci Sports Exerc.* 34: 350–5.

Tudor-Locke C, Bassett DR, Swartz AM, et al. 2004. A preliminary study of one year of pedometer self-monitoring. *Ann Behavior Med* 28(3): 158–62.

Tudor-Locke CE and Myers AM. 2001. Methodological considerations for researchers and practitioners using pedometers to measure physical (ambulatory) activity. *ResQuarter Exerc Sport* 71: 1–12.

Uitenbroek DG. 1993. Seasonal variation in leisure time physical activity. *Med Sci Sports Exerc* 25(6): 755–60.

Utter J, Neumark-Sztainer D, Jeffery R, Story M. 2003. Couch potatoes or french fries: are sedentary behaviors associated with body mass index, physical activity, and dietary behaviors among adolescents? *J Am Diet Assoc.* 103: 1298–305.

U. S. Department of Health and Human Services. 1996. Surgeon General's report on physical activity and health. From the Centers for Disease Control and Prevention. Washington, DC: US Government Printing Office.

Vaz de Almeida MD, Graca P, Afonso C, D'Amicis A, Lappalainen R, Damkjaer S. 1999. Physical activity levels and body weight in a nationally representative sample in the European Union. *Public Health Nutr* 2: 105–13.

Ventham JC and Reilly JJ. 1999. Reproducibility of resting metabolic rate measurement in children. *Br J Nutr.* 81: 435–7.

Warnecke RB, Johnson TP, Chavez N, et al. 1997. Improving question wording in surveys of culturally diverse populations. *Ann Epidemiol.* 7: 334–42.

Washburn RA, Goldfield SR, Smith KW, McKinlay JB. 1990. The validity of self-reported exercise-induced sweating as a measure of physical activity. *Am J Epidemiol* 132: 107–31.

Washburn RA and Montoye HL. 1986. Validity of heart rate as a measure of mean daily energy expenditure. *Exerc Physiol* 2: 161–72.

Wilmore JH and Haskell WL. 1971. Use of the heart rate-energy expenditure relationship in the individualized prescription of exercise. *Am J Clin Nutr* 24: 1186–92.

Wolf AM, Hunter DJ, Colditz GA, et al. 1994. Reproducibility and validity of a self-administered physical activity questionnaire. *Int J Epidemiol* 23: 991–9.

Yore MM, Ham SA, Ainsworth BE, Macera CA, Jones DA, Kohl H. 2005. Occupational Physical Activity: Reliability and Comparison of Activity Levels. *J Phys Act Health* 2(3): 358–65.

3

Establishing Validity and Reliability of Physical Activity Assessment Instruments

David R. Bassett, Jr. and
Eugene C. Fitzhugh

Chapter 2 provided an overview of tools used to assess physical activity and inactivity, including both subjective and objective instruments. Before starting data collection for an epidemiological study, researchers need to decide which instrument to use. Some of the factors that need to be considered before selecting an appropriate assessment tool are discussed in Chapter 2. The chapter mentions validity and reliability as two important factors to evaluate when choosing a physical activity assessment instrument. This chapter provides a more in-depth discussion on validity and reliability of physical activity assessment tools.

In most research applications, researchers should select an existing survey instrument with established validity and reliability, rather than creating new instruments. The benefits of choosing an existing instrument are that it permits comparisons between studies, has higher credibility, and avoids the time and cost of developing a new instrument. However, in a few situations, researchers may desire to develop an original survey instrument. For example, they may want to improve on previous instruments, obtain more detailed information on physical activity, or develop a questionnaire that is culturally relevant for a certain (e.g., minority) population. As part of the process of developing a new instrument, researchers will need to establish the validity and reliability of the new instrument.

The aim of this chapter is to provide an understanding of how to critically evaluate the validity and reliability of survey instruments for measuring physical activity. If an existing instrument were to be chosen, the first step would be to search the literature for studies that have been performed to establish its validity and reliability. If there is sufficient evidence that the chosen instrument is a robust measure of physical activity in the population of interest, then the research can proceed. However, if validity and reliability studies are lacking, then the researchers should conduct studies to address these issues. The results of the validity and reliability studies can be affected by a number of factors, including the type of validation criteria selected, the characteristics of the population being studied, the measurement time frame, and the methods of statistical analysis used. These factors will be discussed in detail in this chapter.

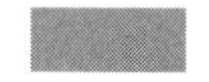

Evaluating Validity of Physical Activity Assessment Instruments

Introduction to Validity

According to Webster, "valid" is defined as "well grounded or justifiable; supported either by objective truth or generally accepted standard or authority" (Grove, 1986). Therefore,

Table 3.1 Types of Validity

Type of validity	*What it ensures*	*How to evaluate this*
Logical validity	Instrument is logically sound, and experts agree that it measures what it is supposed to.	Use an expert panel to evaluate the instrument.
Content validity	Instrument asks about the important content areas.	Check to see if the instrument asks about the content areas that it should.
Construct validity	In cases where a trait cannot be measured directly, but must be estimated indirectly, the instrument is sound in measuring the indirect trait.	Use correlation techniques involving convergent, discriminant, and multiple approaches.
Convergent validity	Instrument is highly correlated to another one that measures the same construct.	Examine relationships between two instruments that purport to measure the same construct.
Discriminant validity	Instrument is unrelated to another one that measures a different construct.	Examine relationships between two instruments that purport to measure different constructs
Criterion-Referenced validity	Instrument compares favorably with a "gold standard."	Determine if the instrument can predict the "gold standard" criterion accurately.
Concurrent validity	Instrument shows agreement with another, generally accepted instrument.	Examine correlation with another instrument with established validity.

Adapted from *Evaluation in Physical Education* (Safrit, 1981). Physical activity refers to any body movements that are produced by skeletal muscles and result in energy expenditure (Caspersen, 1989). In the industrialized world, physical activity is performed in the context of leisure time pursuits, job-related tasks, transportation, household chores (including gardening activities and yardwork), and activities of daily living. The term "exercise" is a subset of physical activity; it refers to activities that are done for the purpose of improving fitness, health, or athletic performance (*see* Chapter 2 for additional discussion).

a valid instrument for assessing physical activity is one that provides a sound measure of physical activity and is backed up by empirical evidence.

Types of Validity

There are many different types of validity, as shown in Table 3.1. Some types of validity are more relevant to psychometric tests, where one must show that an instrument is measuring the variable that it is believed to be measuring. From the viewpoint of physical activity, it is conceptually clear what it is that we are trying to measure. This is because physical activity is a variable that is capable of being directly observed. The most relevant types of validity for the field of physical activity epidemiology are logical, concurrent, and criterion-referenced validity.

Physical activity is a behavior that has multiple dimensions to it. Researchers may be interested in the types of activities that people perform as well as the frequency, intensity, and/or duration of these activities. Energy expenditure from physical activity is a combined measure that reflects all of these dimensions; it is of great interest because of its role in energy balance and prevention of chronic diseases (*see* Chapters 8-12). It is worth noting that the total daily energy expenditure (TDEE) comprises three components: *(a)* energy expenditure from physical activity, *(b)* resting metabolic rate, and *(c)* the thermic effect of feeding.

Researchers may wish to focus on energy expenditure if their primary hypothesis revolves around energy balance or weight control. In other cases, they might specifically want to know about one particular domain of activity (e.g., occupational activity) or they might wish to know the number of minutes spent each day in moderate-intensity physical activity, which is derived from measures of frequency, duration, and intensity. The validation criteria the researchers select will depend on what parameter(s) is of interest.

Validation Criteria for Physical Activity Assessment Instruments

Numerous methods of validating physical activity assessment instruments are available. Epidemiologists investigating physical activity should be aware of these methods, even if they do not plan to conduct the validation studies themselves. Familiarity with validation methods will enable epidemiologists to search the literature and evaluate the research evidence associated with a particular assessment instrument to ensure that the chosen instrument for assessing physical activity is a sound one.

Validation criteria can be divided into two broad categories: direct and indirect. (Note that these terms should not be confused with direct and indirect measures of energy expenditure referred to in Chapter 2). Direct validation criteria are those methods that are well-established to provide rigorous, more objective measures of physical activity but are frequently too time-consuming or expensive to use in large, population-based studies. Further discussion of these criteria is provided below. Indirect validation criteria are physiological variables, such as maximal oxygen uptake or percent body fat, that are influenced by physical activity levels, whether to a smaller or larger extent (Jacobs et al., 1993). Although these indirect criteria provide some support for the soundness of a physical activity assessment instrument, they do not give as strong evidence as the direct validation criteria and will not be discussed further in this chapter.

In this section, we describe direct criterion measures used to examine the validity of physical activity questionnaires used in epidemiologic studies. For each direct validation criterion, we provide examples of studies that have used the particular criterion. These examples will use statistical methods that are described in detail later in this chapter under "Analyzing Validity Data." A complete listing of studies that have used the various criteria to validate different physical activity questionnaires is beyond the scope of this chapter. To obtain more information, the reader should consult textbooks on the measurement of physical activity and energy expenditure (Montoye et al., 1995; Welk, 2002) and a journal supplement that reviews many commonly used physical activity questionnaires (Kriska and Casperson, 1997).

Doubly Labeled Water

Doubly labeled water (DLW) can provide a measure of human energy expenditure under free-living conditions. With this method, energy expenditure is estimated from the rate of metabolic carbon dioxide (CO_2) production. A subject consumes a dose of DLW, which contains higher-than-normal levels of stable isotopes of ^2H_2O and $H_2{}^{18}O$, and within hours the isotopes distribute themselves in equilibrium with body water. A urine sample is collected soon after the equilibration of stable isotopes within the body and then again after 1 to 2 weeks have elapsed. The labeled hydrogen gradually leaves the body as water (^2H_2O), whereas the labeled oxygen is eliminated from the body as water ($H_2{}^{18}O$) and also as carbon dioxide ($C^{18}O_2$). From the difference in the rates of turnover of the isotopes ^2H and ^{18}O in urine, it is possible to compute the rate of CO_2 production, and then caloric expenditure can be estimated (LaMonte et al., 2003; Schoeller, 2002).

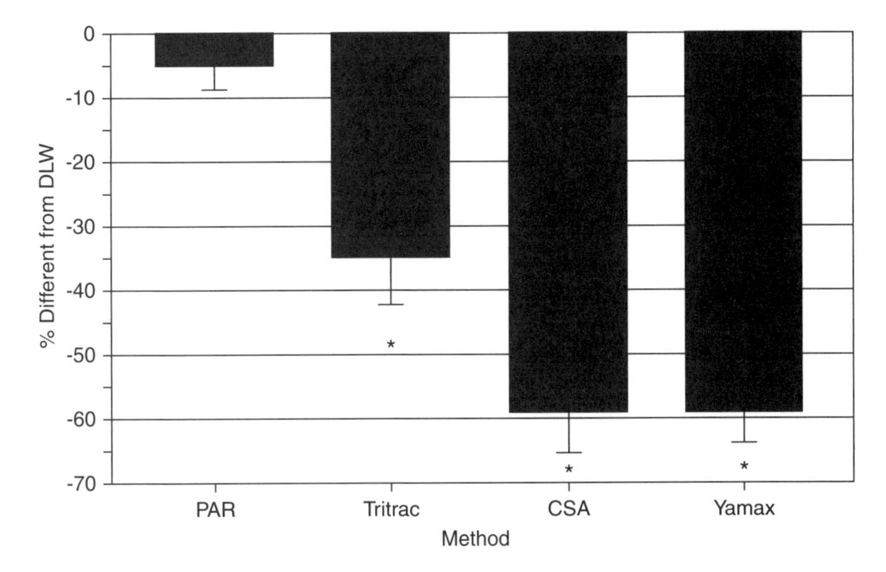

Figure 3.1 Percent difference in the energy expended on physical activity, comparing the doubly labeled water (DLW) technique with the 7-day PAR, the Tritrac, the CSA Actigraph, and the Yamax pedometer in 13 women. Values are mean ± SEM; * $p < 0.05$ compared to DLW. (From Leenders et al., 2001. Evaluation of methods to assess physical activity in free-living conditions. *Med Sci Sports Exerc* 33: 1233–40, with permission.)

An example of this validation technique is provided by Leenders et al. (2001), who examined the validity of the 7-day Physical Activity Recall (PAR) questionnaire and three physical activity monitoring devices (Tritrac accelerometer, CSA Actigraph, and Yamax DW-500 pedometer) in women ages 21 to 37 years using DLW. TDEE was measured over a 7-day period, and body composition, basal metabolic rate (BMR), and peak oxygen consumption were also measured. The energy expended on physical activity was computed by subtracting BMR and the estimated thermic effect of feeding from TDEE. The investigators found that there was no significant difference between the energy expended on physical activity as determined by the 7-day PAR (642 kcal/d) and DLW (798 kcal/d), but the other three methods greatly underestimated the energy expended on physical activity (Fig. 3.1). However, the 7-day PAR significantly overestimated the energy expended on physical activity for less active women and significantly underestimated the energy expended on physical activity for more active women (Fig. 3.2). Therefore, although the 7-day PAR gives an accurate group estimate of the energy expended on physical activity, it may not provide accurate, quantitative information on subgroups of sedentary or highly active women.

Doubly labeled water is a safe, accurate, and objective method of quantifying total energy expenditure in free-living individuals. The primary advantage is that it allows people to go about their daily activities unencumbered by monitors and unburdened by having to complete physical activity recalls for a week or more. Although there is currently no shortage of DLW (D. Schoeller, personal communication 6/22/05), the cost remains high (approximately $500 per adult dose). Furthermore, there are technical difficulties with the analytical procedures needed to measure stable isotopes. A special instrument called a mass ratio spectrophotometer is needed to detect the levels of stable isotopes in body fluids. Hence, only researchers who are thoroughly trained and knowledgeable about sources of error should conduct these studies. Another limitation of this validation criterion is that although it provides accurate data on the TDEE and the energy expended on physical activity, it

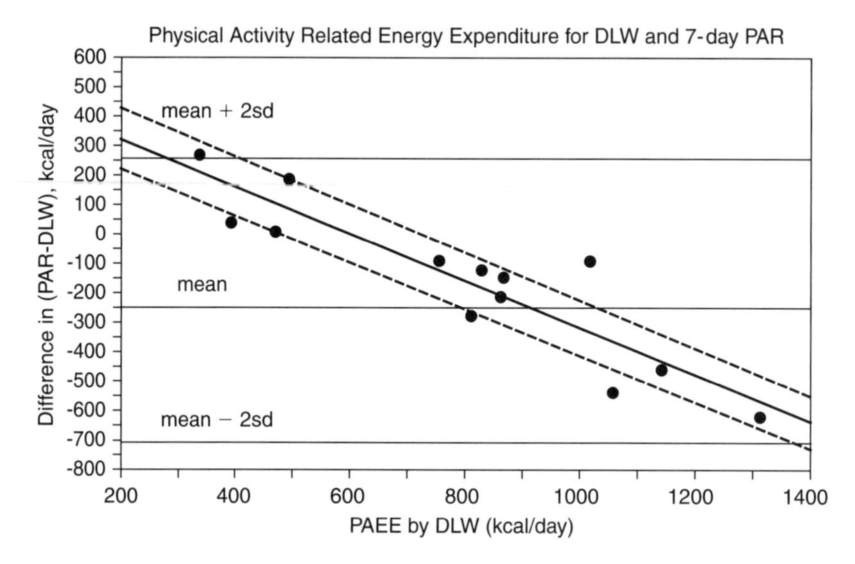

Figure 3.2 Difference between physical activity energy expenditure (PAEE) estimated by the DLW technique and the 7-day PAR, plotted against PAEE estimated by the DLW technique in 13 women. The solid horizontal line represents the mean difference between the two methods, averaged over all women. The solid diagonal line is the line of best fit for the individual data-points, and the dashed line represents the 95% confidence limits. (From Leenders et al., 2001. Evaluation of methods to assess physical activity in free-living conditions. *Med Sci Sports Exerc* 33: 1233–40, with permission.)

cannot determine the pattern of activity over time (e.g., type, intensity, duration, and frequency of physical activity).

Food Intake

Another method for measuring physical activity involves multiple measurements of food intake and body composition. The energy balance equation is a physical law of nature, stating that energy storage is equal to energy intake minus energy expenditure. Therefore, if one knows how much energy an individual consumes over 1 or 2 weeks and how much body fat and lean body mass stores have changed in this period of time, it is possible to compute how much energy was expended. By taking the TDEE and subtracting the resting metabolic rate and an estimate of the thermic effect of food, one can estimate the energy expended on physical activity.

An example of a validation study using the food intake method is that of Albanes et al. (1990). Investigators performed a simultaneous validation study of eight widely used physical activity surveys at the United States Department of Agriculture labs in Beltsville, Maryland (Table 3.2). Twenty-one healthy men ages 28 to 55 years ate their meals at the Human Nutrition Research Center for 7 days, enabling food intake to be quantified. Their body composition changed very little during this period. Physical activity estimates derived from the questionnaires tended to increase with increasing energy intake. Spearman correlations between energy intake and the different physical activity questionnaires ranged from 0.13 for the Minnesota Leisure Time Physical Activity (LTPA) questionnaire to 0.49 for the Harvard Alumni questionnaire; these correlations were higher than those between non-resting energy expenditure and physical activity estimated from the questionnaires. The mean physical activity estimate from the Stanford Five-City Project questionnaire (a 7-day PAR) showed the closest relationship to caloric intake. The questionnaires all had

Table 3.2 Total Energy Intake, Non-Resting Energy Expenditure*, and Physical Activity Estimated From Eight Questionnaires+.

	Energy Intake Level			*All Subjects*
	2400–2800 kcal/day	*3200 kcal/day*	*3600–4000 kcal/day*	*3257 (89) kcal/day*
No. of subjects	5	9	7	21
Non-resting energy expenditure (kcal/day)	1464 (68)	1815 (68)	2318 (76)	1899 (84)
Harvard Alumni (kcal/day)	148 (53)	277 (79)	417 (147)	293 (62)
Pennsylvania Alumni (kcal/day)	3407 (138)	4387 (349)	4688 (197)	4254 (194)
Five-City Project (kcal/day)	2786 (248)	3234 (223)	3272 (238)	3140 (138)
Framingham (kcal/day)	2352 (168)	2780 (252)	3120 (196)	2791 (142)
Minnesota LTPA (kcal/day)	439 (116)	883 (406)	672 (201)	707 (186)
Baecke (index)	6.8 (0.7)	7.5 (0.7)	8.1 (0.5)	7.5 (0.4)
Health Insurance Plan (index)	14.6 (2.3)	18.3 (2.4)	17.0 (1.7)	17.0 (1.3)
Lipid Research Clinics (index)	0.60 (0.40)	0.67 (0.29)	1.29 (0.28)	0.86 (0.19)

Men were divided into three groups according to their level of energy intake. Values are mean (SD).

*Estimated by subtracting resting metabolic rate and the thermic effect of food from total daily energy expenditure (assumed to be total energy intake because body composition changed very little).

+Harvard Alumni and Minnesota LTPA questionnaires estimate leisure-time physical activity; Pennsylvania Alumni, Five-City Project, and Framingham questionnaires estimate total daily energy expenditure; Baecke, Health Insurance Plan, and Lipid Research Clinics questionnaires estimate an index of total daily energy expenditure.

(Adapted from Albanes et al., 1990.)

considerable individual error in their estimates but were generally able to distinguish between groups that varied in terms of the energy expended on physical activity (whether measured as leisure-time physical activity, TDEE, or an index of TDEE).

The food intake method is simple in principle, but it is expensive and relatively few laboratories have the ability to prepare foods and monitor caloric intake with precision. Nevertheless, it is a valid, objective method for assessing the energy expended on physical activity in small groups of free-living subjects, over extended time periods. As with DLW, a limitation of this technique is that the frequency, intensity, duration, and type of physical activity cannot be individually discerned.

Indirect Calorimetry

Indirect calorimetry refers to measurements of energy expenditure made through determining rates of oxygen consumption and carbon dioxide production. Indirect calorimetry is a well-accepted "gold standard" for assessment of the energy expended on physical activity. One method involves having a subject live in a sealed room calorimeter, typically for 24 hours. Although some room calorimeters measure heat production directly, by pumping water through tubes on the interior side of thickly insulated walls and sensing the change in water temperature, most room calorimeters measure energy expenditure by a flow-through system where oxygen uptake and carbon dioxide are monitored continuously. Confining a subject to a room severely restricts the types of activities that can be performed, so this technique is of limited usefulness in validating physical activity assessment instruments intended for use in free-living individuals. Nevertheless, it can provide information on the validity of objective monitoring devices in settings where indoor activities are performed.

A more practical application of indirect calorimetry uses a portable metabolic measurement system, such as the Cosmed K4b2 device (Cosmed, Rome, Italy). With this system, the subject wears a face mask covering the nose and mouth, whereas ventilatory gas exchange is measured via a turbine flow meter and oxygen and carbon dioxide analyzers. By having a subject perform various activities, researchers can determine the accuracy of objective monitoring devices (e.g., pedometers, accelerometers, heart rate [HR] monitors) in a field setting. This is useful in validating physical activity assessment tools (e.g., accelerometers, HR monitors) that measure exercise intensity, as we will discuss later. Limitations to the portable metabolic system are that it is moderately intrusive and it cannot be worn for long periods of time.

Physical Activity Records

With physical activity records (sometimes called diaries), researchers seek to collect physical activity information while (or soon after) an individual engages in various activities. The time of day, the description of the activity, the intensity, and the activity domain are recorded using a paper-and-pencil instrument. Therefore, this method has a high participant burden because subjects must continually record the activities in which they engage.

For example, Ainsworth et al. (1993) used physical activity records to examine the validity of the Harvard Alumni Health Study questionnaire in 78 men and women (ages 21–59 years) with a broad range of activity habits. Physical activity was determined from the sum of energy expended in walking, climbing stairs, and participation in sports and recreation, recalled over the past week. The participants recorded their physical activity for several 2-day periods. Correlations between physical activity, as measured by the questionnaire and the records, were higher for vigorous activities ($r = 0.34$–0.69; $p < 0.05$) than for lighter intensity activities ($r < 0.35$; $p > 0.05$). Energy expended in walking and stair climbing was underestimated by this questionnaire, and non-exercise tasks (e.g., shopping, household chores, occupational jobs, lawn and garden chores) were also underestimated. This resulted in lower total physical activity scores on the questionnaire (1270 metabolic equivalent [MET]·min/week) compared to the records (3856 MET·min/week).

Many earlier physical activity surveys, such as the Harvard Alumni Health Study questionnaire, focused heavily on sports and recreation (and, to some extent, transportation-related activities such as walking). This questionnaire provided a valid estimate of the energy expended in leisure-time physical activity among middle-aged men of upper socioeconomic status, the population for which the questionnaire was designed. However, such surveys may not perform as well in other populations because they do not capture the ubiquitous, lighter intensity activities performed throughout the day (Ainsworth, 2000). Thus, more recent surveys have been developed to capture not only structured exercise but also physical activity conducted in other domains such as domestic chores, transportation, and job-related tasks. However, obtaining adequate subjective recall of non-exercise physical activity, particularly lighter intensity activity, remains a challenge, and future validation studies will need to address this issue.

Physical Activity Logs

Physical activity logs collect information on the type, duration, and intensity of movement, at the end of an observation period (usually a day), as opposed to records where subjects are required to record their activities during or soon after the activity. Typically, participants are given a checklist consisting of a large number of different physical activities. At regular time-intervals, the participants are asked to recall the amount of time they spent on the various activities. The MET level of the activities is typically determined from a compendium of physical activities (Ainsworth et al., 2000b) , allowing the total energy expenditure, as well as the time spent in activities of various intensity categories, to be estimated.

Matthews et al. (2003) examined the validity of the Shanghai Women's Health Study (SWHS) physical activity questionnaire compared to four physical activity logs collected within a 12-month period. Two hundred women (ages 40–70 years) were included in the study. At the end of each observation day, the women were instructed to record in their logs the time spent in a range of activities, including housework, transportation, occupation, and up to 26 different sport, exercise, or recreational activities. The SWHS questionnaire asked about exercise (type, intensity, duration) and non-occupational lifestyle activities. The results of the validation study showed significant correlations between the questionnaire and logs with regard to exercise, for both the first questionnaire administration ($r = 0.50$) and the second questionnaire administration ($r = 0.74$). (The questionnaires were administered 1.5–2.5 years apart.) However, for lifestyle activities, there was low agreement between the questionnaire and logs (with the exception of bicycling). The authors concluded that the SWHS questionnaire is a generally valid measure of exercise behaviors.

Different types of physical activity logs have been developed, with varying levels of respondent burden. Ainsworth et al. (2000a) developed a physical activity log that consists of a list of approximately 50 different activities grouped into general categories (household chores, caring for others, transportation, walking, dancing, sports, conditioning, inactivity, occupation, and volunteering). At the end of the day, participants indicate how much time was spent in each of the categories. In contrast, the physical activity log developed by another researcher (Bouchard et al., 1983) requires participants to list the activity category (1 through 9) performed at regular 15-minute intervals throughout the day. Activity categories are numbered in order of increasing intensity, with examples of specific activities provided for each activity category. Relatively few published studies use physical activity logs as the criterion measure for validation. This may be because logs are self-reporting instruments that fall in between records and questionnaires in terms of respondent burden. Although physical activity logs can lessen concerns about loss of recall over the longer time frame typically used in questionnaires, the logs still rely on subjective recall of past events.

Electronic Pedometers

Pedometers are small, body-borne devices for measuring steps and/or distance. Most pedometers are worn on the belt or waistband, in the mid-line of the thigh. The best pedometers are accurate in their measurement of the number of steps taken (Crouter et al., 2003; Schneider et al., 2003a). Because the number of steps is the most direct expression of what the pedometer actually measures, most researchers express their data as "steps per day" (Tudor-Locke and Myers, 2001). There is wide variation in accuracy among pedometer models (Schneider et al., 2003b), so it is important to choose one that has previously been validated. The Yamax SW-200 step counter (Fig. 3.3) is commonly used in research studies. The New Lifestyles NL-2000 (Fig. 3.4) is another device that is valid for counting steps; it has the ability to store up to 7 days of data. Pedometers have only moderate accuracy for measuring distance, and although the best pedometers estimate the caloric cost of walking reasonably well, they underestimate the cost of other lifestyle activities (Bassett et al., 2000a; Hendelman et al., 2000; Welk et al., 2000). As a result, one study estimated that the Yamax pedometer underestimates 24-hour energy expenditure (determined by DLW) by 59% (Leenders et al., 2001).

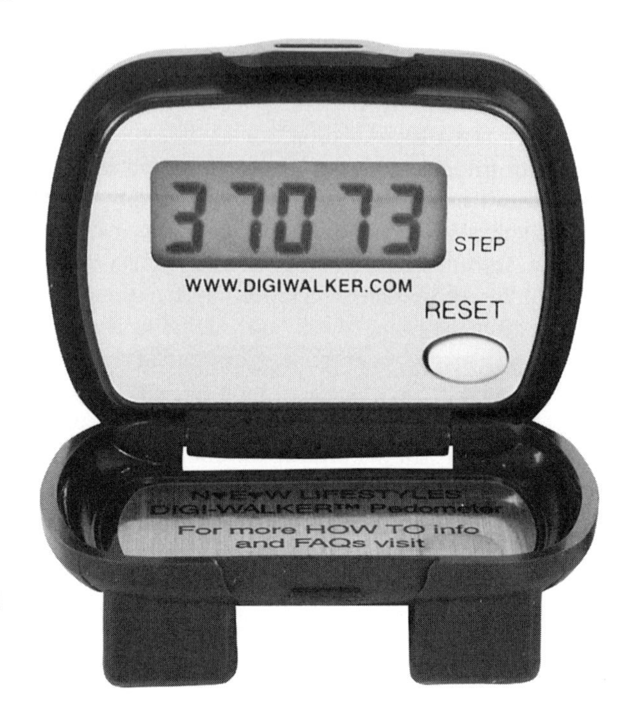

Figure 3.3 Yamax digi-walker SW-200 step counter, the most widely used pedometer in physical activity research. (Photo courtesy of New Lifestyles, Inc., Lee's Summit, MO.)

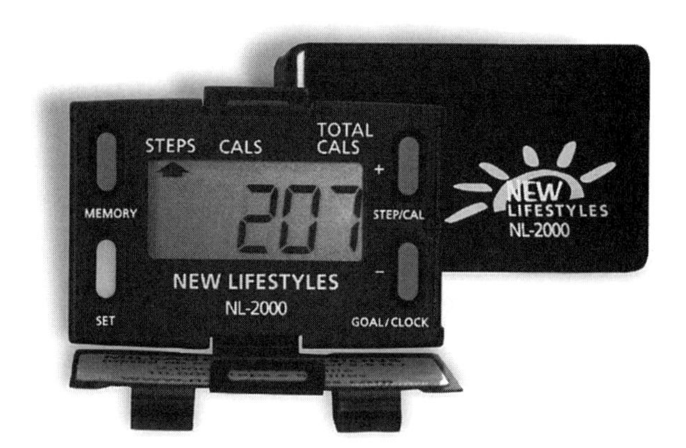

Figure 3.4 New Lifestyles NL-2000 pedometer, a valid device for counting steps. It stores up to 7 days of data in 1-day periods. (Photo courtesy of New Lifestyles, Inc., Lee's Summit, MO.)

In an example of a validation study, Stel et al. (2004) validated the Longitudinal Aging Study Amsterdam Physical Activity (LAPA) Questionnaire using a 7-day diary and a pedometer. The investigators studied a subgroup of 439 older adults enrolled in the Longitudinal Aging Study Amsterdam. Study respondents filled out the LAPA questionnaire, which asked about physical activity in the past 2 weeks, and a 7-day physical activity diary, where they recorded the time spent in various activities (with the 7 days overlapping the time period of the questionnaire). Additionally, participants wore a pedometer for the same 7 days that they kept the 7-day diary. Physical activity data from the LAPA questionnaire was highly correlated with data from the 7-day diary ($r = 0.68$; $p < 0.001$) and moderately correlated with data from the pedometer ($r = 0.56$; $p < 0.001$). The authors concluded that the LAPA physical activity questionnaire is a valid and reliable instrument for classifying physical activity in older people.

A well-known limitation of pedometers is that they fail to record activities such as swimming, rowing, and cycling (Bassett and Strath, 2002). However, pedometers can provide accurate, objective measures of walking-based activities, which are a major source of physical activity, especially in middle-aged and older adults. Pedometers are thus quite useful for validating physical activity survey instruments in these groups. Although the correlations between physical activity as measured by the pedometer and as measured by other direct criterion measures are only in the range of 0.3 to 0.5 when groups with diverse ages and activity levels are examined, pedometers excel at discriminating between sedentary individuals and those who perform various amounts of lifestyle physical activity (Bassett, 2000; Kriska, 2000).

Singe-Site Accelerometers

Accelerometers are small devices, usually worn at the hip, that measure accelerations occurring during body movement. Uni-axial accelerometers such as the Actigraph (Fort Walton Beach, FL; Fig. 3.5) measure acceleration in the vertical direction only. The Actical (Mini-Mitter Co., Sunriver, OR) is an accelerometer capable of detecting accelerations in two planes (Fig. 3.6). Tri-axial accelerometers such as the RT3 Research Tracker (Stayhealthy, Inc. Monrovia, CA) measure accelerations in three planes. The raw acceleration vs. time signal is filtered, integrated, rectified, and averaged over a user-specified time-interval (Chen and Bassett, 2005). The resulting accelerometer value (e.g., acceleration counts per minute) is then stored in a memory chip and can later be downloaded to a computer.

Craig et al. (2003) provided an example of a validation study that used accelerometers. Investigators examined the validity of the International Physical Activity Questionnaire (IPAQ), which was developed in 1999 for the purpose of having a standardized physical activity survey instrument that would be valid across different nations and cultures. Long and short forms of the IPAQ were compared to an objective criterion of body movement obtained with the Actigraph (formerly called the CSA/MTI Actigraph). A large number of adults from many countries were included in this study. Overall, the researchers found fair to moderate agreement between the IPAQ and the Actigraph criterion measure, with a pooled Spearman correlation of 0.33 ($n = 744$ subjects) for the long form and 0.30 ($n = 781$

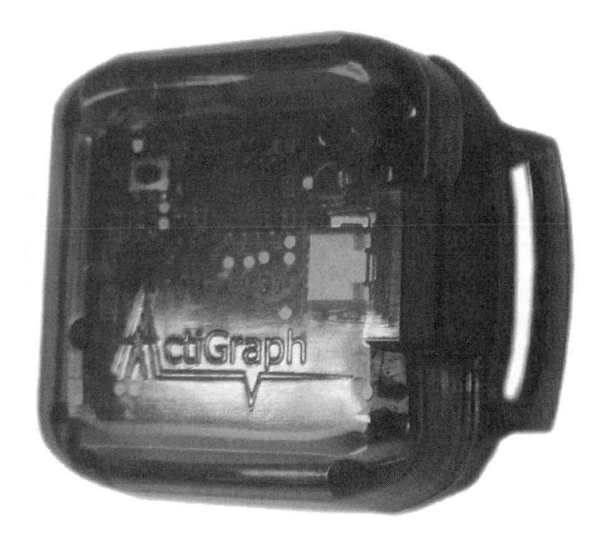

Figure 3.5 Actigraph (formerly CSA/MTI) activity monitor. It contains a uni-axial accelerometer, and when worn on the waist, it responds to and counts vertical accelerations of the trunk during human movements. (Photo courtesy of Actigraph, Inc., Fort Walton Beach, FL.)

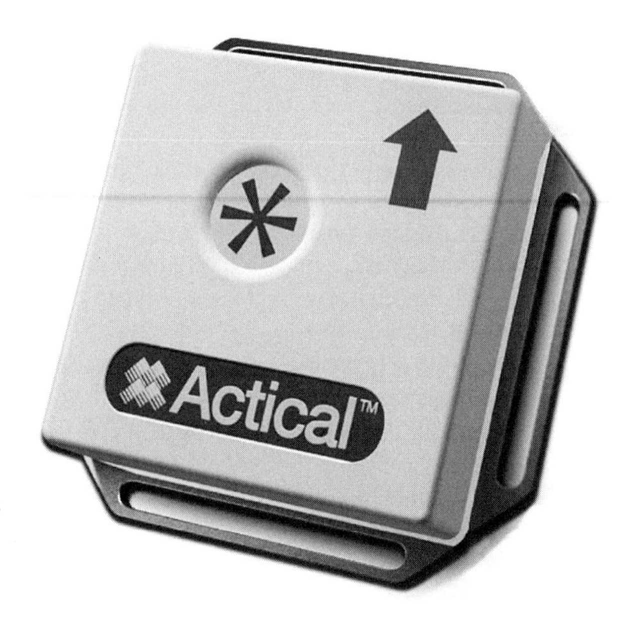

Figure 3.6 Actical activity monitor. This device contains an accelerometer, and when worn on the waist, it responds to and counts vertical accelerations of the trunk in two planes. (Photo courtesy of Mini-Mitter, Inc., Sunriver, OR.)

subjects) for the short form. The authors reported similar correlations between the IPAQ and the Actigraph criterion when assessing the time spent sitting. In each of the 12 countries studied, data were further analyzed to find the percent agreement with regard to the proportion of subjects meeting physical activity recommendations when comparing the IPAQ and the Actigraph. The percent agreement was generally in the range of 0.65 to 0.85 for most of the countries. Therefore, the IPAQ appears to have satisfactory validity when compared to an objective measure of body movement.

Researchers often desire to translate accelerometer data (counts per minute) into units that are more intuitive and meaningful, such as kcal/day of energy expenditure or minutes of moderate physical activity per day. To do this, they rely on single, linear regression equations relating accelerometer scores to, for example, units of energy expenditure (Freedson et al., 1998). These regression equations are typically generated by studies that have performed "metabolic calibrations" of accelerometers in laboratory or field settings (Freedson et al., 1998; Hendelman et al., 2000; Swartz et al., 2000). However, a limitation of the method is that regression equations developed using walking and jogging typically under-predict the energy expenditure of other lifestyle activities, whereas those developed using moderate lifestyle activities (e.g., household chores, occupational tasks, recreation, lawn and garden tasks) over-predict the cost of walking and light activities. Thus, the use of "cut-points" to distinguish light from moderate and moderate from vigorous intensity physical activity has limitations. Depending on which set of cut-points is chosen, the estimated number of minutes spent in moderate activity can vary tremendously (Ainsworth et al., 2000a; Schmidt et al., 2003, Strath et al., 2003).

Accelerometers have two distinct advantages over pedometers: *(a)* vigorous movements result in higher scores than moderate ones, and *(b)* accelerometers can record the minute-by-minute pattern of activity for up to several weeks. A limitation of accelerometers is that, at present, the current methods of estimating "time spent in moderate PA" using counts from the uni-axial accelerometers are not accurate at the individual level (Strath et al., 2002). However, researchers are working hard to improve the prediction of energy expenditure from accelerometers. For example, tri-axial accelerometers appear to provide a better prediction of energy expenditure than uni-axial accelerometers, because they account for changes in direction in the horizontal plane (Westerterp, 1999). Additionally, Crouter et al. (2006) has developed a method of discriminating between Actigraph data points that occur during walking and those obtained during other activities. This method analyzes the variability in counts and relies on the fact that walking results in more consistent counts over time than intermittent, lifestyle activities. Therefore, the regression equations relating counts and energy expenditure are different for walking/jogging and for lifestyle physical activities; thus, by using a two-regression model, a more accurate prediction of energy expenditure can be obtained. Other highly sophisticated Actigraph methods allow for specific types of activities to be identified and may enable even better predictions of energy expenditure in the future (Pober et al., 2004).

Monitoring Heart Rate

The HR is a physiological variable that is strongly related to energy expenditure in graded exercise testing. Thus, HR has long been used to predict energy expenditure during free-living physical activity (Berggren and Christensen, 1950). Because the HR response to a given level of energy expenditure is much lower in aerobically fit individuals, most researchers construct individualized HR-vs.-energy expenditure calibration curves (Ceesay et al., 1989). This method tends to minimize interindividual error in the prediction of energy expenditure compared to the use of raw HR data alone.

Many investigators employ the Flex HR method for a more accurate prediction of energy expenditure, especially during light activities (Ceesay et al., 1989; Emons et al. 1992; Fogelholm et al., 1988; Wareham et al., 1997). Flex HR is usually determined by measuring HRs during lying, sitting, standing, and light exercise (e.g., unloaded cycling) and then computing the mean of the highest resting value and lowest exercise value (Wareham et al., 1997). For HR values falling below the Flex HR, individuals are credited with resting energy expenditure. For HR values above the Flex HR, individual calibration curves are used to predict energy expenditure. The Flex HR method has been validated by comparing it to measures of energy expenditure obtained by indirect calorimetry and DLW, with good agreement obtained (Bitar et al., 1996; Ceesay et al., 1989; Emons et al., 1992).

The Polar S810 heart watch (Polar, Kempele, Finland) is an example of a HR monitor that can store minute-to-minute HR data for several days (Fig. 3.7). The cost is about $379. A transmitter unit strapped to the chest detects heartbeats and sends these data via radio waves to a receiver worn on the wrist. Polar heart watches have been validated against electrocardiographic measures of HR; however, certain radios and computers can affect the radio wave transmission and cause interference (Janz, 2002).

One limitation of the HR method is that it provides no information on the type of physical activity performed. In addition, HR can be influenced by the type of physical activity (arm vs. leg activity; Bassett, 2000) and by factors other than physical activity, such as environmental factors (ambient temperature and humidity), emotion, and body position. Nevertheless, HR monitoring is a fairly good and objective indicator of energy expenditure, and the percentage of maximal HR (or hear rate reserve) is a good estimate of the relative intensity of effort.

Simultaneous Heart Rate–Motion Sensor Technique

Haskell et al. (1993) showed that the simultaneous measurement of HR and motion increases the accuracy of energy expenditure prediction compared to either method used alone.

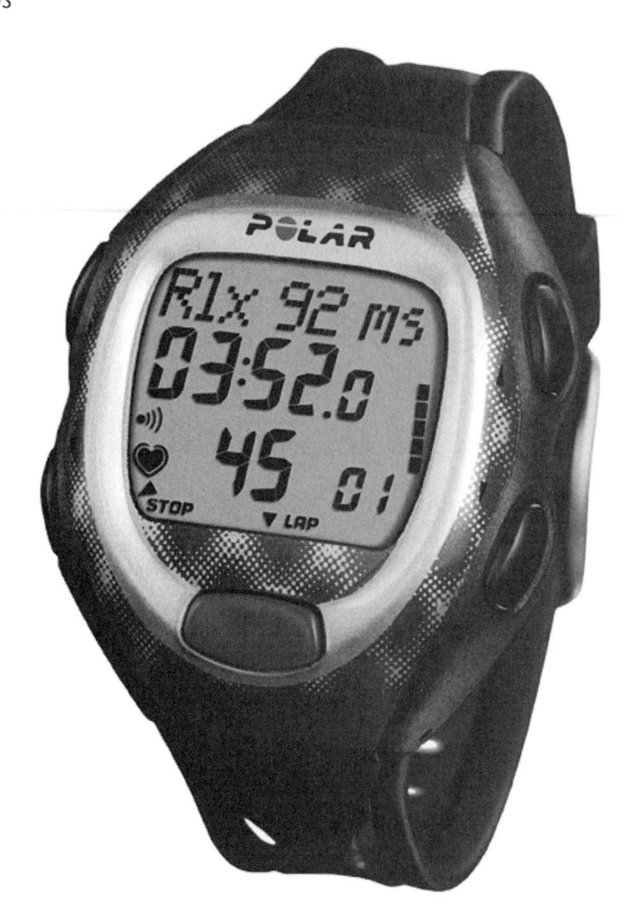

Figure 3.7 Polar S810 heart rate monitor. This device uses a belt worn around the chest to detect heart rate, and data are then transmitted to a wristwatch receiver by telemetry. The heart rate data can be downloaded to a computer for subsequent analysis. (Photo courtesy of Polar, Inc.)

With this validation technique, they proposed that individual calibration curves relating HR and energy expenditure first be established in the laboratory for exercises using the arms and the legs. Then, in free-living situations, motion sensors could be used to discriminate between arm and leg movements, and HR could be used to predict energy expenditure from the corresponding HR-vs.-energy expenditure calibration equations. In essence, this method yields a more accurate prediction than HR measurement alone, because it can screen out HR elevations resulting from factors other than physical activity (such as emotion), and it can also account for the differential HR-vs.-energy expenditure relationship resulting from arm exercise and leg exercise.

Strath et al. (2001) examined the validity of this method in light-to-moderate intensity activities, including 14 activities falling within the general categories of housework, walking, lawn and garden activities, stair climbing, and weight lifting. The simultaneous HR-motion sensor method provided much closer estimates of energy expenditure, as measured using a portable metabolic system (indirect calorimetry), than the CSA Actigraph (Fig. 3.8). In another study, Strath et al. (2002) validated the simultaneous HR–motion sensor method by comparing it to a portable metabolic system in free-living subjects. The simultaneous HR-motion sensor method was found to closely predict energy expenditure as measured with the portable metabolic system. Thus, the authors proposed that the simultaneous HR–motion sensor technique can be used as a criterion measure for measuring time spent in physical activity of different intensity categories.

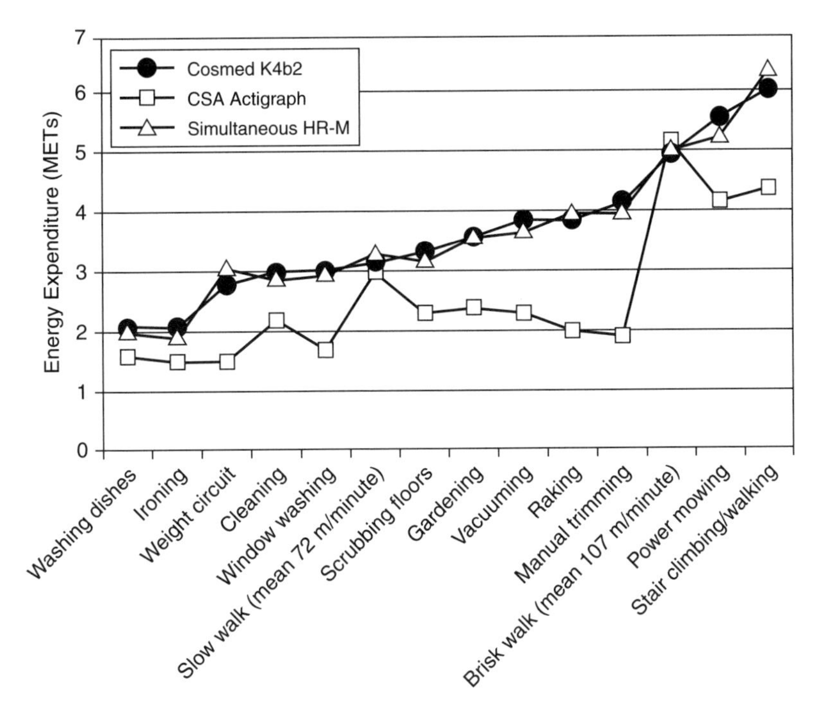

Figure 3.8 Comparison of measured energy expenditure (obtained by using the Cosmed $K4b^2$ portable metabolic system) vs. predicted energy expenditure obtained from the CSA Actigraph (using Freedson's regression equation) and the simultaneous heart rate–motion (HR-M) sensor technique. Note that the CSA Actigraph is valid for predicting the energy cost of walking, but it underpredicts the cost of other lifestyle activities. The simultaneous heart rate–motion sensor method is accurate across a wide range of activities. (Adapted from Strath et al., 2001.)

In another study, Strath et al. (2004) used the simultaneous HR–motion sensor technique to examine the validity of the Harvard Alumni Health Study questionnaire in 25 adults over 7 days. Estimates of the energy expended per day in light, moderate, vigorous, and total physical activity were obtained using the simultaneous HR–motion sensor method. At the end of 7 days, the Harvard Alumni Health Study questionnaire was administered. The correlations between the two methods varied, with vigorous ($r = 0.47$) and total physical activity ($r = 0.35$) showing higher correlations than light ($r = 0.20$) or moderate physical activity ($r = 0.27$). The mean levels of energy expended estimated using the two methods were similar for the categories of moderate and vigorous activities (although individual error scores were large). Light activity was significantly under-reported on the Harvard Alumni Health questionnaire, resulting in an underestimation of total physical activity. The results were consistent with other studies, showing that this physical activity questionnaire is better at measuring vigorous intensity activities than the ubiquitous light-to-moderate intensity activities performed throughout the day (Ainsworth et al., 1993; Bassett et al., 2000b).

Limitations of the simultaneous HR–motion sensor technique are its high cost, the need for individualized HR-vs.-energy expenditure calibration curves, and the time-consuming process of data reduction. At this time, no commercial company has simplified the tedious process of downloading data from the HR monitor, arm accelerometer, and leg accelerometer, nor has any commercial company developed software to predict energy expenditure based on these collective data.

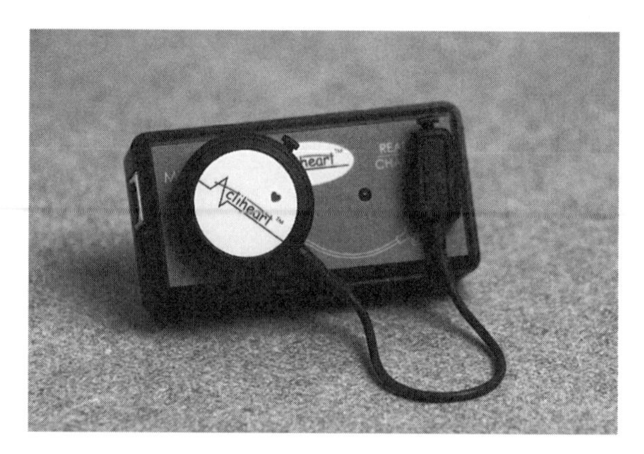

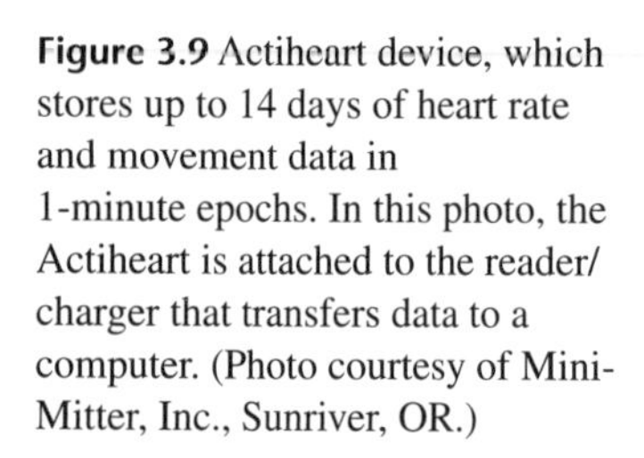
Figure 3.9 Actiheart device, which stores up to 14 days of heart rate and movement data in 1-minute epochs. In this photo, the Actiheart is attached to the reader/charger that transfers data to a computer. (Photo courtesy of Mini-Mitter, Inc., Sunriver, OR.)

The Actiheart (Mini-mitter, Sun River, OR) is a recently developed combined HR monitor-accelerometer weighing 9 g that is worn on the chest (Fig. 3.9). This device can store minute-by-minute data for up to 14 days. Brage et al. (2005) have developed equations to predict energy expenditure from a combination of HR and acceleration data using the Actiheart. Their method is accurate for predicting the energy cost of walking and running, and studies are currently being conducted to establish its validity with regard to other activities. Currently, the cost of the Actiheart is high ($1500 for Actiheart, download unit, and software).

Intelligent Device for Energy Expenditure and Activity Monitor

Recently, a portable device was developed for estimating energy expenditure from a combination of five sensors taped to the thighs, trunk, and feet. The sensors are connected to a small computer worn at the waist by wires. Known as the Intelligent Device for Energy Expenditure and Activity (IDEEA) monitor, it can record posture and body movements, allowing the type of body movement to be assessed (lying, sitting, standing, walking, running, jumping, etc.) and energy expenditure to be estimated. One study tested the ability of the IDEEA monitor to identify 32 common activities falling within one of several general categories (lie, recline, sit, stand, lean) and found that the device was highly successful at discriminating between the different types of activity (Zhang et al., 2003). A second study examined the validity of the IDEEA monitor for measuring energy expenditure by comparing it to indirect calorimetry (Zhang et al., 2004). The IDEEA monitor provided accurate estimates of energy expenditure during common activities (lying, sitting, standing, walking, running). In addition, it accurately estimated 24-hour energy expenditure while the subject lived in a metabolic chamber.

The IDEEA monitor is now considered an accepted method of determining "postural allocation." Therefore, it is useful for validating questions on physical activity survey instruments that ask respondents to recall the amount of time spent lying, sitting, standing, and walking. Researchers are currently examining the validity of the IDEEA monitor over a range of lifestyle, occupational, and leisure-time physical activities. If it lives up to its potential, the IDEEA monitor could be an ideal validation tool for examining not only the energy expended on physical activity but also for examining other dimensions of physical activity (i.e., frequency, intensity, duration, and type).

The main limitations to the IDEEA monitor are the expense (approximately $4,000), the presence of wires and sensors taped to the body, and the need to wear a "handheld computer" at the waist. These additional devices may be distracting and could limit the activities that a person chooses to engage in. However, for validation studies, this level of participant burden may be an acceptable trade-off, considering the quality of the information that can potentially be obtained.

Analyzing Validity Data

Correlation Coefficient

Pearson's correlation coefficient (r), also called the product moment correlation coefficient, is widely used to establish the validity of physical activity assessment instruments. It is a measure of the strength of the association between two variables. Pearson's correlation coefficients range from –1.00 to 1.00. The closer the absolute value of the "r" value is to 1.00, the higher the validity of the PA instrument (Morrow, 2002). (Please refer also to additional discussion in the section on Bland-Altman plots.) Spearman's non-parametric rank statistic can be used in instances where the data are not normally distributed. Like Pearson's r, Spearman's correlation coefficient provides a measure of the strength of an association between two variables.

Analysis of Variance

A repeated measures Analysis of Variance (ANOVA) is often used for examining mean differences between instruments. Where criterion-related validity is being examined, the researcher can simultaneously assess several physical activity assessment instruments and compare them against the "gold standard." A repeated measures ANOVA is then used to determine if there is a significant difference between the criterion and each of the assessment instruments. If an instrument gives values that are significantly higher than the criterion, it is said to overestimate physical activity. On the other hand, if it gives values that are significantly lower than the criterion, it is said to underestimate physical activity.

Bland-Altman Plots

To show that a physical activity instrument is accurate, it is not sufficient to show that a high correlation exists between the instrument and a criterion. For example, you could have a situation where the correlation coefficient is 1.00 but the instrument always yields values that underestimate the true measure by 50%. In addition, accuracy is not guaranteed simply because there is no significant difference between the means of the estimated values and the criterion. This is because a physical activity assessment instrument may greatly overestimate the criterion for some individuals and underestimate it for others. In that case, the instrument would not be accurate (on an individual basis), although the mean scores for the estimate and criterion are close.

A good method of addressing these issues is through the use of a Bland-Altman plot (Bland and Altman, 1986). This method involves plotting the error score (criterion minus estimate) on the y-axis against the mean of the criterion and estimate on the x-axis. Horizontal lines are drawn to depict the mean error and the 95% confidence interval for the individual observations (termed a "95% prediction interval"). Accuracy is ensured if the mean error is close to zero and the 95% prediction interval is tightly grouped around zero.

Percent Agreement

Sometimes researchers are not concerned with whether an instrument correctly measures energy expenditure but only whether it places individuals into the "correct" category of physical activity. An example of this is when investigators are interested in whether subjects do or do not meet the public health recommendation for physical activity, using data collected from questionnaires that ask them to report the time spent in moderate or vigorous physical activity. In the IPAQ validity and reliability study (Craig et al., 2003), the researchers wanted to know how often the IPAQ correctly identified individuals who met (or failed to meet) the minimum standard of 150 minutes of moderate physical activity per week (this is the current recommendation for physical activity; Pate et al., 1995). The Actigraph accelerometer served as the criterion measure for time spent in moderate physical activity. The IPAQ short form correctly classified individuals about 65% to 85% of the time in most countries. Thus, the authors concluded that the questionnaire has acceptable validity relative to an objective measure of physical activity.

Evaluating Reliability of Physical Activity Assessment Instruments

Introduction to Reliability

As mentioned at the beginning of this chapter, physical activity epidemiologists need to know if their instruments are reliable. The reliability of a physical activity assessment instrument refers to the dependability of scores (Safrit, 1981). Reliability is a measure of how consistent an instrument is when administered to the same individual repeatedly or by different investigators. A physical activity assessment instrument can be reliable without being valid (i.e., it consistently gives the same "wrong" number of units of activity), but it cannot be valid without being reliable.

Sources of Variability in Physical Activity Data

When attempting to measure physical activity, it is important to recognize that there are both biological and technical sources of variability. Biological variability is partly the result of inherent fluctuations in a person's level of physical activity. Technical variability refers to, for example, measurement errors that may occur because of poorly worded survey items, variation in the mode of survey administration (e.g., self-administered vs. interviewer-administered), and inadequate levels of subjective recall.

To reduce day-to-day variability occurring when measuring physical activity, researchers typically make measurements over multiple days. On a physical activity survey, this can be accomplished by asking about a "past 7-day" or "past month" time frame. The same purpose can be accomplished by having participants wear objective monitors (e.g., accelerometers) over 1 to 2 weeks. In general, using a measurement time frame such as this yields reliability coefficients that are in the range of 0.65 to 0.85 for most physical activity assessment instruments. Trost et al. (2005) recently concluded that 3 to 5 days of accelerometer monitoring are needed to achieve reliable results in adults. In children and adolescents, longer measurement periods (4–9 days) are needed to achieve an acceptable reliability of 0.80.

However, another threat to reliability comes from seasonal variation in physical activity (for additional discussion, *see* Chapter 2). In temperate North American climates, physical activity levels drop below the year-round average during the cold winter months, and they increase during the warmer summer months. Levin et al. (1999) administered the Minnesota Leisure-Time Physical Activity survey to 76 people every month for 14 months and reported that leisure-time activity was 40% higher in June than in March. Seasonal variation also occurred in a study that entailed 365 days of pedometer monitoring in Tennessee and North Carolina (Tudor-Locke et al., 2004). There are various ways researchers can deal with seasonal fluctuation in physical activity. If the intent is to measure the average physical activity level in the population (e.g., with the Behavioral Risk Factor Surveillance System), then they could conduct their sampling of different individuals throughout the year. However, if the researchers want to estimate an individual's habitual physical activity level to examine relationships with health outcomes, then they could administer the assessment instrument to each person: *(a)* multiple times throughout the year or *(b)* during the spring or fall, when seasonal average resembles the year-round average. The former method has inherent advantages because it will tend to reduce intra-individual variability through averaging of values.

For researchers interested in long-term physical activity levels, there are two basic approaches. First, a physical activity questionnaire that asks about "past-year" activity can be administered repeatedly and the values averaged. Alternatively, the researcher can choose to use a survey that asks about historical physical activity over a period of many years (Winters-Hart et al., 2004).

Types of Reliability

There are several types of reliability that measure different sources of variability in research data. These are outlined in Table 3.3. The main types of reliability we are concerned with in physical activity research are stability (determined by the test–retest method) and interdevice reliability. Split-half reliability, which is frequently assessed in educational testing situations, is not dealt with in this chapter.

Analyzing Reliability Data

Test–Retest Method

In most cases, researchers want to know how reliable (or stable) a measure of physical activity is over time. The test–retest method is a standard procedure for examining this. With this procedure, a survey is administered on two or more occasions, separated by weeks or months. The researchers can then compute an intraclass correlation coefficient (ICC) through the use of repeated measures ANOVA. If the data are skewed (i.e., not normally distributed), then Spearman's correlation coefficient should be used (Craig et al., 2003). Spearman's rho is a non-parametric statistic that is appropriate in this circumstance. In population-based studies, it is typical for physical activity data to be skewed, because some individuals tend to have very high activity levels.

Table 3.3 Types of Reliability

Type of reliability	*What it ensures*	*How to evaluate this*
Stability (test–retest)	Instrument is stable and dependable, when administered to the same person at multiple time points.	Intraclass correlation or Spearman's correlation
Interdevice reliability	Two different devices score the same performance consistently.	Single measure intraclass correlation
Split-half reliability	A test that is administered only once is divided in half, and the two half-tests show internal consistency.	Kuder-Richardson formula (KR-20) Cronbach's

The ICC and Spearman's correlation coefficients can range from 0 to 1.00, and the closer the value is to 1.00, the more reliable it is. In general, reliability coefficients of 0.80 or better are considered good for physical activity assessment instruments. Because true changes in activity levels can occur between testing periods, it is not realistic to expect a value of 1.00, and the longer the intervening time period, the more likely it is that a true change will occur. Note that Pearson's interclass correlation coefficient (r) should not be used for reliability testing, because it reflects the agreement between two different variables, rather than the same variable measured at least twice.

Interdevice Reliability

Sometimes a physical activity researcher is interested in how closely two different devices of the same model (e.g., accelerometers) rate the same person's activity. This is measured by testing the interdevice reliability. To do this, the researcher can measure a person's activity by simultaneously placing two or more accelerometers on the subject. The researcher can then estimate the interdevice reliability using a single-measure ICC.

Summary

In summary, epidemiologists need to be able to document the validity and reliability of the instruments they are using to measure physical activity. This will enable them to understand the strengths and limitations of their studies. Currently, questionnaires are the most common method of assessing physical activity in epidemiological studies. They will continue to be used in the future because of their low cost and ease of administration. However, more expensive and time-consuming methods can, and should, be used to examine the soundness and accuracy of the questionnaires used. Doubly labeled water, energy balance, and indirect calorimetry are the best validation criteria for assessing the total energy expended on physical activity; however, they cannot distinguish between the types of activity performed, their frequency, and duration. Physical activity records and logs are self-reporting instruments that can also be used as validation criteria, with the ability to provide details on the type, intensity, frequency, and duration of physical activity. Finally, HR monitors and movement sensors can be used alone or in conjunction with each other to validate physical activity instruments, after they themselves have been validated against the more expensive "gold standards."

Personal Perspective

Establishing the validity and reliability of physical activity assessment instruments is a continual and ongoing process. Validity cannot be established in a single study; rather, it takes multiple groups working on it to establish the soundness and robustness of a particular instrument (Mahar and Rowe, 2002). Epidemiologists can benefit greatly by knowing the validity and reliability of their questionnaires or surveys; this enables them to understand the strengths and limitations of their studies. In cases where they wish to develop a new survey or validate an existing one, epidemiologists can benefit from collaborating with researchers with expertise in physical activity measurement. For example, let us suppose a team of researchers has developed a new physical activity questionnaire. The new questionnaire could be validated in several ways. It could be compared to DLW to see if it is valid for measuring total energy expenditure. If the questionnaire estimates "time spent in moderate intensity physical activity," then it could be validated against the simultaneous HR–motion sensor technique. Physical activity records or logs could be used to determine if the questionnaire results in accurate, subjective recall of various activities. In addition, the questionnaire would need to be validated in a range of populations varying in age, gender, and ethnicity (if the intent is to use it with diverse groups). The process of establishing validity and reliability truly takes years.

Historically, most physical activity surveys presented people with a list of activities and asked them to recall the frequency and duration of their participation in each activity. However, some of the more recent questionnaires used (e.g., those used for surveillance, such as the Behavioral Risk Factor Surveillance System and IPAQ) simply ask respondents to report how many minutes per day they spend doing moderate or vigorous physical activity. This places the burden of determining intensity, frequency, and duration of physical activity bouts squarely on the respondents' shoulders. Although the new approach made life easier for the researchers who scored the questionnaires, it also raised questions about the validity of this approach! A major impetus for the development of the new questionnaires was the Centers for Disease Control and Prevention and the American College of Sports Medicine recommendation to accumulate 30 minutes of moderate physical activity on most—preferably all—days of the week (Pate et al., 1995). This created an interest in determining how many Americans were meeting the national physical activity recommendation, and attention shifted from the measurement of energy expenditure to a focus on measuring "time spent in moderate physical activity."

There will be many advances within the next 5-10 years that will enable researchers to better measure physical activity. As the cost of technology comes down and the prediction of energy expenditure improves, it will enhance our ability to validate physical activity assessment instruments. In addition, it is certain that objective monitors (e.g., accelerometers), either alone or in conjunction with physical activity surveys, will be used in more epidemiological studies in the future.

References

Ainsworth BE. 2000. Issues in the assessment of physical activity in women. *Res Q Exerc Sport.* 71 (2 Suppl): S37–42.

Ainsworth BE, Bassett DR, Strath SJ, et al. 2000. Comparison of three methods for measuring the time spent in physical activity. *Med Sci Sports Exerc* 32: S457–64.

Ainsworth BE, Leon AS, Richardson MT, Jacobs DR, Paffenbarger RS. 1993. Accuracy of the college alumnus physical activity questionnaire. *J Clin Epidemiol* 46: 1403–11.

Albanes D, Conway JM, Taylor PR, Moe PW, Judd J. 1990. Validation and comparison of eight physical activity questionnaires. *Epidemiology* 1: 65–71.

Bassett DR. 2000. Validity and reliability issues in objective monitoring of physical activity. *Res Quarter Exerc Sport* 71: 30–6.

Bassett DR, Ainsworth BE, Swartz AM, Strath SJ, O'Brien WL, King GA. 2000a. Validity of 4 motion sensors in measuring moderate intensity physical activity. *Med Sci Sports Exerc* 32: S471–80.

Bassett DR, Cureton AL, Ainsworth BE. 2000b. Measurement of daily walking distance- questionnaire versus pedometer. *Med Sci Sports Exerc* 32: 1018–23.

Bassett DR, Strath SJ. 2002. Use of pedometers to assess physical activity. In *Physical Activity Assessments for Health-Related Research*, GJ Welk (Ed.), Champaign, IL: Human Kinetics, pp. 163–77.

Berggren G, Christensen EH. 1950. Heart rate and body temperature as indices of metabolic rate during work. *Arbeitsphysiologie* 14: 255–60.

Bitar A, Vermorel M, Fellmann N, Bedu M, Chamoux A, Coudert J. 1996. Heart rate recording method validated by whole body indirect calorimetry in 10-yr-old children. *J Appl Physiol* 81: 1169–73.

Bland JM, Altman DG. 1986. Statistical methods for assessing agreement between two methods of clinical measurement. *Lancet* 1: 307–10.

Bouchard C, Tremblay A, LeBlanc C, Lortie G, Savard R, Theriault G. 1983. A method to assess energy expenditure in children and adults. *Am J Clin Nutr* 37: 461–7.

Brage S, Brage N, Franks PW, Ekelund U, Wareham NJ. 2005. Reliability and validity of the combined heart rate and movement sensor Actiheart. *Eur J Clin Nutr* 59: 561–70.

Caspersen CJ. 1989. Physical activity epidemiology: concepts, methods, and applications to exercise science. *Exerc Sport Sci Rev* 17: 423–73.

Ceesay SM, Prentice AM, Day KC, et al. 1989. The use of heart rate monitoring in the estimation of energy expenditure: a validation study using whole-body calorimetry. *Br J Nutrition* 61: 175–86.

Chen K, Bassett DR. 2005. The technology of accelerometry-based activity monitors: current and future. *Med Sci Sports Exerc* 37: S490–500.

Craig C, Marshall A, Sjostrom M, et al. 2003. International physical activity questionnaire: 12-country reliability and validity. *Med Sci Sports Exerc* 35: 1381–95.

Crouter SE. 2005. *Measurement of Energy Expenditure during Laboratory and Field Settings*. Ph.D. Dissertation thesis. The University of Tennessee, Knoxville, TN. pp. 1–197.

Crouter SE, Schneider PL, Karabult M, Bassett DR. 2003. Validity of ten electronic pedometers for measuring steps, distance, and kcals during treadmill walking. *Med Sci Sports Exerc* 35: 1455–60.

Emons HJG, Groenenboom DC, Westerterp KR, Saris WHM. 1992. Comparison of heart rate monitoring combined with indirect calorimetry and the doubly labelled water method for the measurement of energy expenditure in children. *Eur J Appl Physiol* 65: 99–103.

Fogelholm M, Hiilloskorpi H, Laukkanen R, Oja P, Lichtenbelt WVM, Westerterp K. 1998. Assessment of energy expenditure in overweight women. *Med Sci Sports Exerc* 30: 1191–7.

Freedson PS, Melanson E, Sirard J. 1998. Calibration of the Computer Science and Applications, Inc. accelerometer. *Med Sci Sports Exerc* 30: 777–81.

Grove PB, ed. 1986. *Webster's Third New International Dictionary of the English Language, Unabridged*. Springfield, MA: Merriam Webster, Inc.

Haskell WL, Yee MC, Evans A, Irby P. 1993. Simultaneous measurement of heart rate and body motion to quantitate physical activity. *Med Sci Sports Exerc* 25: 109–15.

Hendelman D, Miller K, Bagget C, Debold E, Freedson P. 2000. Validity of accelerometry for the assessment of moderate intensity physical activity in the field. *Med Sci Sports Exerc* 32: S442–9.

Jacobs DR, Ainsworth BE, Hartman TJ, Leon AS. 1993. A simultaneous evaluation of 10 commonly used physical activity questionnaires. *Med Sci Sports Exerc* 25: 81–91.

Janz KF. 2002. Use of heart rate monitors to assess physical activity. In *Physical Activity Assessments for Health-Related Research*, GJ Welk (Ed.), Champaign, IL: Human Kinetics. pp. 143–61.

Kriska A. 2000. Ethnic and cultural issues in assessing physical activity. *Res Q Exerc Sport* 71: S47–52.

Kriska AM, Casperson CJ. 1997. A collection of physical activity questionnaires for health-related research (special supplement). *Med Sci Sports Exerc* 29: S1–S205.

LaMonte M, Ainsworth B, Tudor-Locke C. 2003. Assessment of physical activity and energy expenditure. In *Obesity: Etiology, Assessment, Treatment, and Prevention*, RE Anderson (Ed.), Champaign, IL: Human Kinetics pp. 111–40.

Leenders NYJM, Sherman WM, Nagaraja HN, Kien CL. 2001. Evaluation of methods to assess physical activity in free-living conditions. *Med Sci Sports Exerc* 33: 1233–40.

Levin S, Jacobs DR, Ainsworth B, Richardson MT, Leon AS. 1999. Intra-individual variation and estimates of usual physical activity. *Ann Epidemiol* 9: 481–8.

Mahar MT, Rowe DA. 2002. Construct validity in physical activity research. In *Physical Activity Assessments in Health-Related Research*, GJ Welk (Ed.), Champaign, IL: Human Kinetics pp. 51–72.

Matthews CE, Shu XO, Yang G, et al. 2003. Reproducibility and validity of the Shanghai women's health study physical activity questionnaire. *Am J Epidemiol* 158: 1114–22.

Montoye HJ, Kemper HCG, Saris WM, Washburn RA. 1995. *Measuring Physical Activity and Energy Expenditure*. Champaign, IL: Human Kinetics. pp. 1–191.

Morrow JR. 2002. Measurement issues for the assessment of physical activity. In *Physical Activity Assessments for Health-Related Research*, GJ Welk (Ed.), Champaign, IL: Human Kinetics pp. 37–49.

Pate RR, Pratt M, Blair SN, et al. 1995. Physical activity and public health: a recommendation from the Centers for Disease Control and Prevention and the American College of Sports Medicine. *JAMA* 273: 402–7.

Pober DM, Raphael C, Freedson PS. 2004. Novel technique for assessing physical activity using accelerometer data (abstract). *Med Sci Sports Exerc* 36: S198.

Safrit M. 1981. *Evaluation in Physical Education (2nd edition).* Englewood Cliffs, NJ: Prentice-Hall, Inc. pp. 45–118.

Schmidt M, Freedson P, Chasan-Taber L. 2003. Estimating physical activity using the CSA accelerometer and a physical activity log. *Med Sci Sports Exerc* 35: 1605–11.

Schneider PL, Crouter SE, Lukajic O, Bassett DR. 2003a. Accuracy and reliability of ten pedometers for measuring steps over a 400-m walk. *Med Sci Sports Exerc* 35: 1770–84.

Schneider PL, Crouter SE, Lukajic O, Bassett DR. 2003b. Pedometer measures of free-living physical activity: Comparison of 13 models. *Med Sci Sports Exerc* 36: 331–5.

Schoeller DA. 2002. Use of stable isotopes in the assessment of nutrient status and metabolism. *Food Nutr Bull* 23 (3 Suppl): 17–20.

Stel V, Smit J, Pluijm S, Visser M, Deeg D, Lips P. 2004. Comparison of the LASA physical activity questionnaire with a 7-day diary and pedometer. *J Clin Epidemiol* 57: 252–8.

Strath SJ, Bassett DR, Swartz AM. 2003. Comparison of MTI accelerometer cut-points for predicting time spent in physical activity. *Int J Sports Med* 24: 298–303.

Strath SJ, Bassett DR, Swartz AM. 2004. Comparison of the college alumnus questionnaire physical activity index with objective monitoring. *Ann Epidemiol* 14: 409–15.

Strath SJ, Bassett DR, Swartz AM, Thompson DL. 2001. Simultaneous heart rate-motion sensor technique to estimate energy expenditure. *Med Sci Sports Exerc* 33: 2118–23.

Strath SJ, Bassett DR, Thompson DL, Swartz AM. 2002. Validity of the simultaneous heartrate-motion sensor technique for measuring energy expenditure. *Med Sci Sports Exerc* 34: 888–94.

Swartz AM, Strath SJ, Bassett DR, Obrien WL, King GA, Ainsworth BE. 2000. Estimation of energy expenditure using CSA accelerometers at hip and wrist sites. *Med Sci Sports Exerc* 32: S450–6.

Tudor-Locke CE, Bassett DR, Swartz AM, et al. 2004. A preliminary study of one year of pedometer self-monitoring. *Ann Behav Med* 28: 158–62.

Tudor-Locke CE, Myers AM. 2001. Methodological considerations for researchers and practitioners using pedometers to measure physical (ambulatory) activity. *Res Quarter Exerc Sport* 72: 1–12.

Wareham NJ, Hennings SJ, Prentice AM, Day NE. 1997. Feasibility of heart-rate monitoring to estimate the Ely young cohort feasibility study 1994-1995. *Br J Nutr* 78: 889–900.

Welk GJ, ed. 2002. *Physical Activity Assessments for Health-Related Research.* Champaign, IL: Human Kinetics. pp. 1–269.

Welk GJ, Differding JA, Thompson RW, Blair SN, Dziura J, Hart P. 2000. The utility of the Digi-Walker step counter to assess daily physical activity patterns. *Med Sci Sports Exerc* 32: S481–8.

Westerterp K. 1999. Physical activity assessment with accelerometers. *Int J Obes Relat Metab Disord* 23: S45–9.

Winters-Hart C, Brach J, Storti K, Trauth J, Kriska A. 2004. Validity of a questionnaire to assess historical physical activity in older women. *Med Sci Sports Exerc* 36: 2082–7.

Zhang K, Pi-Sunyer FX, Boozer CN. 2004. Improving energy expenditure estimation for physical activity. *Med Sci Sports Exerc* 36: 883–9.

Zhang K, Werner P, Sun M, Pi-Sunyer FX, Boozer CN. 2003. Measurement of human daily physical activity. *Obes Res* 11: 33–40.

4

Current Issues in Examining Dose–Response Relationships Between Physical Activity and Health Outcomes

I-Min Lee

During the initial phase of epidemiologic research on physical activity and health, covering the period between the 1950s and the early 1990s, most efforts focused on determining whether physical activity has any effect on various health outcomes. The chapters in Section II of this book highlight some of this research, which shows that physical activity clearly decreases the risk of many chronic diseases (including cardiovascular disease, diabetes, and certain cancers) and also increases longevity. Having established that physical activity is indeed related to several better health outcomes, likely in causal fashion, researchers in the field, increasingly since the mid-1990s, then began asking more detailed questions about the associations (Haskell, 1994). For example, how much physical activity is needed to decrease the risk of a particular disease? What kinds of activity are necessary? At what intensity must the activity or activities be carried out? For what duration? How often? With incremental increases in physical activity, does benefit also increase commensurately? How much additional benefit is obtained with each unit increase in physical activity? Is there a point beyond which additional activity does not bring additional benefit? These and related questions can be categorized under the broad umbrella of "dose–response" issues.

As the reader will conclude from the chapters in Section II, although epidemiologic research has clearly established an inverse relationship between physical activity and the risk of various chronic diseases, there is far less knowledge regarding the dose–response relationship between physical activity and health. Recently, there have been efforts by researchers in exercise science to improve on this knowledge. An evidence-based symposium held in Hockley Valley, Ontario, Canada in October 2000 convened international leading exercise scientists to determine the dose–response relationship between physical activity and health benefits (Kesaniemi et al., 2001). However, the expert panel arrived at this consensus: "Most of the evidence currently available seems to be related to the effects (benefits or risks) of regular physical activity rather than to the relationship between dose and response." Because of the paucity of data, the consensus panel was unable to describe the dose–response relationship between physical activity and various health outcomes. The panel decided instead to "summarize the evidence for the effects of participation in regular physical activity because the Panel found this useful and necessary to properly understand the dose–response data."

The aim of this chapter, therefore, is to stimulate epidemiologic research on dose–response relationships in physical activity. This chapter discusses issues pertinent to assessing dose–response relationships between physical activity and health outcomes and also provides suggestions for several analytic approaches to help increase our understanding of this topic.

Reasons for The Interest in Dose–Response

There are several reasons why the dose–response relationship between physical activity and health holds interest for both researchers and the public. Perhaps arguably the most important reason is a practical one with considerable public heath implications: knowledge of the dose–response relation provides an understanding of the minimum amount of physical activity necessary for health benefits, and this information can then be translated to recommendations for the public. In the United States, there appears to be little enthusiasm for engaging in physical activity. Although the prevalence of no leisure-time physical activity among adults has declined in recent years, from 29.3% in 1988 to 25.1% in 2002 (Behavioral Risk Factor Surveillance System; Anonymous, 2004), the proportion engaging in regular leisure-time physical activity sufficient to meet recommendations remained low at 28.4% in women and 35.7% in men in 2000 (National Health Interview Survey; Barnes and Schoenborn, 2003). In view of these statistics, it appears unrealistic to expect the public to embrace any physical activity recommendation for high levels of physical activity. A recommendation calling for modest amounts of physical activity, yet sufficient to provide health benefits, is more likely to be palatable to the vast majority of the public. Indeed, the balance between efficacy of recommendations and acceptability was one factor in pushing forward the formulation of a new physical activity recommendation by the Centers for Disease Control and Prevention (CDC) and the American College of Sports Medicine (ACSM) in 1995 (Pate et al., 1995). This 1995 recommendation prescribed a more modest level of physical activity (30 minutes of moderate-intensity physical activity, which can be accumulated in 10-minute bouts, on most days of the week) compared to previous recommendations (20 minutes of vigorous-intensity physical activity, performed continuously, on at least 3 days/week). More information on the evolution of physical activity recommendations over time is provided in Chapter 15.

A second reason why the dose–response relationship is important is that this information is helpful in assessing whether an observed association between physical activity and a particular health outcome is a cause-and-effect association. In epidemiologic research, the "gold standard" of research study designs is the randomized controlled trial (Pocock and Elbourne, 2000). The results from such studies, if well-designed and -conducted, can be taken to reflect a cause-and-effect relationship. However, as can be seen in the chapters in Section II, most epidemiologic studies of physical activity and chronic disease are NOT randomized, controlled trials because of various reasons, including cost and feasibility; rather, the studies are primarily observational epidemiologic studies, either cohort or case–control in study design. Such study designs cannot prove cause-and-effect; however, several supporting criteria, as well as exclusion of alternate explanations for the association observed, can argue for a LIKELY cause-and-effect association (for additional discussion of this topic, please refer to Chapter 10; Hennekens and Buring, 1987). One such supporting criterion is the observation of a dose–response relationship between physical activity and the health outcome studied. However, although the presence of a dose–response relationship strengthens the premise of a causal relation, it is important to note that the absence of a dose–response relationship, by itself, does not rule out a causal relationship.

A third reason for the interest in dose–response relationships is that this knowledge may provide clues to the biology underlying physical activity–disease relationships. For example, Figure 4.1 shows two dose–response curves. The solid line shows the risk of developing

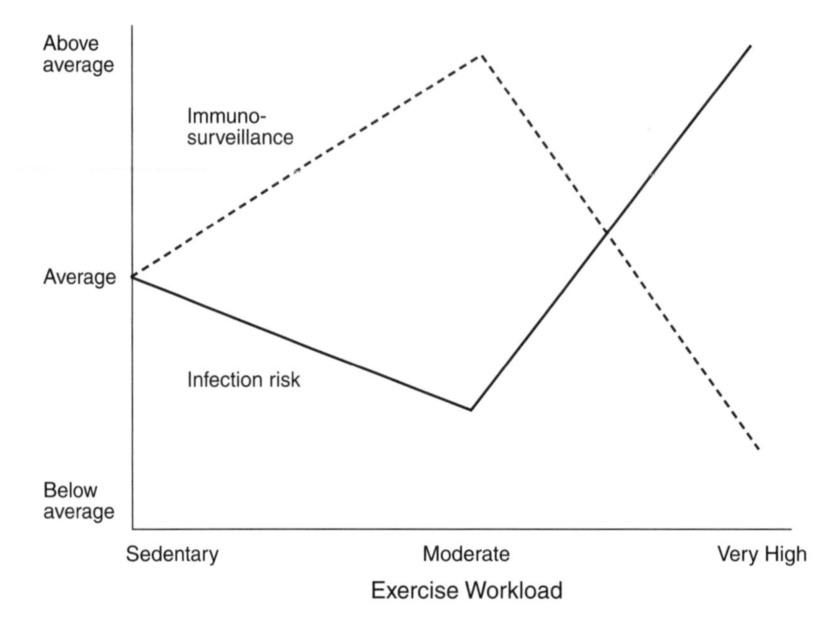

Figure 4.1 Dose–response curves for infection risk and immune function in relation to physical activity levels. (From Nieman 2000, with permission.)

upper respiratory tract infection (URTI) in relation to the amount of physical activity carried out.

The data shown for the solid line indicate that persons who engage in moderate levels of physical activity experience a decreased risk of developing URTI compared with sedentary persons. However, persons who undertake very high levels of physical activity (e.g., overtraining or running a marathon) have increased risks that are even higher than those seen in sedentary individuals.

What might explain this phenomenon? One possible explanation is indicated by the dotted line in Figure 4.1, which shows the dose–response relationship between physical activity and immunosurveillance in the human body. Several immunologic studies indicate that the innate immune system is enhanced by moderate amounts of physical activity; however, following a bout of severe physical exertion, immune function is suppressed for a period of time (Nieman, 2000). Thus, change in immunosurveillance at different levels of physical activity is one plausible explanation for the different susceptibility to URTI.

Definition of Physical Activity when Studying Dose–Response

From many perspectives (e.g., health perspective), the simple definition of physical activity—"any bodily movement produced by skeletal muscles that results in energy expenditure" (Caspersen et al., 1985)—is sufficient. However, when analyzing dose–response relationships, the term "physical activity" is an imprecise one, because it can encompass several related components. An analogy can be made with diet—what is meant when we express interest in the relationship between "diet" and heart disease? *Diet* is an all-encompassing term covering many nutrients and foods. Is the interest in, for example, the amount of saturated fat consumed? Or the number of servings of fruits and vegetables consumed daily?

Similarly, when investigating "physical activity," there can be more precision in specifying the component of interest. From the broadest perspective, the component of interest may be the all-encompassing volume of energy expended (whether this be energy expended on all physical activity or only in certain domains of activity—leisure-time activities, occupational activities, commuting activities, household activities, etc.). Energy expenditure is typically expressed in kilocalories (kcal; or kilojoules, kJ) per unit of time (e.g., a week) or MET-hours per unit of time. Several variables contributing to the volume of energy expended—the kind of activity performed (e.g., walking vs. running), the intensity with which it is performed (e.g., slow- vs. fast-paced walking), the duration of the activity, and the frequency—represent additional components that may be examined for dose–response relationships. Although it may appear to be splitting hairs to be differentiating between the components (after all, more vigorous activities also mean more energy expended, as does longer duration, etc.), there are important implications because some physical activity components can be related to other components. Further rationale for why it is important to distinguish among the different physical activity components is provided in the rest of this chapter.

It is worth noting that most of the epidemiologic research on dose–response relationships between physical activity and health has focused on endurance or aerobic exercise and that limited data are available regarding resistance type or strength training exercise, which can result in different biological responses.

Choice of Physical Activity Component for Study

The choice of the physical activity component to be examined depends on the interest of the investigator. Many contemporary research questions regarding dose–response relationships in physical activity are a consequence of activity recommendations that have changed over time (*see* Chapter 15). For example, when the 1995 recommendation from the CDC and ASCM (Pate et al., 1995) was first released, interest focused on dose–response questions related to the intensity of physical activity. Because this recommendation now allowed for moderate-intensity activity, rather than the vigorous-intensity activity required previously, there was interest in whether moderate-intensity activity is sufficient for health and also whether vigorous-intensity activity conveys additional benefit (if so, how much?). Additionally, the 1995 recommendation included brisk walking as an example of a prescribed moderate-intensity activity; this spawned interest in dose–response relationships with regard to the pace and amount of walking. A particularly controversial issue arising from the 1995 recommendation was the concession sanctioning the accumulation of short bouts of physical activity. This led to the question of the minimum duration (per activity bout) necessary for health benefit, as well as whether and how much additional benefit occurs with longer durations of activity.

Further interest in the dose–response question was stimulated when the Institute of Medicine (IOM) released guidelines in 2002 (IOM, 2002) asking for 60 minutes/day of moderate-intensity physical activity (for further discussion, please refer to Chapter 15). Because this contrasted starkly with the 30 minutes/day required by the 1995 CDC/ACSM recommendation, there is currently intense debate on the dose–response question related to total volume of physical activity, particularly with regard to the maintenance of a healthy body weight.

Thus, the choice of the physical activity component to be examined for dose–response relationships depends largely on the interest of the investigator. Later this chapter discusses issues related to the analyses of several physical activity components.

Inter-Relations Among Physical Activity Components

The inter-relations among physical activity components contribute to the complexity of dose–response analyses. In particular, each of these components of physical activity—kind of activity, intensity, duration, and frequency—contributes to the determination of volume of energy expended. If the appropriate analyses are not carried out, the resulting findings may not provide the correct answer to the research question of interest. This is best illustrated by example. If the research question is "Does greater intensity of physical activity lead to progressively greater reductions in the incidence of disease X?" we could examine the incidence of disease X among persons performing activities of different intensities. If we observed progressively lower rates of the disease with increasingly higher intensities of physical activity, we might conclude that there is an inverse dose–response relationship between intensity of physical activity and the risk of disease X. However, an alternate explanation is possible. Physical activities of greater intensity generate higher energy expenditure (e.g., running costs more energy than walking). It might be the case that there is, indeed, no relationship between *intensity* of physical activity and the risk of disease X but that the inverse relationship merely reflects the inverse dose–response relationship between the *volume* of energy expended and disease X. These different interpretations have important implications. If intensity is important to reduce the incidence of disease X with, for example, a significant reduction in risk only at vigorous intensity of physical activity, then the recommendation should be for patients to engage in vigorous activity. However, if the volume of energy expended were the important component, then the recommendation can be for patients to engage in activities of any intensity so long as the volume of energy expended met the threshold level for risk reduction.

How might we differentiate between these two interpretations of the results? Several analytical approaches are possible, and these are discussed in the section Dose–Response for Intensity of Physical Activity.

Influence of Research Study Design

Whether an investigator selects to use an experimental or observational study design, possible inter-relations among physical activity components need to be considered. In the former study design, control for any inter-related components occurs by designing appropriate intervention arms; in the latter, control occurs during analyses of the observational data.

Continuing with the aforementioned example, suppose an investigator is interested in the dose–response relationship between intensity of physical activity and disease X and chooses to use an experimental design. One possible design may be to have three groups of randomized participants: a control (sedentary) group, group A exercising at moderate intensity, and group B exercising at vigorous intensity. A crucial consideration is this: For how long and how frequently should groups A and B exercise? If both groups exercise for 30 minutes, five times per week, it will be impossible to tease out whether any dose–response relation observed is the result of intensity or volume of energy expended, because group B is exercising at higher intensity and also expending more energy. If the research question of interest is the dose–response relationship of intensity, then the duration and frequency should be manipulated for groups A and B, such that the volume of energy expended is the same for both groups.

As an example, refer to Table 4.1. In this particular study, among the research questions of interest were the effects of moderate and vigorous intensity physical activity on weight loss and cardiorespiratory fitness in overweight, sedentary women (Jakicic et al., 2003).

Table 4.1 Effect of Moderate- and Vigorous-Intensity Physical Activity on Weight Loss and Cardiorespiratory Fitness

	Moderate-intensity group	*Vigorous-intensity group*	*p-value*
Physical activity regimen	Moderate-intensity activity, 40 minutes/day, 5 days/week	Vigorous-intensity activity, 30 minutes/ day, 5 days/week	—
Volume of energy expended, kcal/week	1000	1000	—
Change in weight from baseline	–7.4%	–7.9%	0.85
Change in fitness from baseline	13.5%	18.9%	0.11

(Data from Jakicic et al., 2003.)

For illustrative purposes, data for only two of the four randomized groups are presented in the table.

Note that in addition to the different intensity of physical activity, the duration of physical activity also differed between groups, such that both groups expended the same volume of energy, 1,000 kcal/week. Therefore, any different findings between the groups can be attributed to differences in intensity of physical activity, because the volume of activity was kept constant. As can be seen, the intensity of activity did not appear to matter for weight loss if the volume of activity was controlled (as would be intuitive), with both groups losing about the same amount of body weight at the end of 12 months. Although there was no significant difference regarding improvement in cardiovascular fitness, it appeared that the vigorous group improved somewhat, with the p-value at borderline significance ($p = 0.11$), a finding that also seems intuitive.

It is worth noting that although the randomized, controlled trial generally is considered the "gold standard" of study designs, the data emanating from such studies may be "artificial" for the real world. Participants willing to participate in clinical trials generally tend to be healthier than those who choose not to (for example, Sesso et al., 2002). Additionally, the finite number of intervention arms in a trial examining physical activity doses cannot possibly resemble the many different ways, regarding kinds of activity, intensity, frequency, and duration, that people choose to be active in the real world. Therefore, observational studies provide important, complementary information that often cannot be obtained from randomized trials.

For observational study designs, the investigator cannot control the physical activity parameters but merely observes different physical activity behavior among participants. In these observational studies, therefore, the aim in analyses is to mimic the controlled condition in the randomized trial, such that any inter-relations among the different physical activity components are considered. Details for analyzing several separate physical activity components are provided later in this chapter.

Choosing Cut-Points for Categorizations of Physical Activity Components

When analyzing dose–response relationships for physical activity, physical activity can be treated as a continuous variable or categorized into several groups. Although use of a continuous variable affords greater statistical power, one disadvantage is that the results from these analyses may not be as easy to understand. For example, the finding "risk of disease X decreased 2% for each MET-hour per week increase in physical activity" may be less easily understood compared with "individuals who expended 10–15 MET-hours/week of physical activity, or at least the amount recommended by the CDC/ACSM, had a 25% lower risk of disease X than sedentary individuals." Additionally, most epidemiologic studies have tested for linear trends in dose–response. If the dose–response is not linear, using continuous physical activity data to test for a linear trend will merely yield a non-significant result for linear trend but will not provide additional information on the shape of the curve.

Categorizing physical activity data allows greater flexibility, because this allows the investigator to observe the rates of disease among persons in the different activity categories. The investigator can then decide whether a linear or non-linear trend should be formally assessed. With regard to creating categories of physical activity, the cut-points used by investigators have been arbitrary. (At least two cut-points are needed, giving three categories of physical activity, the minimum needed to evaluate a dose–response.) In observational studies, a popular strategy has been to divide the study population into approximately equal quantiles, such as quartiles (Lee et al., 2001) or quintiles (Manson et al., 2002; Tanasescu et al., 2002). One advantage of this approach is that statistical power is enhanced, because the numbers of health outcomes being evaluated and participants are likely to be fairly evenly distributed among the groups. However, one disadvantage is that the cut-points for the categories may represent awkward breaks, such as quintile groupings of 67.5 or less, 67.5 to 472.5, 472.5 to 980.0, 980.0 to 1,890.0, and greater than 1,890.0 kcal/week (Fried et al., 1998). Additionally, these cut-points imply a high degree of precision in the estimation of physical activity, which is not the case. A further disadvantage of using quantile cut-points is that some investigators have merely referred to their groupings as quantiles without describing the actual levels of physical activity in each quantile (Folsom et al., 1997; Sherman et al., 1994). This hampers the comparison of findings across studies, because it is unclear whether the physical activity quantiles across studies represent the same range of physical activity.

In choosing cut-points, one option may be "natural" breaks based on current issues being debated in the field of exercise science. For example, if the dose–response relationship for the intensity of physical activity is interesting, a reasonable grouping may be light- (not deemed to have cardiovascular benefit), moderate- (currently recommended by the CDC/ACSM; Pate et al., 1995), and vigorous-intensity physical activity (recommendations prior to 1995; e.g., ACSM, 1990). Another area of debate is the minimum duration required for health benefits; if the dose–response in relation to duration is of interest, an option may be these categories: no physical activity; activity in bouts of 10 to less than 20 minutes (the CDC/ACSM recommendation allows accumulated activity in bouts of at least 10 minutes each; Pate et al., 1995); and activity in bouts of 20 minutes or longer (as prescribed by recommendations prior to 1995; e.g., ACSM, 1990). A further "natural" categorization, based on the different amounts of physical activity currently recommended by the CDC/ACSM and the IOM may be less than 30, 30 to 59, and 60 minutes or more of physical activity per day.

A second option for choosing cut-points may be "natural" breaks on the numerical scale. Examples include energy expenditure in 500-kcal/week increments (Paffenbarger et al., 1993) or duration of physical activity bouts in 15-minute increments (Lee et al., 2000). The rationale for using such cut-points is that the categories are easily understood by both the research community and the lay public. Additionally, the hope is that these cut-points represent a balance between not implying too fine a precision in the estimation of physical activity and drawing a fine enough classification to be able to describe the shape of any dose–response relationships that may exist.

Finally, another option for choosing categories may be based on the biological understanding of the disease process. Referring again to Figure 4.1, because the innate immune function seems to be enhanced by moderate levels of physical activity but depressed by exhaustive levels, these same categories (with, perhaps, sedentary persons as the reference) can be an option to study dose–response relationships between physical activity and risk of URTI.

Shape of the Dose–Response Curve

The shape of the dose–response curve is likely to differ for different health outcomes (Kesaniemi et al., 2001). In particular, the minimum amount of physical activity needed to produce benefit is likely different. For example, it is clear that the CDC/ACSM recommendation for 30 minutes/day of moderate-intensity activity reduces the risk of developing cardiovascular disease (*see* Chapter 9). However, higher volume of physical activity may be needed for beneficial changes in certain plasma lipoproteins (Kraus et al., 2002); higher volume also appears necessary to maintain weight loss in previously overweight and obese individuals (Saris et al., 2003). The lipoprotein example illustrates the point that the dose–response relationship between physical activity and a clinical outcome (cardiovascular disease in this example) need not necessarily be identical to that between physical activity and a single risk factor (e.g., high-density lipoprotein) for the clinical outcome, because the clinical outcome has multiple etiologies.

In addition to interest in the minimum effective dose of physical activity for health benefits, it is also of public health and research relevance to understand the shape of the dose–response curve at doses above the minimum. That is, for a particular health outcome, is the dose–response relationship linear in shape (curve A in Fig. 4.2), or is there some other shape (such as curves B and C in Fig. 4.2)? If linear, how steep is the slope? This tells us how much additional benefit might be expected with each incremental increase in level of physical activity.

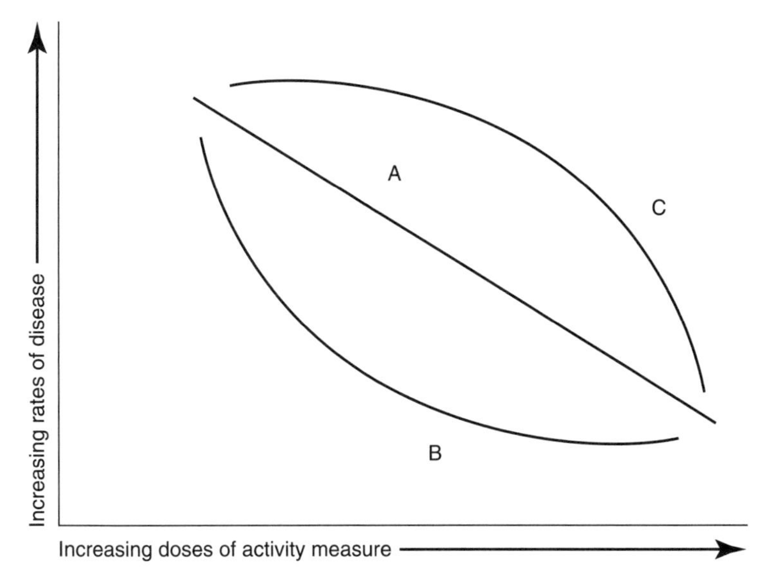

Figure 4.2 Possible dose–response curves between physical activity and health outcomes.

If curve B represents the correct dose–response, then substantial increases in benefit occur with small increases in physical activity. However, if curve C represents the correct shape of the curve, additional benefits accrue only with large increases in physical activity.

When attempting to describe the shape of the dose–response curve, most studies have tested for linear trend across physical activity categories. Commonly, the activity categories are either assigned an ordinal value (e.g., 1–4 for quartiles), and a formal test for linear trend across categories is conducted (Lee et al., 2001), or the median values of the activity categories are used and a similar test for linear trend performed (Hu et al., 2000). (Because most epidemiologic studies use regression models on the logarithmic scale to estimate trends across relative risks, a linear dose–response on the logarithmic scale translates to an exponentially shaped curve on the natural numeric scale. However, with small increases or decreases in relative risks of between 1 and 2 or between 1 and 0.5, linear dose–response relationships on the logarithmic scale also appear linear on the natural scale.)

Although most studies have tested for linear trends in dose–response, this is not the only option. Other shapes of the dose–response curve are possible, and one option to investigate non-linear trends is the use of regression splines (Greenland, 1995). A detailed discussion of the technique is beyond the scope of this chapter. Briefly, this technique allows different shapes of the dose–response curve to occur within the range of physical activity investigated. The different shapes are separated by "knots" or breaks, with the investigator deciding on number of knots (this choice is similar to deciding on cut-points for physical activity categorization). In between knots, the shape of the curve can be parametric (e.g., linear, quadratic, or other higher polynomial) or non-parametric (i.e., with no assumption of the shape of the curve between physical activity and disease rates in this region).

There are few data to inform on the exact shape of the dose–response curves between physical activity and health outcomes. Although individual studies do provide information on the dose–response relationship for participants in that particular study, we need to combine data from all appropriate studies. This is because a single study cannot provide definitive data; rather, the single study should be considered a single piece in a jigsaw puzzle, with many studies needed to complete the picture. Additionally, the range of physical activity in a single study may be limited and not provide a comprehensive understanding of the dose–response relationship across the range of activity carried out by the general population.

The challenge, however, is to combine data from different physical activity studies. A major problem in attempting to synthesize findings is that observational studies have used very different assessments and classifications of physical activity and referent groups, making it virtually impossible to convert the data from different studies into a common scale for direct comparison. (For examples of reviews describing different categories of physical activity used by investigators, *see* Lee and Skerret, 2001 and/or Oguma et al., 2002). This discussion is less germane for randomized trials, where activity levels are dictated by investigators and, hence, generally well-quantified). Thus, investigators have tried, as best they could, to shoehorn the different categories of physical activity into several arbitrary categories to be able to conduct meta-analyses. For example, some investigators have designated three levels of activity (low, moderate, and high) and assigned all levels beyond the third category into the "high" group (Tardon et al., 2005) or assigned the lowest and highest activity levels to the "low" and "high" groups, respectively, with all other activity levels assigned to the "moderate" group (Wendel-Vos et al., 2004). Another strategy has been to plot relative risks as a function of the cumulative percentages of the study sample (i.e., for a study with activity grouped into tertiles, the relative risks would be plotted against 33%, 67%, and 100% of the range of physical activity; for another study with quintiles of activity, they would be plotted against 20%, 40%, 60%, 80%, and 100% of the physical activity range) (Williams, 2001). This clearly illustrates some of the difficulty in

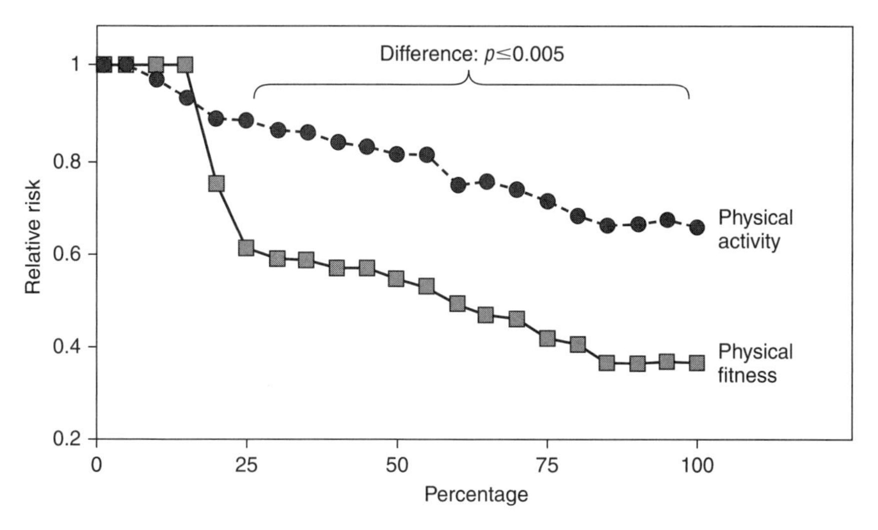

Figure 4.3 Dose–response curves for physical activity and physical fitness in relation to cardiovascular disease. (From Williams 2001, with permission.)

trying to describe dose–response curves for physical activity—What, precisely, does "moderate" translate to in terms of volume of physical activity? Intensity of activity? (It is important not to confuse the term "moderate" used in the meta-analysis with "moderate"-intensity physical activity because they do not have the same meaning.) With the percentage strategy, what does 20%, 40%, and so forth, of the physical activity range mean?

Given these limitations, there are some data from meta-analyses to indicate that the dose–response relationship between physical activity and several health outcomes, such as cardiovascular disease (*see* Fig. 4.3; Williams, 2001), is inverse and linear. However, that for physical fitness and cardiovascular disease does not appear linear over the range of fitness (Fig. 4.3; Williams, 2001).

Population Under Study

The population being investigated can have bearing on the shape of the dose–response curve. Physical activity levels differ according to many characteristics, including sex, age, race, and income (Barnes and Schoenborn, 2003). Additionally, there can be large differences in occupational physical activity, so the range of physical activity carried out by participants in different observational studies can vary. Thus, although investigators have done as best they can with regard to combining physical activity groups across studies in meta-analyses, subjects classified into a particular activity level (e.g., 4th quintile), based on their original study grouping, may not necessarily have similar activity levels. For example, quintiles of leisure-time physical activity were not equivalent among Finnish men (<4.0, 4.1–9.0, 9.1–17.4, 17.5–31.4, and ≥31.5 MET-hours/week; Kujala et al., 1998) and U.S. women (<2.5, 2.5–7.2, 7.3–13.4, 13.5–23.3, and ≥23.4 MET-hours/week; Manson et al., 2002) in two cohort studies. Men in the lowest quintile expended 60% more energy than did the women, yet equivalence of physical activity was assumed, for lack of a simple way of combining data across studies in a meta-analysis of physical activity and cardiovascular disease (Williams, 2001). (Adding to the complexity is that the two studies used different questionnaires to assess activity.)

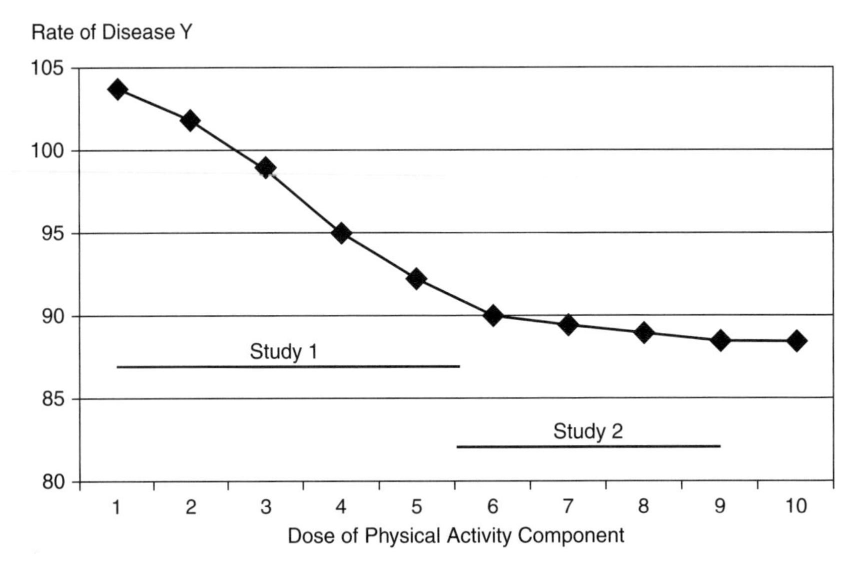

Figure 4.4 Hypothetical dose–response relationship between physical activity and disease Y.

The different ranges of physical activity across various study populations may be one explanation for apparently conflicting findings on dose–response relationships. Suppose Figure 4.4 represents the true dose–response relationship between physical activity and disease Y, and suppose two different studies of dose–response were conducted. In Study 1, investigators happened to enroll participants who engaged in lower levels of physical activity (e.g., women), whereas in Study 2 investigators enrolled participants with higher levels of physical activity (e.g., men).

The data observed in Study 1 would lead investigators to conclude that an inverse, linear dose–response relationship exists, whereas the data from Study 2 would lead to the conclusion that there is little relationship between physical activity and disease Y. Neither study has provided the "right" answer; both have merely observed findings from a different spectrum of the dose–response curve.

Since the 1995 CDC/ACSM recommendation, studies examining whether moderate-intensity physical activity is related to lower risk of several health outcomes (especially cardiovascular disease and all-cause mortality) have not consistently arrived at the same conclusion (Lee, 2004). Some studies have shown benefit even from moderate-intensity activities, whereas others have observed benefit only with vigorous-intensity activities. In general, the studies that have shown moderate-intensity physical activity to be sufficient for health benefits have been studies of women or older men. Referring to the hypothetical Figure 4.4, these studies might have comprised participants similar to those in Study 1 of the figure, where activity levels were low. Because the reference group (assuming the referent to be the lowest activity quantile) is at such a low level of activity, any higher level of activity—even moderate-intensity—is sufficient for benefit. On the other hand, studies noting vigorous activity to be necessary have tended to be studies among middle-aged men. These men might have been those akin to the hypothetical Study 2 participants, where the referent was at a high level of activity, such that much larger increases in intensity of physical activity (e.g., vigorous intensity) may be necessary for additional risk reduction.

Dose–Response for Volume of Physical Activity

The volume of physical activity is the simplest component to analyze in the sense that any assessment of physical activity, no matter how simple, provides some indication of the volume of energy expended. For example, in the U.S. Longitudinal Study of Aging, physical activity was assessed simply as: "Compared with other people your age, would you say that you are physically more active, less active, or about as active?" (Lee, 2000). Response options were: less active, about as active, more active, or a lot more active. Although it is impossible to equate the different activity categories to kilocalories (or MET-hr) of energy expended, it is clear that the categories represent ordered levels of volume of physical activity. This simple assessment was sufficient to reveal an inverse dose–response for mortality (relative risks of 1.40, 1.18, 0.99, and 1.00 [referent], respectively), although the precise levels of physical activity to which the relative risks correspond were unclear.

So categories of physical activity, representing a number of activities (e.g., graded levels of intensity, frequency, or duration) all can be used as proxies for volume of energy expenditure in analysis of the dose–response relationship for volume, even if estimation of the actual energy expended cannot be made. Analyses of any of these components provide an indication of the shape of the dose–response curve, although the scale on the x-axis (volume of physical activity) may not be well-defined. Because of the simplicity with which volume of energy expenditure (or some proxy of this) can be estimated, most of the information that we have on dose–response relationships pertain to the component of volume of energy expended (Lee and Skerrett, 2001).

Of course, some studies will have detailed assessments of physical activity (*see* Chapter 2), so that the volume of energy expended can be calculated. One advantage of using the volume of energy expended as the component of interest is that this allows investigators to combine the myriad activities carried out by free-living persons into a single measure. Two common units used by investigators to estimate volume of energy expenditure are kilocalories (or kilojoules) and MET-hours per unit of time, such as a week. There are advantages and disadvantages to using each. I prefer the unit of kilocalories (or kilojoules; 4.2 kJ = 1 kcal) because this is a widely used unit, easily understood by many, and is the same unit used for food intake. Adding to the ease of understanding is the fact that walking 1 mile at a brisk pace (3–4 mph, as recommended by the CDC/ACSM) expends approximately 100 kilocalories for a 165-lb (75-kg) person (so 2 miles require 200 kilocalories, etc.). Examples of the energy cost, in kilocalories, of common leisure-time activities are provided on pages 289–303 in Paffenbarger and Olsen (1996). The disadvantage is that the energy cost of the same activity, carried out for the same duration, varies according to the weight of the individual, with heavier persons expending more energy. Thus, analyses may be confounded by body weight (i.e., the heavier person with greater energy expenditure may not be more active; he may merely weigh more). However, this problem can be taken care of simply by adjusting for body weight in analyses. This adjustment essentially makes comparisons among persons who weigh the same. Thus, in adjusted analyses, greater kilocalories expended per week among individuals with the same weight has the meaning of greater level of physical activity. One exception to the use of kilocalories is when careful consideration of body weight is important (e.g., in studies of physical activity and weight control); in these situations, use of a unit of energy expenditure that is independent of body weight, such as MET-hours described below, may be preferable.

One example of an analysis of the dose–response relationship between volume of energy expended (in kilocalories per week) and coronary heart disease risk is provided in Table 4.2. These data are for men (mean age: 58 years) in the Harvard Alumni Health Study, and the analysis is adjusted for body mass index (in addition to other potential confounders).

Table 4.2 Dose–Response Relationship Between Volume of Energy Expended and Risk of Coronary Heart Disease, Harvard Alumni Health Study

Energy expended (kcal/week)	*No. of cases*	*Multivariate relative risk**	*95% confidence interval*
<500	438	1.00	(referent)
500–999	429	0.90	0.79–1.03
1000–1999	552	0.81	0.71–0.92
2000–2999	322	0.80	0.69–0.93
≥3000	394	0.81	0.71–0.94
p, linear trend		0.003	

*Adjusted for age, body mass index, smoking, alcohol intake, hypertension, diabetes, and early parental death.

(Data from Sesso et al., 2000.)

The shape of the curve appears to be L-shaped, with risks declining from less than 500 to 1,999 kcal/week, beyond which there is little additional decrease in risk.

The other commonly used unit of energy expenditure is MET-hours. One MET, or metabolic equivalent, is the energy expended during rest. Brisk walking (3–4 mph) requires 4 METs, or four times the resting metabolic rate. Thus, walking 3.5 miles in 1 hour will expend 4 MET-hours of energy. (A list of activities and their energy cost in METs is provided in Ainsworth et al. [1993], with an update in Ainsworth et al. [2000]). This unit of energy expenditure, while less likely to be understood by the general population, has the advantage of being independent of body weight. So a normal-weight person and an obese person walking 3.5 miles in 1 hour will each expend 4 MET-hours of energy.

One example of an analysis using MET-hours per week is provided in Chapter 9, Figure 9.2. The data are from men in the Health Professionals' Follow-up Study (age: 40–75 years). The findings, compared with the Harvard Alumni Health Study, are very similar between quintiles 1 and 4. In quintile 5, however, there is a further reduction in risk among the health professionals (as contrasted with a leveling of the curve among Harvard alumni), so that the dose–response curve looks more linear than that seen among the Harvard alumni. The range of physical activity in the two studies is comparable (Harvard alumni: <500 to ≥3,000 kcal/week; health professionals: ≤6.32 to ≥41.99 MET-hours/week, which corresponds to approximately <500 to >3,300 kcal/week).

Dose–Response for Intensity of Physical Activity

At the time of the 1995 CDC/ACSM physical activity recommendation, there were few epidemiologic data specifically addressing whether moderate-intensity physical activity is sufficient for health benefits (Pate et al., 1995). However, there existed a large body of literature showing that greater volume of energy expended is associated with lower risk of chronic diseases—particularly cardiovascular disease. Given the physical activity behavior of the U.S. population (Anonymous, 2001), it was assumed that in these studies much of the energy expended must have come from moderate-intensity activity, because only a small proportion of the population engages in vigorous-intensity activity. Thus, the 1995 recommendation allowed for moderate-intensity activity.

However, an alternate explanation for the epidemiologic observations is possible. Higher intensity activities cost more energy than lower intensity ones. Therefore, individuals with high volumes of energy expenditure may also be more likely to participate in vigorous activities, compared with those expending less energy. For example, among men in the most active quintile of total energy expenditure in the Harvard Alumni Health Study, 43.5% of total energy expended was derived from vigorous activities, as contrasted to 32.1% among men in the second quintile (Lee et al., 1995). Therefore, the observed association between greater volume of energy expended and lower rates of cardiovascular disease may have been driven primarily by vigorous-intensity activities. This alternate explanation is an illustration of one issue discussed earlier: the inter-relations among physical activity components. In this case, intensity and volume are inter-related. Careful analysis is required to separate the effect of intensity independent of its contribution to the volume of energy expended.

Another factor to consider is that persons who engage in vigorous activities also may be more likely to engage in moderate activities (e.g., persons who enjoy sports may be more likely to walk for transportation and when running errands, etc., compared with inactive persons). Therefore, in analysis of dose–response relationships for intensity of physical activity, confounding by activities of a different intensity also needs to be considered. If interest is in the dose–response for moderate-intensity activity, then vigorous activities should be taken into account.

The issues discussed in the preceding paragraphs—confounding by volume of energy expended and by activities of other intensities—are analogous to confounding by total energy intake and by other nutrients in studies of diet. Intakes of many nutrients in a free-living population are positively correlated with total energy intake (e.g., someone with a large total caloric intake also will consume larger amounts of fat, protein, and carbohydrate compared with someone with a small total caloric intake). The nutrients themselves also may be correlated—a person consuming large amounts of red meat will have high intakes of both protein and saturated fat. Thus, an observation of increased risk of heart disease with, for example, higher protein intake, may not be real but merely reflect a true positive association with high caloric intake. Or the association may be reflecting the correlation between protein and saturated fat, and it may be the saturated fat that is responsible for the increased risk, not the protein. Analytic methods that have been developed to control for such confounding in dietary studies can be adapted for studying physical activity.

One method of analysis that can assess the dose–response for intensity of physical activity, independent of the volume of energy expended, is the standard multivariate model. In this regression model, adjustment is made for the volume of energy expended, and terms related to intensity of physical activity are entered at the same time. If, however, the physical activity variables are highly correlated, then statistical concerns may arise with simultaneous inclusion of the variables in the same regression model because divergent results can be obtained. Some researchers have suggested that variables with correlation coefficients of more than approximately 0.60 not be included at the same time in a single model (Willett, 1998).

One example of use of the standard multivariate model is taken from the Health Professionals' Follow-up Study (Tanasescu et al., 2002) and is shown in Table 4.3.

In this analysis, in addition to adjusting for standard potential confounders, the investigators have adjusted for the volume of energy expended, in MET-hours per wk. Their findings showed an inverse dose–response relationship between intensity of physical activity and coronary heart disease rates, independent of the fact that higher intensity activities cost more energy. Moderate-intensity activities were not associated with significantly greater benefit compared with light-intensity activities, but vigorous activities were.

Another method borrows from the "energy decomposition" or "energy partition" method used in dietary studies (Willett, 1998). This allows comparison of the effects of the energy expended on activities of different intensities. In such an analysis, terms representing the

Table 4.3 Dose–Response Relationship Between Intensity of Physical Activity, Independent of Volume of Energy Expended, and Risk of Coronary Heart Disease, Health Professionals' Follow-Up Study (Standard Multivariate Model)

Intensity of physical activity	*Low*	*Moderate*	*Vigorous*	*p, linear trend*
No. of cases	482	911	307	—
Person-years	88,374	251,489	135,892	—
Relative risk*	1.00	0.94	0.83	0.02
(95% confidence interval)	(referent)	(0.83–1.04)	(0.74–0.97)	

*Adjusted for volume of energy expended (MET-hours/week) as well as age, smoking, alcohol intake, nutrient intake, family history of myocardial infarction, body mass index, diabetes, hypercholesterolemia, and hypertension.

(Data from Tanasescu et al., 2002.)

energy expended on activities of different intensity are entered simultaneously in a regression model. For example, in the Harvard Alumni Health Study, investigators were interested in the associations of vigorous and non-vigorous intensity physical activity with all-cause mortality, apart from their contributions to total energy expenditure (Lee et al., 1995). Subjects were classified into groups based on the energy expended on vigorous and on non-vigorous activities, and terms representing both kinds of energy expenditure were entered simultaneously into a regression model (Table 4.4).

In this analysis, the results for the association of vigorous energy expenditure with mortality are not confounded by the energy expended on non-vigorous activities (and vice versa). The trend across vigorous activities is significant (*p* for linear trend = 0.001), and that for non-vigorous activities is not (*p* for linear trend = 0.32). It is not sufficient merely to note that the former is significant and the latter not (Willett, 1998). The lack of significance for non-vigorous activities might simply reflect less precise reporting of these activities compared with vigorous activities. What is important is whether the two trends differ from

Table 4.4 Independent Dose–Response Relationships of Vigorous and Non-Vigorous Intensity Physical Activity With All-Cause Mortality, Harvard Alumni Health Study ("Energy Decomposition" Model)

Vigorous energy expenditure, kcal/week	*<150*	*150–399*	*400–749*	*750–1,499*	*≥1,500*	*p, linear trend*
No. of deaths	1,282	998	379	250	388	—
Relative risk, B1*	1.00	0.88	0.91	0.87	0.86	0.001
95% confidence interval	referent	0.81–0.96	0.81–1.02	0.76–1.00	0.76–0.96	—
Non-vigorous energy expenditure, kcal/week	*<150*	*150–399*	*400–749*	*750–1,499*	*≥1,500*	*P, linear trend*
No. of deaths	386	579	691	713	928	—
Relative risk, B2*	1.00	0.98	1.09	1.08	1.05	0.32
95% confidence interval	referent	0.86–1.11	0.96–1.23	0.96–1.23	0.93–1.18	—
P (B1–B2)	—	0.19	0.04	0.02	0.02	0.001

*Adjusted for age, body mass index, smoking, hypertension, diabetes, early parental death, as well as energy expended on activities of the other intensity.

(Data from Lee et al., 1995.)

each other. If the trends differ significantly, this indicates that the two kinds of energy expenditure (vigorous and non-vigorous) are different in their effect on mortality rates, independent of their contribution to the total volume of energy expended. In Table 4.4, the two trends do differ significantly ($p = 0.001$). This indicates that vigorous physical activity is needed to decrease mortality rates among these men and that non-vigorous activity is not sufficient. (As an aside, this may result from the nature of the population, as discussed previously. Additionally, light- and moderate-intensity activities were grouped together to form non-vigorous activities. The lack of an association for these activities may be because any benefit of moderate activities is diluted by the lack of effect for light activities.)

If interest is in a particular level of physical activity—for example, 1,500 kcal/week or more—the same principle applies. It is not sufficient to observe that the relative risk for vigorous energy expenditure at this level is significant (relative risk = 0.86; 95% confidence interval, 0.76–0.96) while that for non-vigorous energy expenditure is not significant (corresponding data, 1.05 [0.93–1.18]). What is important is whether the relative risks of 0.86 and 1.05 differ significantly from each other, as indicated by p(B1-B2) in Table 4.4 (they do; p(B1-B2) = 0.02).

A third approach taken by investigators to prevent confounding by activities of a different intensity is restriction—that is, examining participants who engage in only one kind (intensity) of activity (thereby preventing confounding by activities of other intensities). For example, additional analyses of the study shown in Table 4.4 separately examined *(a)* Harvard alumni who participated only in vigorous activities and *(b)* Harvard alumni who only participated in moderate activities (data not shown; Lee et al., 1995). The former analyses are less commonly conducted, because few persons exercise vigorously but engage in no moderate activity. However, the latter analyses have been performed frequently in recent years. In particular, there has been a great deal of interest in walking, a common moderate-intensity activity (national data indicate that 34% of U.S. adults walk regularly, and another 45.6% walk on an occasional basis; Eyler et al., 2003).

In the Women's Health Study, investigators investigated the role of moderate-intensity physical activity in preventing coronary heart disease by examining the association of walking with coronary heart disease risk among women who did not engage in any vigorous activities (to prevent confounding by vigorous activities; Lee et al., 2001). Table 4.5 shows the association of time spent walking and risk of coronary heart disease among women who did not participate in vigorous activities. Women who walked for as little as an hour a week had lower risks compared with those who did not walk regularly.

Table 4.5 Dose–Response Relationship Between Walking and Risk of Coronary Heart Disease, Women's Health Study (Restriction Model)*

Time spent walking per week	*No. of cases*	*Multivariate relative risk†*	*95% confidence interval*
No regular walking	68	1.00	(referent)
1–59 min	45	0.86	0.57–1.29
1.0–1.5 hr	19	0.49	0.28–0.86
≥2 hr	28	0.48	0.29–0.78
p, linear trend		<0.001	

*Analyses restricted to women who did not participate in vigorous activities.

†Adjusted for age; randomized treatment assignment; smoking; intake of alcohol, saturated fat, fiber, and fruits and vegetables; menopausal status; hormone therapy; and parental history of myocardial infarction at <60 years of age.

(Data from Lee et al., 2001)

In this study, investigators examined, separately, whether the time spent walking, the pace of walking, or both was important in predicting lower rates of coronary heart disease. In this particular group of women, it was the time spent walking that was more important (p for linear trend = 0.01), and the pace did not matter (p for linear trend = 0.55) once time was accounted for (data not shown).

In another study, the Nurses' Health Study, investigators examined the relationship between walking, assessed in MET-hours per week and categorized into quintiles, and risk of coronary heart disease among women who did not participate in vigorous activities (Manson et al., 1999). The relative risks (95% confidence intervals) associated with increasing quintiles were 1.00 (referent), 0.78 (0.57–1.06), 0.88 (0.65–1.21), 0.70 (0.51–0.95), and 0.65 (0.47–0.91), respectively (p for linear trend = 0.02). Significantly lower risks were observed beginning at the fourth quintile, representing 3.9–9.9 MET-hours/wk, or approximately 1–2.5 hours/week of brisk walking. Note that the categorization of walking in this study (MET-hours/wk) does not distinguish between the pace and time of walking. Strolling at less than 2 mph (2 METs) for 5 hours will generate 10 MET-hours of energy, as will brisk walking at 3 to 4 mph (4 METs) for 2.5 hours. Thus, it is unclear from this analysis whether it is the time spent, the pace of walking, or both that is important for decreased risk of coronary heart disease.

Dose–Response for Duration (Frequency) of Physical Activity

As mentioned previously, a highly controversial element of the 1995 CDC/ACSM recommendation was acceding that physical activity can be accumulated in short bouts over the day, as opposed to the previous requirement for it to be completed in a single bout. At the time of the recommendation, only two randomized trials in men were available, showing that accumulated short bouts of activity were sufficient to improve cardiovascular fitness and risk factors (Pate et al., 1995). Since, there have been other trials in both men and women to support this finding (Hardman, 2001; Kohl et al., 2006). Most of the trials have focused on weight loss and/or increased physical fitness as the outcomes of interest; a few trials have investigated improvement in cardiovascular risk factors. Generally, "short" bouts in these trials referred to activity sessions lasting 10 to 15 minutes.

Because these studies were randomized trials, the trials could be designed such that the intervention groups exercised in bouts of different duration but with all groups expending the same volume of energy. (This is accomplished by altering the frequency; e.g., three 10-minute bouts, two 15-minute bouts, or one 30-minute bout). Thus, the trials can show the effect of various activity durations, independent of their contribution to energy expenditure.

With regard to chronic disease outcomes, randomized trials are not well-suited to examine these long-term outcomes because of cost and feasibility restraints. Observational epidemiologic studies have investigated different durations of physical activity in relation to mortality and chronic disease outcomes (Lee and Skerrett, 2001). However, almost all of these studies have not accounted for the volume of energy expended; thus, it is difficult to separate the effect of duration from the volume of energy expenditure (a person who exercises for a longer duration will also expend more energy). That is, these studies cannot answer this question: For two individuals expending the same volume of energy, does it matter if one accomplishes this by exercising, for example, 30 minutes in a single session every day, 5 days/week, vs. another who accomplished this by exercising 15 minutes twice a day, 5 days/week?

Only one study has attempted to answer this question in relation to a chronic disease outcome, coronary heart disease (Lee et al., 2000). In the Harvard Alumni Health Study, participants reported their sports and recreational activities, and the duration per episode

Table 4.6 Dose–Response Relationship Between Duration of Physical Activity Bouts and Risk of Coronary Heart Disease, Harvard Alumni Health Study

Duration (minutes)	*No. of cases*	*Age-adjusted relative risk (95% confidence interval)*	*Age- and energy-adjusted relative risk* (95% confidence interval)*
No sports or recreation	155	1.00 (referent)	1.00 (referent)
1–15	24	0.85 (0.55–1.31)	0.94 (0.61–1.47)
16–30	61	0.76 (0.57–1.03)	0.92 (0.65–1.30)
31–45	32	0.85 (0.58–1.24)	1.07 (0.68–1.67)
46–60	55	0.80 (0.59–1.10)	1.02 (0.69–1.50)
>60	155	0.78 (0.62–0.98)	1.05 (0.73–1.40)
p, linear trend		0.04	0.68

*Adjusted for age and volume of energy expended.

(Data from Lee et al., 2000.)

of activity. Obviously, the men engaged in different activities for varying lengths of time. Investigators classified participants according to the longest duration per episode of activity, assuming that if there was increased benefit with longer duration, the longest duration would be most relevant. Table 4.6 shows the age-adjusted relative risks for coronary heart disease associated with different duration of participation in leisure activities (men with no sports or recreational activities might have climbed stairs, which was assumed to take minimal amount of time). The age-adjusted findings show a significant inverse dose–response relationship between duration of activity and risk of developing coronary heart disease (p for linear trend = 0.04).

However, as discussed earlier, do these findings mean that longer durations are more beneficial or that longer durations simply expend more energy (and we have clear data showing that greater volume of energy expended is associated with lower risk)? To answer this, the investigators next adjusted for the volume of energy expended. Table 4.6 shows that there was no longer an association with duration once volume of energy expenditure was controlled for (p for linear trend = 0.68), implying that it is the volume of energy expended that is important and not the duration. Further adjustment for other confounders did not change this result. These findings lend support to the CDC/ACSM recommendation that allows for physical activity to be accumulated in short bouts throughout the day. (As an aside, an alternate explanation for the results in Table 4.6 could be misclassification—if duration were less well-measured than volume of energy, the findings above could also occur). It is worth noting that the available data showing health benefits of accumulated bouts of physical activity have generally considered "short" bouts to be episodes of 10 to 15 minutes. There are almost no data examining bouts shorter than 10 minutes.

Although the preceding discussion covers duration of activity, it also indirectly relates to frequency of participation because for activities of a particular intensity, the combined contribution of duration and frequency yields energy expended. Thus, analyses that account for duration of activity and volume of energy expended have implicitly included frequency.

Future Directions

It is clear from the available evidence that there is an inverse dose–response relationship between physical activity and many different health outcomes. However, the details surrounding this relationship remain unclear. Future research should be more specific regarding which component of physical activity is of interest and should consider the methodologic issues discussed in this chapter. With regard to the volume of energy expenditure in relation to health outcomes, the shape of the curve, the minimum amount required for a benefit, and the point beyond which potential harm occurs all need to be clarified. There is little information regarding whether higher intensity of physical activity confers added benefit to health outcomes, above its contribution to the volume of energy expended. The kinds of physical activity that have been studied in the epidemiologic literature have largely been endurance or aerobic kinds of activity, with few data on resistance and strength training exercise. Additionally, the majority of studies have focused on leisure-time physical activity, with fewer data on occupational activity, and fewer still addressing household and transportation activity. With regard to short, accumulated bouts of activity vs. a single, longer bout of equivalent energy expenditure, there are hardly any data pertaining to bouts shorter than 10 minutes. It is impossible to address this question with any precision in observational studies, so well-designed experimental studies are needed. Finally, investigators should bear in mind that the answers to the aforementioned questions may be—in fact, are likely to be—different for different health outcomes (whether risk factors or clinical outcomes).

Personal Perspective

At first glance, it is somewhat surprising that with the large body of research on physical activity and health available, we know so little about dose–response relationships. However, on more detailed examination, it is apparent that there are many issues that prevent a straightforward interpretation of the data on hand. This chapter discusses several of the issues and provides some suggestions for addressing the complexities in studies of dose–response relationships. The reader will note that focus has been placed on the lower end of the dose–response curve, rather than the upper end. This emphasis is for public health reasons because the majority of the U.S. population is sedentary, rather than to imply that there are no health effects at the upper end. In fact, there are risks—such as musculoskeletal injuries and sudden cardiac death (*see* Chapters 13 and 14)—with high levels of physical activity, especially among individuals unaccustomed to physical activity.

It is heartening to note that studies specifically addressing moderate-intensity physical activity and short, accumulated bouts of activity support the 1995 CDC/ACSM physical activity recommendation. The majority of these studies were conducted *after* the 1995 CDC/ACSM prescription was formulated. This recommendation departed sharply from previous ones and was based on the available literature then, as well as some educated "hunches" of the expert panel writing the prescription, to formulate a palatable activity recommendation. In hindsight, the experts did get it right.

References

ACSM. 1990. American College of Sports Medicine position stand. The recommended quantity and quality of exercise for developing and maintaining cardiorespiratory and muscular fitness in healthy adults. *Med Sci Sports Exerc* 22: 265–74.

Ainsworth BE, Haskell WL, Leon AS, et al. 1993. Compendium of physical activities: classification of energy costs of human physical activities. *Med Sci Sports Exerc* 25: 71–80.

Ainsworth BE, Haskell WL, Whitt MC, et al. 2000. Compendium of physical activities: an update of activity codes and MET intensities. *Med Sci Sports Exerc* 32: S498–504.

Anonymous. 2001. Physical activity trends—United States, 1990–1998. *MMWR* 50: 166–9.

Anonymous. 2004. Prevalence of no leisure-time physical activity—35 States and the District of Columbia, 1988–2002. *MMWR* 53: 82–6.

Barnes PM, Schoenborn CA. 2003. *Physical activity among adults: United States, 2000. Advance data from vital and health statistics; no. 333*. Hyattsville, MD: National Center for Health Statistics.

Caspersen CJ, Powell KE, Christenson GM. 1985. Physical activity, exercise, and physical fitness: definitions and distinctions for health-related research. *Public Health Rep* 100: 126–31.

Eyler AA, Brownson RC, Bacak SJ, Housemann RA. 2003. The epidemiology of walking for physical activity in the United States. *Med Sci Sports Exerc* 35: 1529–36.

Folsom AR, Arnett DK, Hutchinson RG, Liao F, Clegg LX, Cooper LS. 1997. Physical activity and incidence of coronary heart disease in middle-aged women and men. *Med Sci Sports Exerc* 29: 901–9.

Fried LP, Kronmal RA, Newman AB, et al. 1998. Risk factors for 5-year mortality in older adults: the Cardiovascular Health Study. *JAMA* 279: 585–92.

Greenland S. 1995. Dose-response and trend analysis in epidemiology: alternatives to categorical analysis. *Epidemiology* 6: 356–65.

Hardman AE. 2001. Issues of fractionization of exercise (short vs long bouts). *Med Sci Sports Exerc* 33: S421–7; discussion S52–3.

Haskell WL. 1994. J.B. Wolffe Memorial Lecture. Health consequences of physical activity: understanding and challenges regarding dose-response. *Med Sci Sports Exerc* 26: 649–60.

Hennekens CH, Buring JE. 1987. *Epidemiology in medicine*. Boston/Toronto: Little, Brown and Company.

Hu FB, Stampfer MJ, Colditz GA, Ascherio A, Rexrode KM, et al. 2000. Physical activity and risk of stroke in women. *JAMA* 283: 2961–7.

IOM. 2002. *Food and Nutrition Board, Institute of Medicine. Dietary reference intakes for energy, carbohydrate, fiber, fat, fatty acids, cholesterol, protein, and amino acids (macronutrients)*. Washington, DC: National Academies Press.

Jakicic JM, Marcus BH, Gallagher KI, Napolitano M, Lang W. 2003. Effect of exercise duration and intensity on weight loss in overweight, sedentary women: a randomized trial. *JAMA* 290: 1323–30.

Kesaniemi YK, Danforth E, Jr., Jensen MD, Kopelman PG, Lefebvre P, Reeder BA. 2001. Dose-response issues concerning physical activity and health: an evidence-based symposium. *Med Sci Sports Exerc* 33: S351–8.

Kohl HW III, Lee I-M, Vuori IM, Wheeler FC, Bauman A, Sallis JF. 2006. Physical activity and public health: The emergence of a sub-discipline report from the International Congress on Physical Activity and Public Health. *J Physical Activity Health* 3: 344–64.

Kraus WE, Houmard JA, Duscha BD, et al. 2002. Effects of the amount and intensity of exercise on plasma lipoproteins. *N Engl J Med* 347: 1483–92.

Kujala UM, Kaprio J, Sarna S, Koskenvuo M. 1998. Relationship of leisure-time physical activity and mortality: the Finnish twin cohort. *JAMA* 279: 440–4.

Lee IM. 2004. No pain, no gain? Thoughts on the Caerphilly study. *Br J Sports Med* 38: 4–5.

Lee IM, Hsieh CC, Paffenbarger RS, Jr. 1995. Exercise intensity and longevity in men. The Harvard Alumni Health Study. *JAMA* 273: 1179–84.

Lee IM, Rexrode KM, Cook NR, Manson JE, Buring JE. 2001. Physical activity and coronary heart disease in women: is "no pain, no gain" passe? *JAMA* 285: 1447–54.

Lee IM, Sesso HD, Paffenbarger RS, Jr. 2000. Physical activity and coronary heart disease risk in men: does the duration of exercise episodes predict risk? *Circulation* 102: 981–6.

Lee IM, Skerrett PJ. 2001. Physical activity and all-cause mortality: what is the dose-response relation? *Med Sci Sports Exerc* 33: S459–71; discussion S93–4.

Lee Y. 2000. The predictive value of self assessed general, physical, and mental health on functional decline and mortality in older adults. *J Epidemiol Community Health* 54: 123–9.

Manson JE, Greenland P, LaCroix AZ, et al. 2002. Walking compared with vigorous exercise for the prevention of cardiovascular events in women. *N Engl J Med* 347: 716–25.

Manson JE, Hu FB, Rich-Edwards JW,, et al. 1999. A prospective study of walking as compared with vigorous exercise in the prevention of coronary heart disease in women. *N Engl J Med* 341: 650–8.

Nieman DC. 2000. Is infection risk linked to exercise workload? *Med Sci Sports Exerc* 32: S406–11.

Oguma Y, Sesso HD, Paffenbarger RS, Jr., Lee IM. 2002. Physical activity and all cause mortality in women: a review of the evidence. *Br J Sports Med* 36: 162–72.

Paffenbarger RS, Jr., Hyde RT, Wing AL, Lee IM, Jung DL, Kampert JB. 1993. The association of changes in physical-activity level and other lifestyle characteristics with mortality among men. *N Engl J Med* 328: 538–45.

Paffenbarger RS, Jr., Olsen E. 1996. *Lifefit: An effective exercise program for optimal health and a longer life*. Champaign, IL: Human Kinetics.

Pate RR, Pratt M, Blair SN, et al. 1995. Physical activity and public health. A recommendation from the Centers for Disease Control and Prevention and the American College of Sports Medicine. *JAMA* 273: 402–7.

Pocock SJ, Elbourne DR. 2000. Randomized trials or observational tribulations? *N Engl J Med* 342: 1907–9.

Saris WH, Blair SN, van Baak MA, et al. 2003. How much physical activity is enough to prevent unhealthy weight gain? Outcome of the IASO 1st Stock Conference and consensus statement. *Obes Rev* 4: 101–14.

Sesso HD, Gaziano JM, VanDenburgh M, Hennekens CH, Glynn RJ, Buring JE. 2002. Comparison of baseline characteristics and mortality experience of participants and nonparticipants in a randomized clinical trial: the Physicians' Health Study. *Control Clin Trials* 23: 686–702.

Sherman SE, D'Agostino RB, Cobb JL, Kannel WB. 1994. Physical activity and mortality in women in the Framingham Heart Study. *Am Heart J* 128: 879–84.

Tanasescu M, Leitzmann MF, Rimm EB, Willett WC, Stampfer MJ, Hu FB. 2002. Exercise type and intensity in relation to coronary heart disease in men. *JAMA* 288: 1994–2000.

Tardon A, Lee WJ, Delgado-Rodriguez M, et al. 2005. Leisure-time physical activity and lung cancer: a meta-analysis. *Cancer Causes Control* 16: 389–97.

Wendel-Vos GC, Schuit AJ, Feskens EJ, et al. 2004. Physical activity and stroke. A meta-analysis of observational data. *Int J Epidemiol* 33: 787–98.

Willett W. 1998. *Nutritional epidemiology, second edition*. New York, NY: Oxford University Press, pp. 273–301.

Williams PT. 2001. Physical fitness and activity as separate heart disease risk factors: a meta-analysis. *Med Sci Sports Exerc* 33: 754–61.

5

Individual Responses to Physical Activity

The Role of Genetics

Tuomo Rankinen and
Claude Bouchard

As evidenced by several consensus meetings and expert panel reports (NIH, 1996; Bouchard, 2001; Bouchard and Blair, 1999; Leon, 1997; U.S. Department of Health and Human Services, 1996), the body of scientific evidence regarding the effects of physical activity level and sedentary behavior on risk factors for common diseases, health outcomes, and mortality rates is already impressive and growing. However, the effects of regular exercise and habitual physical activity have been almost always tested and reported in terms of main effects and group differences. Consequently, the interpretations and conclusions have been based on the average effects observed in groups of subjects. Although means and main effects are effective and convenient ways to summarize large amount of data, they do not reflect the extent to which the members of the group do not follow the pattern suggested by the group mean. In fact, there are considerable individual differences in risk factor responses to regular physical activity, even when all subjects are exposed to the same volume of exercise, adjusted for their own tolerance level (Bouchard and Rankinen, 2001).

The concept of heterogeneity in responsiveness to standardized exercise programs was first introduced in the early 1980s (Bouchard, 1983). A series of carefully controlled and standardized exercise training studies conducted with young and healthy adult volunteers showed that the individual differences in training-induced changes in several physical performance and health-related fitness phenotypes were large, with the range between low and high responders reaching several-fold (Bouchard, 1983; Bouchard, 1995; Bouchard et al., 1992; Lortie et al., 1984; Simoneau et al., 1986). However, the most extensive data on the individual differences in trainability come from the HERITAGE Family Study, where 742 healthy but sedentary subjects followed a highly standardized, well-controlled, laboratory-based endurance training program for 20 weeks. The average increase in maximal oxygen consumption (VO_{2max}), a measure of cardiorespiratory fitness, was 384 mL of O_2 with a standard deviation (SD) of 202. The training responses varied from no change to increases of more than 1000 mL of O_2 per minute (Bouchard et al., 1999; Bouchard and Rankinen, 2001; Skinner et al., 2000). A similar pattern of variation in training responses was observed for other phenotypes, including plasma lipid levels and submaximal exercise heart rate and blood pressure (Bouchard and Rankinen, 2001; Leon et al., 2000; Wilmore et al., 2001). For example, systolic blood pressure (SBP) and diastolic blood pressure (DBP) measured

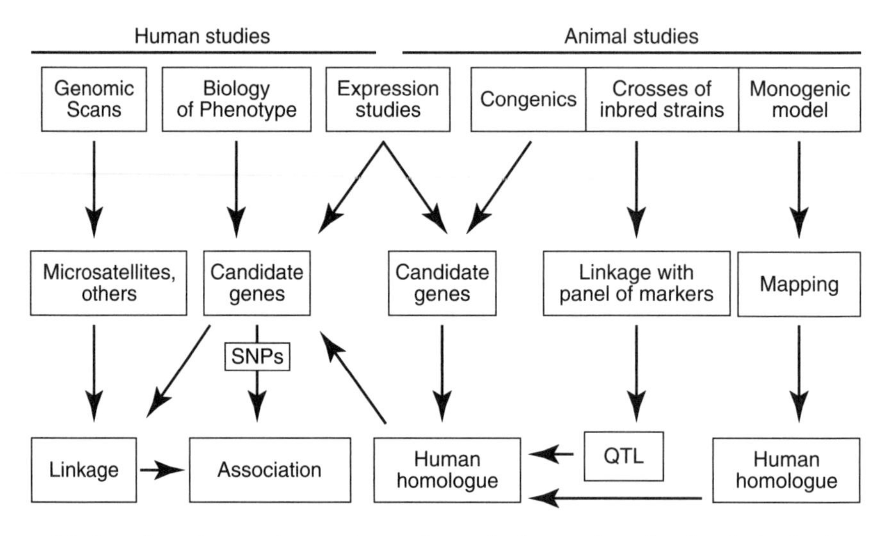

Figure 5.1 Overview of research strategies used to study the genetic and molecular basis of complex multifactorial phenotypes.

during steady-state submaximal (50 W) exercise decreased, by and average of 7 and 3.5 mmHg, respectively, in response to exercise training (Wilmore et al., 2001). However, the responses varied from marked decreases (SBP > 25 mmHg and DBP > 12 mmHg) to no changes or, in some cases, even to slight increases (Bouchard and Rankinen, 2001; Wilmore et al., 2001). Similar heterogeneity in responsiveness to exercise training has been reported in other populations (Hautala et al., 2003; Kohrt et al., 1991).

This kind of variation is an example of normal biological diversity, is observed in most populations, is beyond measurement error and day-to-day fluctuation, and is potentially very informative in terms of the adaptive mechanisms involved (Bouchard and Rankinen, 2001; Shephard et al., 2004). However, we are only now beginning to understand the factors contributing to these interindividual differences. The purpose of this chapter is to provide an overview of the basic study designs and research methods that can be used to investigate the genetic basis of human heterogeneity in the ability to benefit from a physically active lifestyle and to summarize the key findings regarding the genetics of physical activity levels and responsiveness to regular exercise.

Study Designs and Research Methods for Genetic Research

Figure 5.1 presents the most common research strategies to investigate the genetic basis of multifactorial phenotypes. Both human studies and animal models or a combination of both can be used to identify the genes underlying quantitative phenotypes. In humans, statistical analyses based on the paradigms of genetic epidemiology traditionally have been used to investigate the contribution of genetic determinants to quantitative phenotypes and test hypotheses regarding a variety of general and specific models of inheritance. More recently, molecular studies based on random genetic markers or candidate genes have been used increasingly in linkage and association studies designed to identify genes contributing to phenotypes. These complementary approaches are reviewed in the following sections.

Assessment of Familial Aggregation

The first step in the study of the genetic basis of a quantitative multifactorial phenotype is to determine whether or not the phenotype aggregates in families. The presence of familial aggregation, or familiality, can be demonstrated by the higher occurrence of a trait or a disease within families of affected cases, as compared to the families of healthy controls or to the population at large. If a reliable estimate of the trait prevalence in the general population is available, the familial aggregation (familial risk) of a discrete trait can be expressed by the lambda coefficient:

$$\lambda_R = P(A|R)/P(A),$$

where P(A) is the population prevalence of the trait, and P(A|R) is the trait prevalence among relatives of an affected proband (Risch, 1990). For quantitative traits, the lambda coefficient is defined as:

$$\lambda_R(h,1) = P_R(1|h)/P(1),$$

where P(1) is the probability that a randomly selected person in the general population has a trait value in the 1th segment of the trait distribution, and $P_R(1|h)$ is the probability that a person has a trait value in the 1th segment given that a relative of type R has a trait value in the hth segment (Gu and Rao, 1997). Familial risk ratios for physical fitness phenotypes have been reported for a stratified sample of the Canadian population (Katzmarzyk et al., 2000).

If reliable general population trait prevalence estimates are not available, then the presence of familial aggregation for quantitative traits can be tested by comparing the phenotypic variance within families to the variance between families using a one-way analysis of variance. A significantly higher between-family than within-family variance (significant *F*-ratio) suggests that individuals of the same family are more similar than individuals of different families, which in turn suggests familial resemblance.

Assessment of Heritability

After showing that a particular trait aggregates in families, the next step is to quantify the estimated contribution of genetic factors to the familial aggregation. The genetic analysis of multifactorial phenotypes is based on a partitioning of the total phenotypic variance (V_P) into genetic and environmental components as follows:

$$V_P = V_G + V_C + V_E,$$

where V_G is the genetic component of the variance, V_C is the common (shared) environmental variance, and V_E is the residual or non-shared environmental variance. These variance components can be further partitioned to include specific components such as gene–environment interaction (GxE), gene–gene interactions, or epistasis or dominance deviations. The heritability (h^2) of the trait is defined as the proportion of total phenotypic variance explained by the genetic factors ($h^2 = V_G/V_P$). However, sometimes the genetic and shared environmental components of variance are difficult to differentiate (e.g., in nuclear family data). In these cases, the heritability estimate is the combined effect of genes and shared environment on a phenotype and is referred to as the maximal heritability estimate.

The components of variance can be estimated from phenotypic covariance between pairs of relatives. The expected additive genetic, dominance and shared environmental covariances for different types of relative pairs are summarized in Table 5.1. The heritability estimates are based on comparisons of phenotypic similarities between pairs of relatives with different level of biological relatedness. For example, biological siblings, who share

Table 5.1 Expected Covariances for Different Types of Relative Pairs

	Coefficient for		
Types of relatives	*Additive genetic*	*Dominance*	*Shared environment*
Spouse–spouse	0	0	1
Parent–child (living together)	1/2	0	1
Full sibs (living together)	1/2	1/4	1
Full sibs (living apart)	1/2	1/4	0
Half-sibs (living together)	1/4	0	1
Half-sibs (living apart)	1/4	0	0
Aunt/uncle–niece/nephew	1/4	0	0
First cousins (living apart)	1/8	0	0
Dbl. first cousins (living apart)	1/4	1/16	0
DZ twins (living together)	1/2	1/4	1
MZ twins (living together)	1	1	1

about 50% of their genes identical by descent (IBD), should be phenotypically more similar than their parents (biologically unrelated individuals) if genetic factors contribute to the trait of interest. Similarly, a greater phenotypic resemblance between identical twins (100% of genes IBD) than between fraternal twins (50% of genes IBD) suggests a genetic contribution to the phenotype.

The estimation of maximal heritability from the family data is based on fitting various familial correlation models. In addition to a full model, which includes all available familial correlations, several reduced models are tested. The reduced models test specific null hypotheses by restricting some of the covariances (e.g., no sibling resemblance, no spouse resemblance, no sex differences in parents or offspring). The most parsimonious model (or a combination of models) is selected based on the Akaike's Information Criterion (Akaike, 1974), and the familial correlations (r) from this model are used to estimate the maximal heritability of the trait. A commonly used equation to calculate heritabilities (h^2) in nuclear family data is:

$$h^2 = (r_{sibling} + r_{parent\text{-}offspring})(1 + r_{spouse}) / (1 + r_{spouse} + 2r_{spouse}r_{parent\text{-}offspring})$$

It is important to note that heritability is a ratio of variances and, therefore, depends on changes in either the numerator or the denominator. Heritability is also a population measure and does not apply to given individuals. Moreover, estimates of heritability for a given phenotype are likely to vary among populations depending on genetic and environmental characteristics.

Study Designs Used to Assess Heritability

Estimation of the heritability of multifactorial phenotypes requires data on various kinds of relatives with different degrees of relatedness. Several designs are available to assess the heritability of quantitative phenotypes in humans, but they fall into one of the following broad categories: twin studies, adoption studies, and family studies.

Twin Studies The classical twin design has been the most widely used to assess the heritability of a phenotype. The aim of the twin method is to compare the resemblance of identical (monozygotic; MZ) twins to fraternal (dizygotic; DZ) twins. MZ twins are genetically identical because they originate from the division of one zygote, whereas DZ twins share only about one-half of their genes IBD. Thus, any difference in the resemblance between MZ and DZ twin pairs is ascribed to genetic factors, assuming that both types of twins are exposed to similar environmental conditions. This assumption is the most critical, is seldom met, and represents a major limitation of the twin method.

The analysis of twin data was traditionally based on analysis of variance (ANOVA). If genetic factors are involved in determining the phenotype under study, then the within-pair variance will be lower for MZ twins than for DZ twins. The *F*-ratio of the ANOVA is thus used to test for the presence of a genetic effect. The resulting estimate of genetic variance can also be used to estimate the heritability of the phenotype. Several methods have been proposed to estimate heritability from twin data, and the most widely used and simplest method estimates heritability as twice the difference between the MZ and DZ intraclass correlations:

$$h^2 = 2[r_{MZ} - r_{DZ}].$$

Twin data are now explored with more complex modeling and variance decomposition methods. The total V_P is decomposed to V_G, V_C, V_E components, and the genetic heritability is defined as the proportion of total V_P explained by V_G (V_G/V_P). An example of a basic univariate path model to estimate the variance components is shown in Figure 5.2. The V_C is assumed to affect phenotypic covariance similarly in both types of twins, whereas the effect of V_G on covariance is two times greater in MZ twins compared to DZ pairs. Hypotheses about genetic and non-genetic effects can be tested using a number of structural equation modeling-based software that have been developed or modified to deal specifically with twin data and continuous or discrete traits (e.g., LISREL [Cardon et al., 1991] and MX [Neale et al., 2003]).

Several extensions of the classical twin method can be used to assess genetic and environmental sources of variation in a quantitative phenotype. One extension includes data on the spouses and offspring of adult twins, the twin-family method. In contrast to the classical twin method, the twin-family method provides more information on environmental sources of variance and on the role of assortative mating in familial resemblance. It thus increases the external validity of the heritability estimates. Another extension of the twin method compares twins discordant for exposure to a factor in the environment. This is the co-twin control method. It is an ideal design to control for host characteristics like age, sex, and genetic composition and is a powerful approach to estimate the effects of an environmental factor on a phenotype.

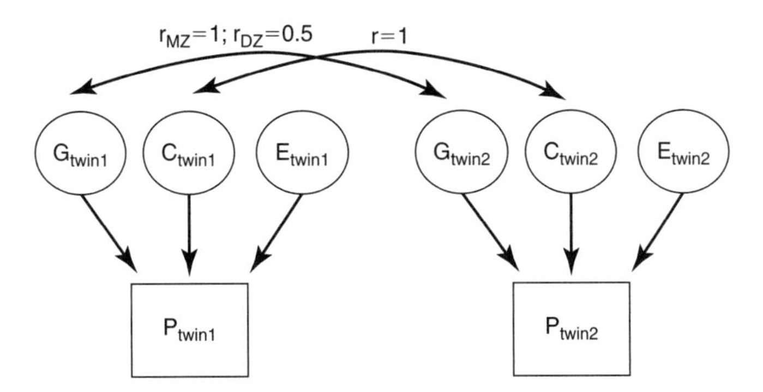

Figure 5.2 An example of a basic univariate genetic path model in monozygotic (MZ) and dizygotic (DZ) twins. Phenotypic variance (P) is affected by genetic (G), common environmental (C), and unique environmental (E) components of variance. Genetic component of phenotypic covariance is assumed to be two times greater in MZ than in DZ pairs ($r_{MZ} = 1$ vs. $r_{DZ} = 0.5$), whereas covariance resulting from common environmental factors is equal in both types of twins.

Data on twins reared apart can also be used in combination with twins reared together to assess heritability. This design alleviates some of the limitations of the classical twin method because twins reared apart do not share a common postnatal life environment in the strict sense. The correlation between MZ twins reared apart can potentially provide a more direct estimate of heritability.

Despite its limitations, the twin method represents a powerful design to detect the presence of a genetic effect in a quantitative phenotype. However, twins share prenatal as well as postnatal environments to a unique extent and may not be representative of the population at large. In particular, the environmental component shared by MZ brothers and sisters may be quite different from that shared by DZ twins. Heritability estimates derived from twin data should be interpreted with caution and should be considered as upper-bound estimates of the heritability of a phenotype.

Adoption Studies The study of adopted children and their foster and biological parents is a powerful design to assess genetic and cultural heritabilities. Resemblance between an adopted child and members of his/her biological family is attributable largely to the genes they share in common, whereas resemblance between an adopted child and his/her adoptive family primarily results from a shared environment. If data on an adoptee's biological parents are not available, then the study design is referred to as a partial adoption design. In the partial adoption study, the resemblance between biological and adopted siblings living in the same family environment is compared. For example, the absence of a significant correlation between adoptive parents and their adopted children combined with a significant correlation between the same parents and their biological children suggests that the phenotype under study is more influenced by genetic factors than by the family environment.

Although adoption studies offer an attractive design to assess heritability, they have limitations. One important variable to control in adoption studies is age at adoption. Ideally, adoption should have occurred immediately after birth so that the resemblance between the adoptee and his/her biological parent can be defined as entirely genetic and not be confounded by any effect of familial environment. It is often advisable to adjust the correlations for age at adoption and to test whether or not they are different from the non-adjusted correlations. An assumption underlying the adoption design includes the absence of selective placement of adoptees, which occurs when adoption agencies try to match adoptive parents and biological parents on a variety of characteristics (e.g., socioeconomic status, complexion, and others). In addition, it is assumed that adoptive families are an unbiased sample of the population. This is clearly not the case because adoptive families are not randomly selected.

Family Studies Family studies, including nuclear families (parents and their offspring) and extended pedigrees (plus grandparents, cousins, uncles/aunts, etc.), are the most widely used designs to investigate the genetic basis of quantitative phenotypes. One major advantage of this design is that families are typically more representative of the population at large than fixed sets of relatives like twins or adoptees. However, data on nuclear families alone do not contain sufficient information to estimate separately and to quantify the relative contribution of genetic and shared environmental components of variance and can only be used to assess familiality—that is, the fraction of phenotypic variance attributable to the combined effects of all familial influences.

Molecular Genetic Studies

Once the familial aggregation and heritability of the phenotype have been established, the next challenge is to identify the genes and mutations that contribute to the trait heritability. The following provides a brief overview of the common types of DNA sequence variations, followed by the descriptions of study designs and research strategies for linkage and association studies with DNA sequence variants.

DNA Sequence Variation

The major source of genetic variation is the variety of heritable changes (mutations) in the nucleotide sequence of the DNA. These changes may vary from a substitution of a single base to a loss or gain of entire chromosomes or large chromosomal regions. Mutations that occur in the germline cells can be transmitted to future generations, whereas somatic cell mutations are restricted to a single individual and the population of cells derived from the mutated cell. Large-scale germline chromosomal abnormalities are relatively rare but they usually show a clear phenotype, which is generally pathogenic and often lethal. Large-scale somatic mutations are more common and often occur in tumor cells.

Small-scale mutations can be grouped into three mutation classes: *(1)* base substitutions, *(2)* deletions, and *(3)* insertions (Fig. 5.3). Base substitutions usually change a single base (single-nucleotide polymorphisms; SNPs). Synonymous or silent substitutions are the most frequently observed in coding DNA. They do not change an amino acid in the final gene product. However, they may have functional consequences by changing the splicing pattern of the gene. Non-synonymous substitutions result in an altered codon that specifies either a different amino acid (a missense mutation) or a termination codon (a nonsense mutation). A missense mutation can induce either a conservative or non-conservative amino acid substitutions. A conservative substitution does not significantly change the chemical

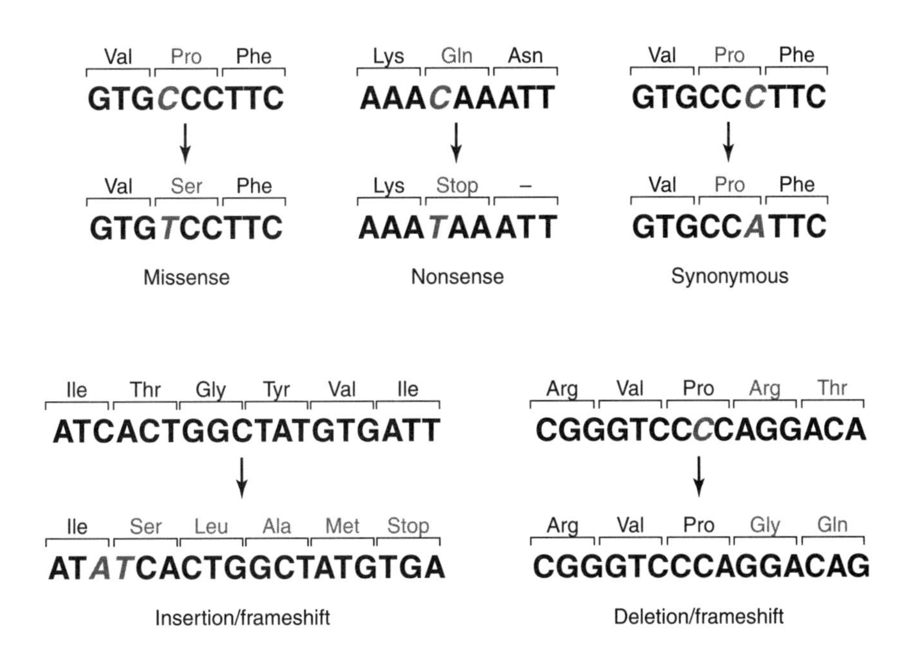

Figure 5.3 The main classes of small-scale mutations. The upper panel presents single base substitutions, where a change of a single nucleotide induces either a change in amino acid (missense) or a premature stop codon (nonsense) or has no effect on the gene product (synonymous/silent). The lower panel shows examples of small-scale insertion (left) and deletion (right) mutations that alter the translational reading frame of the gene (frameshift). Polymorphic nucleotides and resulting changes in amino acids are indicated with gray font. (Reproduced with permission from Rankinen and Bouchard, 2005.)

properties of the amino acid encoded by the new codon, whereas the amino acid introduced by a non-conservative substitution has different chemical characteristics. Therefore, non-conservative substitutions are more likely to change the properties of the gene product than conservative substitutions. Deletions and insertions refer to the removal or addition, respectively, of one or a few nucleotides from the DNA sequence. These variations are relatively common in non-coding DNA. They are less frequent in exons where they may introduce frameshifts (i.e., they alter the normal translational reading frame of the gene and thereby change the final gene product; Fig. 5.3).

Small-scale mutations used to be viewed as functionally significant only if they affected the amino acid sequence. However, silent substitutions in exons as well as mutations in the non-coding sequence may also have strong effects on gene transcription and on the final gene product. Mutations in the 5′ regulatory region may disrupt transcription factor binding sites, response elements, or enhancer or silencer sequences and thereby affect the rate at which a gene is transcribed. Although the 3′ untranslated region of a gene is typically not as critical for its expression control as the coding and promoter regions, it contains sequence elements affecting nuclear transport, polyadenylation, subcellular targeting, and stability of messenger RNA (mRNA; Conne et al., 2000). Mutations in these sequences, therefore, can also influence gene transcription and translation. Both synonymous and non-synonymous substitutions in the coding sequence may alter splicing sites between coding and non-coding regions and splicing enhancers and silencers with potentially dramatic effects on the mature polypeptide (Fig. 5.4; Cartegni et al., 2002).

Association Studies

Most of the published physical activity-related molecular genetic studies have utilized a candidate gene approach—that is, a gene has been targeted based on its potential physiological and metabolic relevance to the trait of interest. The study designs are typically either case–control or cross-sectional cohort studies with unrelated subjects. Statistical tests for

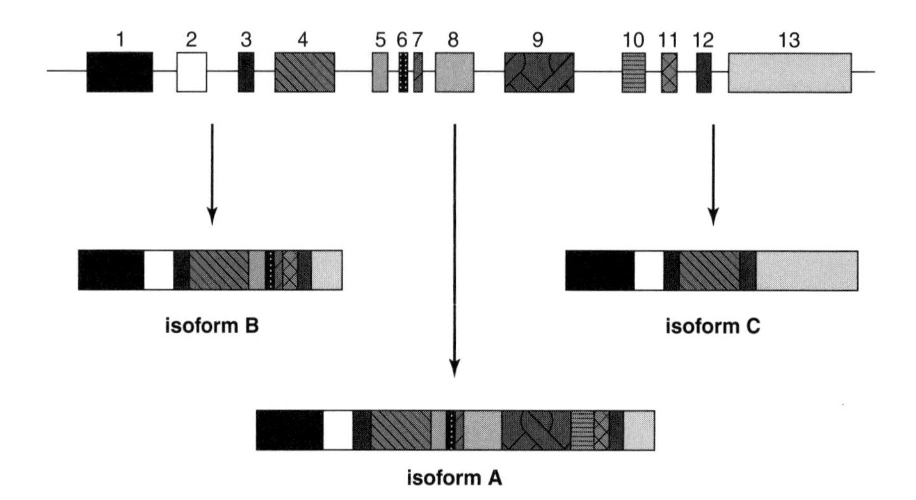

Figure 5.4 An example of alternative splicing. A gene consisting of 13 exons encodes three distinct messenger RNAs. Isoform A contains all 13 exons, whereas exons 8 through 10 and 5 through 11 are spliced off from isoforms B and C, respectively. Isoform C also utilizes an alternative stop codon. (Reproduced with permission from Rankinen and Bouchard, 2005.)

an association are based on the comparison of allele and genotype frequencies of genetic markers between two groups of subjects, one having the phenotype of interest (e.g., high endurance athletes—that is, the "cases") and the other not (the "controls"). With continuous traits, the test is done by comparing mean phenotypic values across genotype groups or between carriers and non-carriers of a specific allele defined by a SNP or an insertion/deletion polymorphism.

The advantage of the association studies is that they do not necessarily require family data, and therefore, recruitment of the subjects and data collection are less time-consuming than in the family and twin studies. However, a potential problem in cohort studies with unrelated subjects is an increased risk of false-positive findings resulting from population stratification. Population stratification refers to an existence of distinct subpopulations within the study cohort. If the subpopulations differ from each other or from the rest of the cohort in terms of allele frequencies *and* phenotypic values, they may produce a statistically significant association between a DNA sequence variant and a phenotype, even if such an association does not exist. The stratification is clearly a problem when a study cohort includes subjects from different ethnic groups. However, to what extent stratification affects cohorts sampled from a single ethnic group is still unclear and remains a topic of lively debate. Nevertheless, several statistical methods have been developed to detect and control for population stratification in cohort studies.

In the late 1990s, concerns over population stratification bias prompted development of family-based association studies. Because the segregation of chromosomes to gametes during meiosis is a random process, the transmission of alleles from parents to offspring is also random. Transmission of a specific allele to children with a specific trait (e.g., disease, high body mass index [BMI], etc.) more often than would be expected by chance alone would indicate that the allele is associated with and potentially contributes to the phenotypic variation. Statistical models testing the preferential transmission of alleles to affected children are called transmission disequilibrium tests (TDTs). Because the TDT models utilize the randomness of allele transmission within families, they are not affected by the population substructures. The original TDT models were developed to use parent–child trios (mother, father, and affected child). However, these models have been extended to families with multiple offspring and to quantitative traits.

Linkage Studies

An alternative strategy to identify genes affecting a given phenotype relies on linkage analysis. The basic idea of genetic linkage is to test if a genetic locus is transmitted from parents to children together with a trait (or another genetic locus) of interest. The process is fairly straightforward when the trait is influenced by only one (major) gene. In these cases, the underlying genetic architecture can be deduced by observing the transmission of the trait in affected families. However, multifactorial and oligogenic traits such as exercise and health phenotypes rarely follow a specific and simple inheritance model.

For these traits, the statistical testing of linkage is performed by using either a regression-based method or by a variance components modeling. Briefly, in the Elston regression method, the phenotypic resemblance of siblings is modeled as the mean-corrected cross-product of the sibs' trait values. In the variance component linkage methods, the total V_P is decomposed into additive effects of a trait locus, a residual familial background, and a residual non-familial component. The phenotypic covariance of the sibling pairs is modeled as a function of allele sharing or IBD. The linkage testing is performed using likelihood ratio test contrasting a null hypothesis model of no linkage with an alternative hypothesis model in which the variance caused by the trait locus is estimated.

The major conceptual difference between linkage and association is that association targets a specific allele or a genotype at a given gene locus whereas linkage refers to a chromosomal region rather than a specific gene or mutation. Thus, the linkage analysis can be used to identify chromosomal regions that harbor gene(s) affecting the phenotype (quantitative trait loci; QTL), even if there is no *a priori* knowledge of the existence of such genes. By definition, the linkage analysis always requires family or pedigree data. In addition, the basic observation unit is a pair of relatives (usually siblings) rather than an individual subject. Therefore, data collection is more challenging than in case–control and cohort studies with unrelated subjects.

The identification of a QTL is only the first step in the gene discovery process. Because linkage analysis provides information about a genomic region, a typical QTL may span several millions of DNA basepairs and may contain dozens or even hundreds of genes. The procedure used to identify the causal gene(s) within a QTL is called positional cloning, and the principal steps of the positional cloning strategy are summarized in Figure 5.5. Briefly, the initial detection of the QTL is followed by the addition of more microsatellite markers (dense mapping) within the chromosomal region with a view to narrow down the size of the

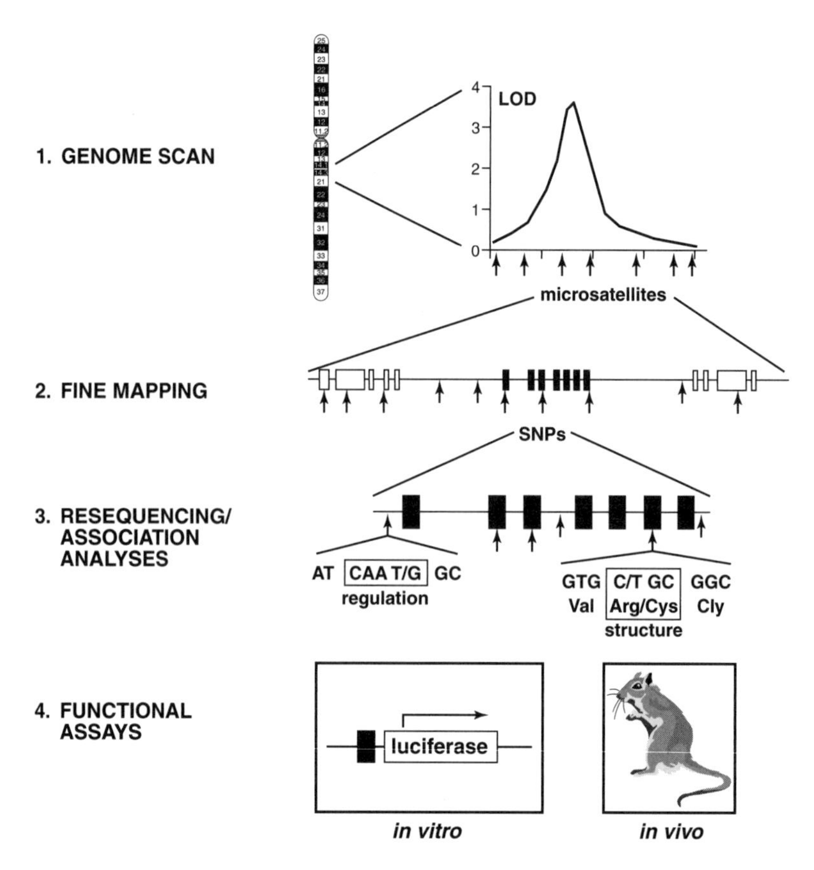

Figure 5.5 Schematic presentation of the positional cloning strategy. The initial genome-wide linkage scan is followed by fine mapping with additional microsatellite and single nucleotide polymorphism (SNP) markers. Genes showing significant associations with the SNPs are then resequenced to identify all relevant DNA sequence variants in the study population. The relevance of the uncovered mutations is verified with additional association studies in other populations (replications) and using *in vitro* and *in vivo* functional studies. (The figure is modified from Boerwinkle et al., 2000.)

target region as much as possible using linkage analysis. Once the resolution limit of the linkage approach is reached, the next step involves fine mapping using association analyses with SNPs. The rationale of fine mapping is that the greater number of SNPs used and the greater sensitivity of the association tests allow more detailed information about the region to be derived. Even if the SNPs used for fine mapping do not include the specific DNA sequence variant(s) affecting the trait, they can provide useful leads regarding the underlying causal mutation(s). The closely located, yet functionally neutral, SNPs may cosegregate with the trait-influencing DNA variant and thereby be part of a haplotype that also contains the causal allele. This phenomenon is called allelic association or linkage disequilibrium and is part of the theoretical basis for association mapping.

Once the results from association analyses are deemed strong enough, the next step is to screen by sequencing the candidate gene for DNA sequence variants. The confirmation of the relevance of detected mutations generally includes additional association studies in the original and other populations, as well as functional assays *in vitro* (expression studies in different cell lines) and *in vivo* (transgenic and knock-out animal models). The positional cloning approach has been used successfully to identify genes causing several diseases, such as long QT syndrome 1 (Wang et al., 1996) and autosomal dominant familial polymorphic ventricular tachycardia (Laitinen et al., 2001; Swan et al., 1999). Both traits are characterized by increased incidence of cardiac events during exercise. The positional cloning efforts of the response to exercise QTLs in the HERITAGE Family Study are designed to yield a panel of new candidate genes that are being investigated for their roles in the adaptation to regular exercise.

Gene–Environment Interactions

The contributions of genetic and environmental factors to the phenotypic variance are frequently viewed as separate and independent components. This polarization is further fueled by the "nature vs. nurture" debate popularized by the lay media. However, geneticists have recognized for a long time that there are complex interactions between genes and environments. The concept has been well-documented in plant and animal genetics. There is also plenty of evidence of gene–environment interactions from genetic epidemiology studies. Such studies have repeatedly emphasized that some genotypes are particularly sensitive to selected environmental factors.

Thus far, we have dealt with the heterogeneity of the responsiveness to regular exercise in terms of interindividual differences in changes in risk factors. Epidemiologists also face the fact that despite the general inverse relationship between physical activity level and the risk for a given chronic disease, some physically active individuals still develop the disease, whereas some sedentary people do not. The interactions between genetic and environmental factors can manifest themselves in several ways. Figure 5.6 presents one possible scenario applied to gene–fitness interactions on health outcomes. Subjects who lack the genetic risk factor and are physically fit (i.e., exercise regularly or are physically active) have the lowest risk of disease. In subjects with increased genetic risk, being fit can potentially prevent or delay the onset of the disease, prevent the complications of the disease, or increase the subject's responsiveness to treatment. On the other hand, unfit or sedentary people may have an increased risk of morbidity in general, but with a genetic predisposition the disease may manifest itself at an earlier age, have more severe complications, and be more resistant to treatment. These examples underline the idea that a state (such as fitness) or a behavior (such as physical activity) can potentially compensate a genetic predisposition to a disease. Thus, it is both clinically and physiologically meaningless to argue whether a multifactorial disease has a genetic or an environmental origin. To better understand the

		Genetic predisposition	
		No	Yes
Low fitness or sedentary behavior	No	• No disease, or late onset • No complications • Good response to treatment	• Average or late onset • Minor complications • Good response to treatment
	Yes	• Average or early onset • Moderate to severe complications • Impaired or normal response to treatment	• Early onset • Severe complications • Resistant to treatment

Figure 5.6 A schematic presentation of possible genotype–fitness interaction effects on the risk level for a multifactorial disease.

dynamics of the complex network of factors contributing to hypertension, it is necessary to investigate them together and to account for the gene–environment interactions in addition to the main effects.

Genotype–environment interactions can be tested using several types of study designs. In observational studies, the key requirement is that both the genotype (DNA sequence variant) and the interacting environmental/behavioral phenotype (e.g., physical activity level, dietary intake) be reliably quantified. An example of such an approach comes from the San Luis Valley Diabetes Study, in which 397 Hispanics and 569 non-Hispanic Caucasians were followed for 14 years. During the follow-up, the frequency of the T/T genotype of the C–480T polymorphism in the hepatic lipase (LIPC) gene locus was higher among the 91 cases of coronary heart disease (CHD), and the CHD-free survival during the follow-up among the T/T homozygotes was significantly worse than in the C/C homozygotes and the C/T heterozygotes. Interestingly, the increased CHD risk associated with the T/T genotype was observed in the sedentary or moderately active subjects but not in subjects who participated in vigorous physical activities (Hokanson et al., 2003).

Similarly, King and coworkers investigated the risk of breast and ovarian cancer associated with the mutations in the *BRCA1* and *BRCA2* genes in Ashkenazi Jewish women (King et al., 2003). Although mutations in both genes significantly increase the risk of breast cancer, the results suggest that physical activity and body weight modify the penetrance of the disease. Mutation carriers who were physically active as teenagers were diagnosed with breast cancer significantly later in life (i.e., older age of onset) than those who were sedentary. In the sedentary group, 60% and 95% of the women were diagnosed with breast cancer by the age of 45 and 55 years, respectively, whereas the corresponding ages in the physically active women were 53 and 73 years (King et al., 2003). Similarly, women who were overweight at menarche and were heavier at age 21 years had earlier age of breast cancer onset among the carriers of *BRCA1* and *BRCA2* mutations.

Another option for testing genotype–environment interactions is to change one environmental/behavioral characteristic in a systematic and controlled fashion and then document the contribution of the genotype to the interindividual differences in response. Such an approach has been used to investigate the role of genotype in the responsiveness of body composition and metabolic phenotypes to long-term negative and positive energy balance in identical twins (Bouchard et al., 1990; Bouchard et al., 1994) and the genetic basis of cardiovascular and metabolic responsiveness to endurance training in nuclear families (Bouchard et al., 1995). In the negative energy balance trial, seven pairs of young adult male MZ twins exercised on cycle ergometers twice a day, 9 of 10 days, over a period of 93 days while being kept on a constant daily energy and nutrient intake. The mean total

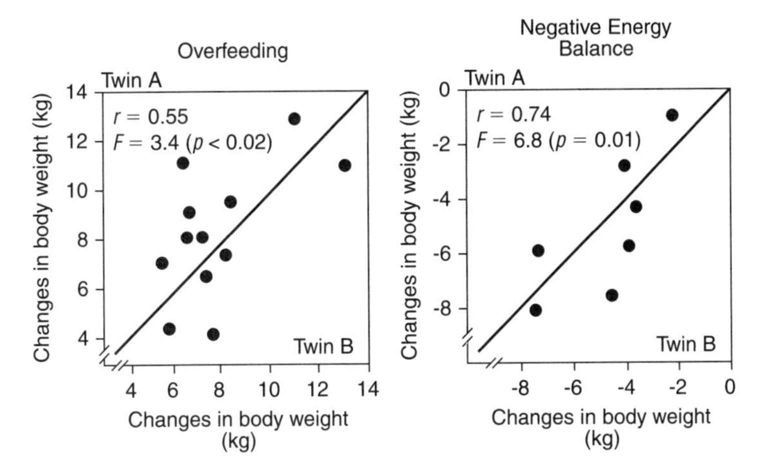

Figure 5.7 Intrapair resemblance in the response of identical twins to long-term changes in energy balance. Left, 12 pairs of identical twins were submitted to an 84,000-kcal energy intake surplus over 100 days. Right, seven pairs were subjected to a negative energy balance protocol caused by exercise. The energy deficit was 58,000 kcal over 93 days. (Reproduced with permission from Bouchard et al., 1990 and Bouchard et al., 1994.)

energy deficit caused by exercise above the estimated energy cost of body weight maintenance reached about 58,000 kcal (244 MJ). The mean body weight loss was 5.0 kg (range: 1 kg to about 8 kg). However, although there were large individual differences in response to the negative energy balance, subjects with the same genotype were more alike in body composition changes than subjects with different genotypes. The F-ratio of the between-pair to the within-pair variances reached 6.8 for body weight and 14.1 for body fat, and the intraclass correlation coefficients were 0.74 and 0.87, respectively (Figure 5.7). Similar findings were reported when 12 pairs of young, lean identical twins were overfed by a standardized amount of calories over a period of 100 days (Figure 5.7).

Genetics of Physical Activity and Sedentarism

The majority of the physical activity-related genetic studies in humans have focused on the biological responses to regular physical activity and exercise training, whereas the genetic background of physical activity as a behavior has received less attention. However, although both environmental and social factors have major influence on the habitual physical activity levels, both twin and family studies support the notion that genetic factors are also involved. Studies in MZ and DZ twins have consistently reported greater intraclass correlations for activity traits in MZ than in DZ twins (Table 5.2). Similarly, family studies have reported greater between-family than within-family variance in phenotypes reflecting physical activity level or sedentarism. Heritability estimates have ranged from 30% to 83% in twin studies and from 10% to 30% in studies with nuclear families.

Data on the molecular genetics of physical activity levels in humans remain scarce. However, animal studies provide some examples as to how genes may affect physical activity patterns. For example, mice lacking the dopamine transporter gene exhibit marked hyperactivity (Gainetdinov et al., 1999), whereas dopamine receptor D2 (DRD2)-deficient mice are characterized by reduced physical activity levels (Kelly et al., 1998). Another example of the potential involvement of a gene in physical activity regulation comes from

Table 5.2 Summary of Intraclass Correlations From Twin Studies for Physical Activity Level and Physical Activity-Related Phenotypes

			Number of pairs		*Correlation coefficients*		
Physical activity trait	*Age*	*Sex*	*MZ*	*DZ*	*MZ*	*DZ*	*Reference*
Total physical activity	>18	Male	1537	3507	0.57	0.26	(Kaprio et al., 1981)
Sports participation	18–22	Male	249	241	0.89	0.60	(Koopmans et al., 1994)
		Female	329	303	0.85	0.72	
Leisure-time physical activity outside the school	16	Male	147	191	0.72	0.45	(Aarnio et al., 1997)
	16	Female	231	179	0.64	0.41	
Intermittent moderate activities	33–51	Male	1006	530	0.38	0.12	(Lauderdale et al., 1997)
Jogging / running (>10 miles/week)					0.53	0.07	
Strenuous racquet sports (>5 h/week)					0.52	0.28	
Bicycling (>50 miles/ week)					0.58	0.14	
Swimming (>2 miles/week)					0.39	0.35	
Sports participation	15	Male	17	19	0.66	0.62	(Beunen and Thomis, 1999)
		Female	17	19	0.98	0.71	
Sports participation index	12–25	Male	85	68	0.82	0.46	(Maia et al., 2002)
		Female	118	85	0.90	0.53	
Leisure-time physical activity		Male	85	68	0.69	0.22	
		Female	118	85	0.72	0.56	
Self-rated ability on athletic competition	27–80	Male	226	202	0.50[a]	0.26[a]	(McGue et al., 1993)
	27–86	Female	452	345			
Perceived athletic self-competence	10–18	Male	45	49	0.58[a]	0.23[a]	(McGuire et al., 1994)
	10–18	Female	47	48			

[a]Coefficients adjusted for sex.

the fruit fly (*Drosophila melanogaster*). These insects exhibit two distinct activity patterns related to food-search behavior; rovers move about twice the distance while feeding compared to sitters. This activity pattern is genetically determined and is regulated by the *dg2* gene, which encodes a cyclic guanosine monophosphate-dependent protein kinase (PKG) (Osborne et al., 1997). PKG activity is significantly higher in wild-type rovers than in wild-type and mutant sitters, and activation of the *dg2* gene reverts foraging behavior from a sitter to a rover. Furthermore, overexpression of the *dg2* gene in sitters changed their behavior to the rover phenotype (Osborne et al., 1997).

Only a few association studies on DNA sequence variation in candidate genes and physical activity traits are available in humans. The candidate genes with positive findings that have been investigated with an *a priori* hypothesis include DRD2, angiotensin-converting enzyme (ACE), and leptin receptor (LEPR) (Simonen et al., 2003; Stefan et al., 2002; Winnicki et al., 2004). In both the Québec Family Study (QFS) and the HERITAGE Family Study cohorts, a C/T transition in codon 313 of the *DRD2* gene was associated with physical activity levels in

Caucasian women (Simonen et al., 2003). The T/T homozygote women of the QFS reported significantly less weekly activity during the previous year than the heterozygotes and the C/C homozygotes. Similarly, among Caucasian women in the HERITAGE Family Study, the T/T homozygotes showed lower sports and work indices, derived from the ARIC-Baecke physical activity questionnaire, than the other genotypes (Simonen et al., 2003).

In Pima Indians, a glutamine (Gln) to arginine (Arg) substitution in codon 223 of the *LEPR* gene was associated with total physical activity level, calculated by dividing 24-hour energy expenditure by sleeping energy expenditure, measured in a respiratory chamber. The Arg233Arg homozygotes showed about 5% lower physical activity level than the Gln223Gln homozygotes (Stefan et al., 2002). In a group of never-treated stage I hypertensives, the *ACE* I/D genotype and marital status were the strongest contributors to their physical activity status. The frequency of the D/D genotype was significantly higher in the sedentary patients than among active patients. Approximately 76% of the D/D homozygotes were sedentary, whereas the corresponding frequency in the I-allele homozygotes was 48% (Winnicki et al., 2004).

The only genome-wide linkage scan for physical activity traits published so far was carried out in the QFS cohort (Simonen et al., 2003). The scan was based on 432 polymorphic markers genotyped in 767 subjects from 207 families. Physical activity measures were derived from a 3-day activity diary (and classified according to total daily activity, inactivity, and moderate-to-strenuous activity phenotypes) and an 11-item questionnaire (weekly physical activity during the past year). The strongest evidence of linkage ($p = 0.0012$) was detected on chromosome 2p22–p16 with the physical inactivity phenotype. Suggestive linkages were also found on 13q22 with total daily activity and moderate-to-strenuous activity phenotypes and on 7p11 with both inactivity and moderate-to-strenuous activity. In addition, weekly activity during the past year showed suggestive evidence of linkage on 11p15 and 15q13, inactivity on 20q12, and moderate-to-strenuous activity on 4q31 and 9q31 (Simonen et al., 2003). These observations suggest that several regions of the nuclear genome encode genes contributing to human variation in physical activity level or the inclination to be sedentary.

Genetics and Responsiveness to Exercise Training

The heritability of VO_{2max} in the sedentary state has been estimated from a few twin and family studies, the most comprehensive of these being the HERITAGE Family Study (Bouchard et al., 1998). An analysis of variance revealed a clear familial aggregation of VO_{2max} in the sedentary state. The variance in VO_{2max} (adjusted for age, sex, body mass, and body composition) was 2.7 times greater between families than within families, and about 40% of the variance in VO_{2max} was accounted for by family lines. Maximum likelihood estimation of familial correlations (spouse, four parent-offspring, and three sibling correlations) revealed a maximal heritability of 51% for VO_{2max}. However, the significant spouse correlation indicated that the genetic heritability was less than 50% (Bouchard et al., 1998). Data from the twin studies have yielded very similar heritability estimates, ranging from 25% to 66% (Bouchard et al., 1986; Fagard et al., 1991; Sundet et al., 1994).

In pairs of MZ twins, the VO_{2max} response to standardized training programs showed six to nine times more variance between genotypes (between pairs of twins) than within genotypes (within pairs of twins) (Bouchard et al., 1992). Thus, gains in absolute VO_{2max} were much more heterogeneous between pairs of twins than within pairs of twins. In the HERITAGE Family Study, the increase in VO_{2max} in 481 individuals from 99 two-generation families of Caucasian descent showed 2.6 times more variance between families than within families, and the model-fitting analytical procedure yielded a maximal heritability estimate of 47% (Bouchard et al., 1999).

In addition to VO_{2max}, the heritability of training-induced changes in several other phenotypes, such as submaximal aerobic performance (Perusse et al., 2001), resting and submaximal exercise blood pressure, heart rate, stroke volume and cardiac output (An et al., 2003; An et al., 2000; An et al., 2000; Rice et al., 2002), body composition, and body fat distribution, (Perusse et al., 2000; Rice et al., 1999), and plasma lipid, lipoprotein, and apolipoprotein levels (Rice et al., 2002) have been investigated in the HERITAGE Family Study. The maximal heritabilities for these traits ranged from 25% to 55%, further confirming the contribution of familial factors to the person-to-person variation in responsiveness to endurance training.

Candidate Gene Studies

The evidence from the genetic epidemiology studies suggests that there is a genetically determined component affecting exercise-related phenotypes. However, because these traits are complex and multifactorial in nature, the search for genes and mutations responsible for the genetic regulation must target not only several families of phenotypes but also consider the phenotypes in the sedentary state and in response to exercise training. It is also obvious that the research on molecular genetics of exercise-related phenotypes is still in its infancy. We have begun the publication in *Medicine and Science in Sports and Exercise* of an annual review on the Human Gene Map for Performance and Health-Related Fitness phenotypes (Rankinen et al., 2001). The 2005 update of the map included 165 gene entries and QTL on the autosomes and 5 on the X chromosome (Rankinen et al., 2006a) for physical performance and health-related fitness phenotypes. As a comparison, the latest version of a similar map for obesity-related phenotypes included more than 600 loci (Rankinen et al., 2006b). These numbers demonstrate that relatively little has been accomplished to date. For example, no gene contributing to human variation in endurance performance has been identified as a result of studies based on model organisms. Now that we have entered the era in which the human, mouse, and rat genomic sequences have become available, the field of exercise science and sports medicine will need to devote more attention to molecular and genetic research.

The 2005 update of the Human Gene Map for Performance and Health-Related Fitness (Rankinen et al., 2006a) included 29 autosomal genes from 66 studies with evidence of associations with cardiorespiratory endurance or muscular strength phenotypes. A clear favorite gene among exercise scientists has been the *ACE* gene, which was investigated in 28 reports. A 287-basepair insertion (I)/deletion (D) polymorphism in intron 16 of the *ACE* gene was first reported to be strongly associated with plasma ACE activity in 1990 (Rigat et al., 1990). The ACE activity was lowest in subjects with two copies of the I allele (I/I homozygotes), highest in the D/D homozygotes, and intermediate in the I/D heterozygotes.

In exercise-related studies, the I-allele has been reported to be more frequent in Australian elite rowers and in Spanish endurance athletes than in sedentary controls (Alvarez et al., 2000, Gayagay et al., 1998). Similarly, British long-distance runners tended to have a greater frequency of the I-allele than sprinters (Myerson et al., 1999). In a group of post-menopausal women who were selected on the basis of their physical activity levels (sedentary, recreationally active, endurance athletes), the I/I genotype was associated with greater VO_{2max} and maximal arterial-venous oxygen difference compared to the D/D homozygotes (Hagberg et al., 1998). The I-allele was also associated with greater increase in muscular endurance and efficiency after 10 weeks of physical training in British Army recruits (Montgomery et al., 1998; Williams et al., 2000; Woods et al., 2002).

In contrast, the frequency of the D-allele was found to be higher in elite swimmers than in sedentary controls (Woods et al., 2001). Moreover, in almost 300 sedentary but healthy white offspring from the HERITAGE Family Study, the D/D homozygotes showed the greatest improvements in VO_{2max} and maximal power output following a controlled and supervised 20-week endurance training program (Rankinen et al., 2000). Furthermore, some studies have suggested that the D-allele is associated with greater muscular strength gains in response to resistance training (Folland et al., 2000). It should also be noted that there are several reports showing no associations between the ACE genotype and performance phenotypes (Rankinen et al., 2000; Sonna et al., 2001; Taylor et al., 1999).

The observations on the *ACE* gene need to be put in perspective. It is clear that the statistical evidence for an association or against an association is not very strong in the published reports to date. As noted before (Cardon and Palmer, 2003), the most likely explanation for seemingly inconsistent results from association studies in different populations is typically the overinterpretation of marginal statistical evidence. Therefore, the available data are still too sparse and fragmented to fully evaluate what role the *ACE* gene plays in the variation of human physical performance level.

The genetic data hold great promise to help us understand why some individuals respond favorably to exercise training in terms of reduction of chronic disease risk factor levels, whereas others do not. Here again, we rely on the 2005 update of the Human Gene Map for Performance and Health-Related Fitness. It includes 31 genes from 46 studies that have been investigated in relation to exercise training-induced changes in hemodynamic (11 genes, 15 studies), body composition (15 genes, 19 studies), plasma lipid and lipoprotein (7 genes, 10 studies), and hemostatic (3 genes, 3 studies) phenotypes. The genes associated with body composition, plasma lipid, and hemostatic phenotype training responses were all based on a single study. However, with hemodynamic phenotypes, some candidate gene findings have been replicated in at least two studies. For example, an association between blood pressure training response and the angiotensinogen (AGT) M235T polymorphism has been reported both in the HERITAGE Family Study and the DNASCO study (Rankinen et al., 2000; Rauramaa et al., 2002). In Caucasian HERITAGE males, the AGT M235M homozygotes showed the greatest reduction in submaximal exercise DBP following a 20-week endurance training program (Rankinen et al., 2000), whereas in middle-aged Eastern Finnish men, the M235M homozygotes had the most favorable changes in resting SBP and DBP during a 6-year exercise intervention trial (Rauramaa et al., 2002).

Similarly, an association between the ACE I/D polymorphism and training-induced left ventricular (LV) growth has been reported in two studies (Montgomery et al., 1997; Myerson et al., 2001). In 1997, Montgomery and coworkers reported that the ACE D-allele was associated with greater increases in LV mass and septal and posterior wall thickness after 10 weeks of physical training in British Army recruits (Montgomery et al., 1997). In 2001, the same group reported a new study using a similar training paradigm in British Army recruits (Myerson et al., 2001). The cohort included 62 ACE I/I and 79 ACE D/D homozygotes, and the training-induced increase in LV mass was 2.7 times greater in the D/D genotype compared to the I/I homozygotes. Interestingly, the association between the ACE genotype and LV mass response was not affected by angiotensin II type 1 receptor inhibitor (Losartan) treatment (Myerson et al., 2001).

Linkage Studies

The HERITAGE Family Study is the first and, thus far, the only study employing a family design in exercise-related questions (Bouchard et al., 1995). To date, six genome-wide linkage scans dealing with 16 endurance training response and 7 acute exercise response

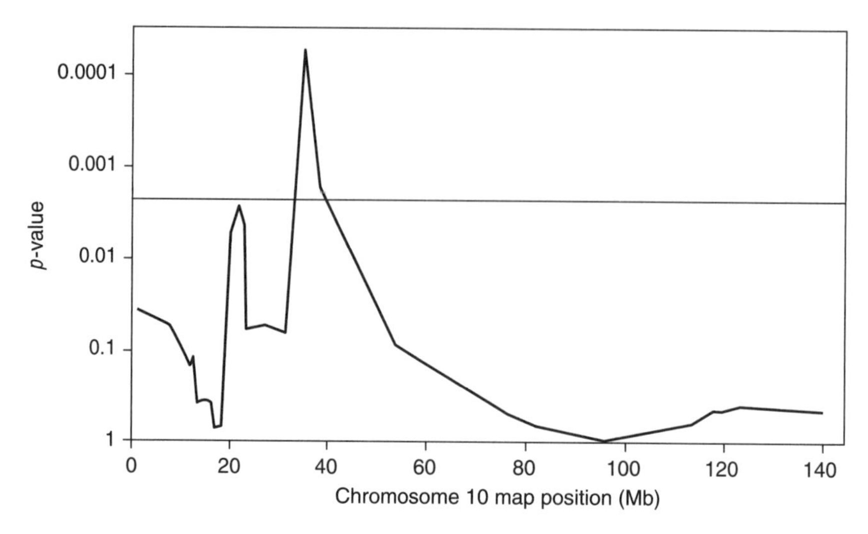

Figure 5.8 A quantitative trait locus for submaximal exercise (50 W) stroke volume training response on chromosome 10 in the HERITAGE Family Study. *p*-values from the regression-based multipoint linkage analysis are presented on the *y*-axis, and chromosomal location derived from the Location Database are presented on the *x*-axis. The reference line indicates the criteria for promising linkage ($p < 0.0023$). (For further details, *see* reference Rankinen et al., 2002.)

phenotypes have been published (Bouchard et al., 2000; Chagnon et al., 2001; Rankinen et al., 2002; Rankinen et al., 2001; Rice et al., 2002; Rice et al., 2002).

Figure 5.8 provides an example of a QTL for endurance training-induced changes in submaximal exercise stroke volume on chromosome 10. The QTL covers approximately 15 million basepairs in the short arm of chromosome 10 (10p11.2) and the maximum linkage (Logarithm of Odds (LOD) = 1.96) was detected with a microsatellite marker, D10S1666 (Rankinen et al., 2002). Promising linkages were also found on chromosome 8q24.3 for submaximal exercise SBP training response and on 10q23–q24 for SBP measured during submaximal exercise at 80% of VO_{2max} (Rankinen et al., 2001). In addition, promising evidence of linkage was reported for training-induced changes in fat mass and percent body fat on chromosomes 1q31.1, 11q13.4–q21 and 18q21–q23, and for BMI and fat-free mass training responses on 5q21.1 and 12q23.2, respectively (Chagnon et al., 2001).

Personal Perspectives

The data reviewed herein suggest a number of thoughts regarding research on physical activity-related traits in epidemiological studies. First, it is fair to conclude that a sedentary lifestyle has negative consequences on risk factors for a number of chronic diseases, a variety of health outcomes, and longevity (Rankinen and Bouchard, 2007). The same observations have been made for a low level of cardiorespiratory fitness. In contrast, moderate to high levels of physical activity or fitness are associated with a more favorable risk profile and reduced risks for morbidities and premature death.

However, although these findings are based on mean effects, the importance of individual differences is suggested by the data of almost all studies but is seldom addressed. This has led to overly pessimistic interpretations of the consequences of a sedentary mode of life but is equally important to overinterpretation of the data supporting the notion that physical activity has favorable influences on health outcomes. As a result of the completion of the HERITAGE Family Study, it is clear that there is considerable human heterogeneity in responsiveness to regular exercise despite the fact that all participants were exposed to the same volume of exercise adjusted for their own tolerance level.

Thus, more than 20 years after we introduced the concept of human heterogeneity in responsiveness to standardized exercise programs, we have conclusive evidence that this phenomenon is pervasive. It is present in men and women, in young adults and middle-aged people, and in African-Americans and Caucasians. This heterogeneity in the ability to benefit from a physically active lifestyle is well beyond measurement errors and normal day-to-day variation in the traits considered. Another unique contribution of the HERITAGE Family Study has been to show conclusively that for relevant response phenotypes adjusted for age, gender, and ethnic background, there is familial aggregation such that low responders tend to cluster in some families, whereas high responders aggregate in others. This pattern suggests a contribution of genetic factors to the individual differences in response to regular exercise. Genetic epidemiology and molecular genetic studies performed on the HERITAGE Family Study cohort have indeed demonstrated that it was the case. Some of this evidence has been reviewed in this chapter. One extremely important observation is that the low responders for one response trait are not necessarily low responders for other traits. The underlying biology for this complex phenomenon remains to be described.

We now believe that there are compelling reasons for epidemiologists to account for individual differences in their models and incorporate genetic information in studies designed to understand the relationships between physical activity or fitness traits and health or disease traits. Family-based designs would often be more powerful and epidemiologists should use such designs more frequently. The statistical models are obviously more complex, but they offer an opportunity to account for the effects of family lines and maternal or paternal effects as well as for the testing of hypotheses about genetic effects and segregation patterns. It would also be desirable to go one step further and to incorporate candidate genes and DNA sequence variants in studies on the epidemiology of physical activity traits. The availability of cost-effective high throughput genotyping technologies makes this possible with little DNA material.

Although the research on molecular genetics of physical activity, health-related fitness, and health-related outcomes is still in its infancy, we need to recognize early that some alleles at key genes are likely to play an important role in the ability to benefit from regular exercise. The sooner we incorporate this advance in our thinking and move in the direction of fully integrated molecular epidemiology research, the sooner we will be able to understand the true relation between a sedentary lifestyle or poor fitness and the risk of disease. Moving along this path will provide some of the building blocks that are necessary to bring us eventually to the era of individualized, and hopefully more efficacious, public health recommendations and preventive medicine measures.

References

Aarnio M, Winter T, Kujala UM, Kaprio J. 1997. Familial aggregation of leisure-time physical activity—a three generation study. *Int J Sports Med* 18: 549–56.

Akaike H. 1974. A new look at the statistical model identification. *IEEE Trans Automat Control* 19: 716–23.

Alvarez R, Terrados N, Ortolano R, et al. 2000. Genetic variation in the renin-angiotensin system and athletic performance. *Eur J Applied Physiol* 82: 117–20.

An P, Perusse L, Rankinen T, et al. 2003. Familial Aggregation of Exercise Heart Rate and Blood Pressure in Response to 20 Weeks of Endurance Training: The HERITAGE Family Study. *Int J Sports Med* 24: 57–62.

An P, Rice T, Gagnon J, et al. 2000. Familial Aggregation of Stroke Volume and Cardiac Output During Submaximal Exercise: The HERITAGE Family Study. *Int J Sports Med* 21: 566–72.

An P, Rice T, Perusse L, et al. 2000. Complex segregation analysis of blood pressure and heart rate measured before and after a 20-week endurance exercise training program: The HERITAGE Family Study. *Am J Hypertens* 13: 488–97.

Beunen G, Thomis M. 1999. Genetic determinants of sports participation and daily physical activity. *Int J Obes Relat Metab Disord* 23 (Suppl 3): S55–63.

Boerwinkle E, Hixson JE, Hanis CL. 2000. Peeking under the peaks: following Up genome-wide linkage analyses. *Circulation* 102: 1877–8.

Bouchard C. 1983. Human adaptability may have a genetic basis. In F Landry, (Ed.), *Risk reduction and health promotion. Proceedings of the 18th annual meeting of the Society of Prospective Medicine*, Ottawa: Canadian Public Health Association, pp. 463–76.

Bouchard C. 1995. Individual differences in the response to regular exercise. *Int J Obes Relat Metab Disord* 19: S5–8.

Bouchard C. 2001. Physical activity and health: introduction to the dose-response symposium. *Med Sci Sports Exerc* 33: S347–50.

Bouchard C, An P, Rice T, et al. 1999. Familial aggregation of VO_{2max} response to exercise training: results from the HERITAGE Family Study. *J Applied Physiol* 87: 1003–8.

Bouchard C, Blair SN. 1999. Introductory comments for the consensus on physical activity and obesity. *Med Sci Sports Exerc* 31: S498–501.

Bouchard C, Daw EW, Rice T, et al. 1998. Familial resemblance for VO_{2max} in the sedentary state: the HERITAGE family study. *Med Sci Sports Exerc* 30: 252–8.

Bouchard C, Dionne FT, Simoneau JA, Boulay MR. 1992. Genetics of aerobic and anaerobic performances. *Exerc Sport Sci Rev* 20: 27–58.

Bouchard C, Leon AS, Rao DC, Skinner JS, Wilmore JH, Gagnon J. 1995. The HERITAGE family study. Aims, design, and measurement protocol. *Med Sci Sports Exerc* 27: 721–9.

Bouchard C, Lesage R, Lortie G, et al. 1986. Aerobic performance in brothers, dizygotic and monozygotic twins. *Med Sci Sports Exerc* 18: 639–46.

Bouchard C, Rankinen T. 2001. Individual Differences in Response to Regular Physical Activity. *Med Sci Sports Exerc* 33: S446-S51.

Bouchard C, Rankinen T, Chagnon YC, et al. 2000. Genomic scan for maximal oxygen uptake and its response to training in the HERITAGE Family Study. *J Applied Physiol* 88: 551–9.

Bouchard C, Tremblay A, Despres JP, et al. 1990. The response to long-term overfeeding in identical twins. *N Engl J Med* 322: 1477–82.

Bouchard C, Tremblay A, Despres JP, et al. 1994. The response to exercise with constant energy intake in identical twins. *Obes Res* 2: 400–10.

Cardon LR, Fulker DW, Joreskog KG. 1991. A LISREL 8 model with constrained parameters for twin and adoptive families. *Behav Genet* 21: 327–50.

Cardon LR, Palmer LJ. 2003. Population stratification and spurious allelic association. *Lancet* 361: 598–604.

Cartegni L, Chew SL, Krainer AR. 2002. Listening to silence and understanding nonsense: exonic mutations that affect splicing. *Nat Rev Genet* 3: 285–98.

Chagnon YC, Rice T, Perusse L, et al. 2001. Genomic scan for genes affecting body composition before and after training in Caucasians from HERITAGE. *J Applied Physiol* 90: 1777–87.

Conne B, Stutz A, Vassalli JD. 2000. The 3′ untranslated region of messenger RNA: A molecular 'hotspot' for pathology? *Nat Med* 6: 637–41.

Fagard R, Bielen E, Amery A. 1991. Heritability of aerobic power and anaerobic energy generation during exercise. *J Applied Physiol* 70: 357–62.

Folland J, Leach B, Little T, et al. 2000. Angiotensin-converting enzyme genotype affects the response of human skeletal muscle to functional overload. *Exp Physiol* 85: 575–9.

Gainetdinov RR, Wetsel WC, Jones SR, Levin ED, Jaber M, Caron MG. 1999. Role of serotonin in the paradoxical calming effect of psychostimulants on hyperactivity. *Science* 283: 397–401.

Gayagay G, Yu B, Hambly B, et al. 1998. Elite endurance athletes and the ACE I allele—the role of genes in athletic performance. *Human Genetics* 103: 48–50.

Gu C, Rao DC. 1997. A linkage strategy for detection of human quantitative-trait loci. I. Generalized relative risk ratios and power of sib pairs with extreme trait values. *Am J Hum Genet* 61: 200–10.

Hagberg JM, Ferrell RE, McCole SD, Wilund KR, Moore GE. 1998. V02 max is associated with ACE genotype in postmenopausal women. *J Applied Physiol* 85: 1842–6.

Hautala AJ, Makikallio TH, Kiviniemi A, et al. 2003. Cardiovascular autonomic function correlates with the response to aerobic training in healthy sedentary subjects. *Am J Physiol Heart Circ Physiol* 285: H1747–52.

Hokanson JE, Kamboh MI, Scarboro S, Eckel RH, Hamman RF. 2003. Effects of the hepatic lipase gene and physical activity on coronary heart disease risk. *Am J Epidemiol* 158: 836–43.

Kaprio J, Koskenvuo M, Sarna S. 1981. Cigarette smoking, use of alcohol, and leisure-time physical activity among same-sexed adult male twins. *Prog Clin Biol Res* 69: 37–46.

Katzmarzyk PT, Perusse L, Rao DC, Bouchard C. 2000. Familial risk ratios for high and low physical fitness levels in the Canadian population. *Med Sci Sports Exerc* 32: 614–9.

Kelly MA, Rubinstein M, Phillips TJ, et al. 1998. Locomotor activity in D2 dopamine receptor-deficient mice is determined by gene dosage, genetic background, and developmental adaptations. *J Neurosci* 18: 3470–9.

King MC, Marks JH, Mandell JB. 2003. Breast and ovarian cancer risks due to inherited mutations in BRCA1 and BRCA2. *Science* 302: 643–6.

Kohrt WM, Malley MT, Coggan AR, et al. 1991. Effects of gender, age, and fitness level on response of V02max to training in 60–71 yr olds. *J Appl Physiol* 71: 2004–11.

Koopmans JR, Van Doornen LJP, Boomsma DI. 1994. Smoking and sports participation. In U Godlbourt, U De Faire, K Berge (Eds.), *Genetic factors in coronary heart disease*. Lancaster: Kluwer Academic, pp. 217–35.

Laitinen PJ, Brown KM, Piippo K, et al. 2001. Mutations of the cardiac ryanodine receptor (RyR2) gene in familial polymorphic ventricular tachycardia. *Circulation* 103: 485–90.

Lauderdale DS, Fabsitz R, Meyer JM, Sholinsky P, Ramakrishnan V, Goldberg J. 1997. Familial determinants of moderate and intense physical activity: a twin study. *Med Sci Sports Exerc* 29: 1062–8.

Leon A, (Ed.) 1997. *Physical activity and cardiovascular health: a national consensus*. Champaign, IL: Human Kinetics Publishers.

Leon AS, Rice T, Mandel S, et al. 2000. Blood lipid response to 20 weeks of supervised exercise in a large biracial population: the HERITAGE Family Study. *Metabolism* 49: 513–20.

Lortie G, Simoneau JA, Hamel P, Boulay MR, Landry F, Bouchard C. 1984. Responses of maximal aerobic power and capacity to aerobic training. *Int J Sports Med* 5: 232–6.

Maia JA, Thomis M, Beunen G. 2002. Genetic factors in physical activity levels. A twin study. *Am J Prev Med* 23: 87–91.

McGue M, Hirsch B, Lykken DT. 1993. Age and the self-perception of ability: a twin study analysis. *Psychol Aging* 8: 72–80.

McGuire S, Neiderhiser JM, Reiss D, Hetherington EM, Plomin R. 1994. Genetic and environmental influences on perceptions of self-worth and competence in adolescence: a study of twins, full siblings, and step- siblings. *Child Dev* 65: 785–99.

Montgomery HE, Clarkson P, Dollery CM, et al. 1997. Association of angiotensin-converting enzyme gene I/D polymorphism with change in left ventricular mass in response to physical training. *Circulation* 96: 741–7.

Montgomery HE, Marshall R, Hemingway H, et al. 1998. Human gene for physical performance. *Nature* 393: 221–2.

Myerson S, Hemingway H, Budget R, Martin J, Humphries S, Montgomery H. 1999. Human angiotensin I-converting enzyme gene and endurance performance. *J Applied Physiol* 87: 1313–6.

Myerson SG, Montgomery HE, Whittingham M, et al. 2001. Left Ventricular Hypertrophy With Exercise and ACE Gene Insertion/Deletion Polymorphism: A Randomized Controlled Trial With Losartan. *Circulation* 103: 226–30.

Neale MC, Boker SM, Xie G, Maes HH. 2003. *Mx: Statistical Modeling*. Richmond, VA: Virginia Commonwealth University, Department of Psychiatry.

NIH. 1996. Physical activity and cardiovascular health. NIH Consensus Development Panel on Physical Activity and Cardiovascular Health. *JAMA* 276: 241–6.

Osborne KA, Robichon A, Burgess E, et al. 1997. Natural behavior polymorphism due to a cGMP-dependent protein kinase of Drosophila. *Science* 277: 834–6.

Perusse L, Gagnon J, Province MA, et al. 2001. Familial aggregation of submaximal aerobic performance in the HERITAGE Family study. *Med Sci Sports Exerc* 33: 597–604.

Perusse L, Rankinen T, Zuberi A, et al. 2005. The human obesity gene map: the 2004 update. *Obes Res* 13: 381–490.

Perusse L, Rice T, Province MA, et al. 2000. Familial aggregation of amount and distribution of subcutaneous fat and their responses to exercise training in the HERITAGE family study. *Obes Res* 8: 140–50.

Rankinen T, An P, Perusse L, et al. 2002. Genome-Wide Linkage Scan for Exercise Stroke Volume and Cardiac Output in the HERITAGE Family Study. *Physiol Genom* 10: 57–62.

Rankinen T, An P, Rice T,, et al. 2001. Genomic scan for exercise blood pressure in the Health, Risk Factors, Exercise Training and Genetics (HERITAGE) Family Study. *Hypertension* 38: 30–7.

Rankinen T, Bouchard C. 2005. Genes, Genetic Heterogeneity, and Exercise Phenotypes. In FC Mooren, K Volker (Ed.), *Molecular and Cellular Exercise Physiology*. Champaign, IL: Human Kinetics, pp. 39–54.

Rankinen T, Bouchard C. 2007. Invited commentary: Physical activity, mortality, and genetics. *Am J Epidemiol* 166: 260–2.

Rankinen T, Bray MS, Hagberg JM, et al. 2006. The human gene map for performance and health-related fitness phenotypes: the 2005 update. *Med Sci Sports Exerc* 38: 1863–88.

Rankinen T, Gagnon J, Perusse L, et al. 2000. AGT M235T and ACE ID polymorphisms and exercise blood pressure in the HERITAGE Family Study. *American J Physiol: Heart Circulatory Physiol* 279: H368–74.

Rankinen T, Perusse L, Gagnon J, et al. 2000. Angiotensin-converting enzyme I/D polymorphism and trainability of the fitness phenotypes. The HERITAGE Family Study. *J Applied Physiol* 88: 1029–35.

Rankinen T, Perusse L, Rauramaa R, Rivera MA, Wolfarth B, Bouchard C. 2001. The human gene map for performance and health-related fitness phenotypes. *Med Sci Sports Exerc* 33: 855–67.

Rankinen T, Wolfarth B, Simoneau JA, et al. 2000. No association between the angiotensin-converting enzyme ID polymorphism and elite endurance athlete status. *J Applied Physiol* 88: 1571–5.

Rankinen T, Zuberi A, Chagnon YC, et al. 2006b. The human obesity gene map: the 2005 update. *Obesity (Silver Spring)* 14: 529–644.

Rauramaa R, Kuhanen R, Lakka TA, et al. 2002. Physical exercise and blood pressure with reference to the angiotensinogen M235T polymorphism. *Physiol Genom* 10: 71–7.

Rice T, An P, Gagnon J, et al. 2002. Heritability of HR and BP response to exercise training in the HERITAGE Family Study. *Med Sci Sports Exerc* 34: 972–9.

Rice T, Chagnon YC, Perusse L, et al. 2002. A genomewide linkage scan for abdominal subcutaneous and visceral fat in black and white families: The HERITAGE Family Study. *Diabetes* 51: 848–55.

Rice T, Despres JP, Perusse L, et al. 2002. Familial aggregation of blood lipid response to exercise training in the health, risk factors, exercise training, and genetics (HERITAGE) Family Study. *Circulation* 105: 1904–8.

Rice T, Hong Y, Perusse L, et al. 1999. Total body fat and abdominal visceral fat response to exercise training in the HERITAGE Family Study: evidence for major locus but no multifactorial effects. *Metabolism* 48: 1278–86.

Rice T, Rankinen T, Chagnon YC, et al. 2002. Genomewide linkage scan of resting blood pressure: HERITAGE Family Study. Health, Risk Factors, Exercise Training, and Genetics. *Hypertension* 39: 1037–43.

Rigat B, Hubert C, Alhenc-Gelas F, Cambien F, Corvol P, Soubrier F. 1990. An insertion/deletion polymorphism in the angiotensin I-converting enzyme gene accounting for half the variance of serum enzyme levels. *J Clin Invest* 86: 1343–6.

Risch N. 1990. Linkage strategies for genetically complex traits. I. Multilocus models. *Am J Hum Genet* 46: 222–8.

Shephard RJ, Rankinen T, Bouchard C. 2004. Test-retest errors and the apparent heterogeneity of training response. *Eur J Appl Physiol* 91: 199–203.

Simoneau JA, Lortie G, Boulay MR, Marcotte M, Thibault MC, Bouchard C. 1986. Inheritance of human skeletal muscle and anaerobic capacity adaptation to high-intensity intermittent training. *Int J Sports Med* 7: 167–71.

Simonen RL, Rankinen T, Perusse L, et al. 2003. A dopamine D2 receptor gene polymorphism and physical activity in two family studies. *Physiol Behav* 78: 751–7.

Simonen RL, Rankinen T, Perusse L, et al. 2003. Genome-wide linkage scan for physical activity levels in the Quebec Family study. *Med Sci Sports Exerc* 35: 1355–9.

Skinner JS, Wilmore KM, Krasnoff JB, et al. 2000. Adaptation to a standardized training program and changes in fitness in a large, heterogeneous population: the HERITAGE Family Study. *Med Sci Sports Exerc* 32: 157–61.

Sonna LA, Sharp MA, Knapik JJ, et al. 2001. Angiotensin-converting enzyme genotype and physical performance during US Army basic training. *J Applied Physiol* 91: 1355–63.

Stefan N, Vozarova B, Del Parigi A, et al. 2002. The Gln223Arg polymorphism of the leptin receptor in Pima Indians: influence on energy expenditure, physical activity and lipid metabolism. *Int J Obes Relat Metab Disord* 26: 1629–32.

Sundet JM, Magnus P, Tambs K. 1994. The heritability of maximal aerobic power: a study of Norwegian twins. *Scand J Med Sci Sports* 4: 181–5.

Swan H, Piippo K, Viitasalo M, et al. 1999. Arrhythmic disorder mapped to chromosome 1q42-q43 causes malignant polymorphic ventricular tachycardia in structurally normal hearts. *J Am Coll Cardiol* 34: 2035–42.

Taylor RR, Mamotte CD, Fallon K, van Bockxmeer FM. 1999. Elite athletes and the gene for angiotensin-converting enzyme. *J Applied Physiol* 87: 1035–7.

US Department of Health and Human Services. 1996. *Physical Activity and Health: A Report of the Surgeon General*. Atlanta, GA: US Dept of Health and Human Services, Centers for Disease Control and Prevention, National Center for Chronic Disease Prevention and Health Promotion.

Wang Q, Curran ME, Splawski I, et al. 1996. Positional cloning of a novel potassium channel gene: KVLQT1 mutations cause cardiac arrhythmias. *Nature Genetics* 12: 17–23.

Williams AG, Rayson MP, Jubb M, et al. 2000. The ACE gene and muscle performance. *Nature* 403: 614.

Wilmore JH, Stanforth PR, Gagnon J, et al. 2001. Heart rate and blood pressure changes with endurance training: The HERITAGE Family Study. *Med Sci Sports Exerc* 33: 107–16.

Winnicki M, Accurso V, Hoffmann M, et al. 2004. Physical activity and angiotensin-converting enzyme gene polymorphism in mild hypertensives. *Am J Med Genet A* 125: 38–44.

Woods D, Hickman M, Jamshidi Y, et al. 2001. Elite swimmers and the D allele of the ACE I/D polymorphism. *Human Genetics* 108: 230–2.

Woods DR, World M, Rayson MP, et al. 2002. Endurance enhancement related to the human angiotensin I-converting enzyme I-D polymorphism is not due to differences in the cardiorespiratory response to training. *Eur J Applied Physiol* 86: 240–4.

6

Design of Present-Day Epidemiologic Studies of Physical Activity and Health

I-Min Lee and
Ralph S. Paffenbarger Jr.

Over the span of more than a half-century, beginning with the pioneering investigations by Professor Jeremy Morris (*see* Chapter 1), many epidemiologic studies have contributed to the large body of evidence we have today on the benefits of physical activity for health (which outweigh, by a large margin, some well-documented adverse effects, including those discussed in Chapters 13 and 14). Although it is impossible to reference all epidemiologic studies describing the health benefits of physical activity in this textbook, numerous examples of the studies have been cited in the different chapters. The aim of this chapter is primarily to provide an in-depth discussion of two large, present-day prospective cohort studies—one in men (the Harvard Alumni Health Study) and one in women (the Nurses' Health Study)—that have published several important findings related to physical activity and health. These two studies will be used as exemplars to illustrate important principles in the design, conduct, and analyses of data from epidemiologic studies investigating physical activity as a predictor of health outcomes. This chapter also goes on to discuss, more briefly, other selected ongoing, prospective cohort studies to provide additional illustrations of several of the main principles. As a further resource for investigators interested in designing physical activity questionnaires, we refer the reader to a journal supplement that describes physical activity questionnaires used by epidemiologic studies with findings published in 1995 or earlier, which documents the reliability and validity of each questionnaire for measuring physical activity (Kriska and Caspersen, 1997).

The Harvard Alumni Health Study

Design and Rationale

The Harvard Alumni Health Study, established by Professor Ralph Paffenbarger Jr., was initiated in the early 1960s to investigate predictors of coronary heart disease (CHD) incidence and mortality, with physical inactivity as a risk factor of particular interest. At that time, the studies of Morris et al. (*see* Chapter 1) indicated that men with higher levels of *occupational* physical activity suffered less CHD and less severe disease when it occurred (Morris et al., 1953). However, occupational physical activity was on the wane even then, with increasingly fewer individuals engaging in hard physical labor on the job. Professor Paffenbarger was interested in whether *leisure-time* physical activity also was associated with the same risk reduction for CHD as occupational activity.

After initial explorations, Professor Paffenbarger decided on college alumni as an appropriate group of subjects for a prospective cohort study of the predictors of CHD risk. In particular, Harvard University alumni were deemed ideal for several reasons. First, investigators hoped to establish a prospective study in which subjects could be followed for many years, with minimal losses to follow-up to avoid biased results. Preliminary work in the 1950s had indicated that the alumni office at Harvard University kept careful records on the whereabouts of students who had graduated (subsequent research in recent years has shown this to continue to hold true; Lee et al., 2000). Second, to conduct a large study at low cost, investigators wanted to collect information by mail and surmised that Harvard alumni would be well-educated and interested regarding health matters, thereby being able to provide accurate health information on mailed questionnaires. Validation studies subsequently conducted (e.g., comparing alumni self-reports of chronic diseases with physicians' records) have proved this assumption correct. Third, available in the Harvard University archives were data from a standardized medical anamnesis and physical examination that students were obliged to undergo when they entered the university, 12 to 46 years prior to the initiation of the prospective cohort study. This allowed for a retrospective component to the study, affording investigators the opportunity to explore host and environmental data, recorded years in advance of the clinical onset of CHD, as predictors of disease. Thus, the Harvard Alumni Health Study can be considered a "bidirectional" study, with retrospective and prospective components.

Subjects in this study comprise men who matriculated at Harvard University as undergraduates between 1916 and 1950 (no women were admitted then). Data from the medical examination at university entry are available for approximately 33,000 men; the first health questionnaire was mailed to surviving alumni of the relevant classes in either 1962 or 1966, and approximately 22,000 men responded.

A criticism that has been directed at this study, as well as the Nurses' Health Study described later, is that subjects are not representative of the general population. This is certainly true; however, although the select group of participants may limit the generalizability of findings, it does not invalidate them. That is, the observations regarding physical activity and decreased risk of many chronic diseases are valid within the study and also valid for similar populations. Extending the findings to other population groups—although biologically plausible—would ideally be supported by empirical observations in these other groups. When the study was initiated, the choice of Harvard alumni, as described earlier, was based on practical considerations—particularly the need for high rates of follow-up to ensure the validity of results.

Assessment of Physical Activity

Because Harvard alumni are likely to hold white-collar occupations with little physical activity on the job, investigators were interested in collecting information primarily on leisure-time physical activities (including sports and recreational activities), as well as walking and stair-climbing that occurred on-the-job or in the course of commuting. Figure 6.1 shows the Harvard Alumni Health Study physical activity questionnaire, sometimes called the "Paffenbarger survey (or questionnaire)." Additionally, it has been referred to as the College Alumni Health Study physical activity questionnaire because Professor Paffenbarger also initiated a similar prospective cohort study among alumni from the University of Pennsylvania using the same questionnaire (Helmrich et al., 1991; Sesso et al., 1998). The questionnaire asks about alumnus' usual pattern of stair-climbing and walking and also asks participants to list the sports and recreational activities performed during the past week, as well as their frequency and duration.

1. How many flights of stairs do you usually climb up each day? __________
   (Let 1 flight = 10 steps)

2. How many city blocks or their equivalent do you regularly walk each day? __________
   (Let 12 blocks = 1 mile)

3. List any sports or recreation you have participated in during the past week. Please include only the time you were physically active (i.e., actual playing time in jogging, bicycling, swimming, brisk walking, gardening, carpentry, calisthenics, etc.)

Sport, recreation, or other physical activity	Number of times in week	Average time per episode	
		Hours	Minutes
1.			
2.			
3.			
4.			
5.			

(Additional examples of physical activity questionnaires used by epidemiologic studies, with documentation of their reliability and validity, can be found in Kriska & Caspersen 1997.)

Figure 6.1 Harvard Alumni Health Study Physical Activity Questionnaire.

To estimate the energy expended on physical activities, we sum the energy expended on walking, stair-climbing, and participation in sports and recreational activities. Walking one block daily rates 56 kilocalories per week (kcal/week); climbing up and down one flight of stairs daily burns 14 kcal/week (Bassett et al., 1997). The energy expended on each sport or recreation is estimated by considering its energy cost (Ainsworth et al., 1993a) and the frequency and duration of participation over the past week. To estimate total energy expenditure, we then sum kilocalories per week from walking, stair-climbing, and all sports and recreational activities. (Further discussion of our preference to use kilocalories per week, rather than another measure of energy expenditure such as metabolic equivalent [MET]-hours per week, as well as the advantages and disadvantages, is provided in Chapter 4.)

Reliability and Validity of Physical Activity Assessment

The reliability and validity properties of the Harvard Alumni Health Study physical activity questionnaire have been extensively investigated; these studies are summarized in Table 6.1. With regard to reliability, investigators have noted reliability to be higher over the short term than the long term. Test-retest correlation coefficients on the order of 0.7 to 0.8 have been observed over 4 weeks (Ainsworth et al., 1993b) compared to 0.4 to 0.5 over 8 months to 1 year (Jacobs et al., 1993). The lower reliability over longer periods of time is likely to result partly from true changes in physical activity. In a study that examined test-retest correlation coefficients over a 7- to 12-week period, participants who reported that their activity had remained unchanged showed higher coefficients compared to all participants in the study (Washburn et al., 1991). Additionally, in another study of postmenopausal women, whose physical activity patterns might have been more stable over time than in younger participants, a test-retest correlation of better than 0.7 was observed over 1 year (LaPorte et al., 1983). With regard to any differences between men and women, there have not been large differences noted in reliability for total energy expenditure (i.e., energy expended on walking, climbing stairs, and participation in sport/recreational activities). However, for sports and recreational activities, reliability appears to be better among men (Ainsworth et al., 1993b); this may result partly from greater participation in such activities by men than women.

Table 6.1 Harvard Alumni Health Study Physical Activity Questionnaire: Reliability and Validity Studies

Reference	*Subjects*	*Methods of comparison*	*Main results*
Reliability studies			
LaPorte et al., 1983	59 postmenopausal women	Test–retest over 1 year	Correlation coefficient: stairs = 0.54* walking = 0.42* total activity = 0.73*
Cauley et al., 1987	14 postmenopausal women	Test–retest over 4 weeks	Correlation coefficient: stairs = 0.89* walking = 0.97* total activity = 0.76*
Washburn et al., 1991	633 men and women, 25–65 years	Test–retest over 7–12 weeks	Correlation coefficient: all = 0.58* those reporting unchanged activity over this period (n = 264) = 0.69*
Rauh et al., 1992	45 Latino men and women, 18–55 years	Test–retest over 2 weeks	Correlation coefficient: stairs = 0.68* walking = 0.23 sports/recreation = 0.67* total activity = 0.34*
Ainsworth et al., 1993b	28 men and 50 women, 21–59 years	Test–retest over 1, 7, and 8 months	Correlation coefficient for total activity: 1 month = 0.72* 7 months = 0.34* 8 months = 0.43*
Jacobs et al., 1993	103 men and women, 20–59 years	Test-retest over 1 and 12 months	Correlation coefficient for total activity: 1 month = 0.72* 12 months = 0.50*
Validity studies			
Siconolfi et al., 1985	36 men and 32 women, 20–70 years	VO_{2max}	Correlation coefficient: overall = 0.29* men = 0.26 women = 0.08
Cauley et al., 1987	255 postmenopausal women	Large-scale integrated activity monitor	Correlation coefficient: daytime activity = 0.95–0.97* evening activity = 0.70–0.72*
Albanes et al., 1990	21 men, 28–55 years	Measured energy intake over 10 weeks (men were weight stable)	Spearman r = 0.49 (no significance level provided)
Washburn et al., 1991	732 men and women, 25–65 years	HDL cholesterol, BMI	Correlation coefficient: HDL cholesterol = 0.18* (men); 0.23* (women) BMI = –0.11 (men); –0.17* (women)

Continued

Table 6.1 Harvard Alumni Health Study Physical Activity Questionnaire: Reliability and Validity Studies (*Continued*)

Rauh et al., 1992	45 Latino men and women, 18–55 years	Accelerometer	Correlation coefficient = 0.34*
Ainsworth et al., 1993b	28 men and 50 women, 21–59 years	Physical activity records, VO_2 peak, % body fat	Correlation coefficient: records, men = 0.65* records, women = 0.54* VO_2 peak, men = 0.58* VO_2 peak, women = 0.53* % body fat, men = –0.36 % body fat, women = –0.36*
Jacobs et al., 1993	103 men and women, 20–59 years	14 four-week physical activity histories, accelerometer, VO_{2max}, % body fat	Spearman's *r*: 4-week activity histories = 0.31* accelerometer = 0.30* VO_{2max} = 0.52* % body fat = –0.30*
Bassett et al., 2000	48 men and 48 women, 25–70 years	Pedometer	Spearman's *r* for walking: men = 0.35* women = 0.48*
Bonnefoy et al., 2001	19 men, 66–82 years	VO_{2max}, DLW	Spearman's *r*, comparing: sports/recreation and VO_{2max} = 0.42 all activities and VO_{2max} = 0.17 sports/recreation and DLW = 0.67* all activities and DLW = 0.37
Strath et al., 2004	12 men and 13 women, 20–56 years (8% African-American)	Simultaneous heart-rate motion sensor	Spearman's *r*: light = 0.29 (men), 0.10 (women) moderate = 0.26 (men), 0.29 (women) vigorous = 0.42* (men), 0.59* (women) all = 0.34 (men), 0.36 (women)

Abbreviations: BMI: body mass index; DLW: doubly labeled water.
*$p < 0.05$

Validation studies of the Harvard Alumni Health Study physical activity questionnaire (Table 6.1) have mostly been conducted in subjects ages 20 to 70 years, with one study focusing on subjects older than age 65 years (Bonnefoy et al., 2001). Subjects primarily have been Caucasian, although studies have also been conducted in African-Americans (Strath et al., 2004) and Latinos (Rauh et al., 1992). Comparison methods used to assess validity have included physical activity records or histories, physiologic measures influenced by physical activity (e.g., VO_2 max, a measure of physical fitness; high-density lipoprotein [HDL] cholesterol; body fat), measured energy intake in the face of constant weight, mechanical or electronic devices that measure movement (e.g., pedometers, accelerometers), and doubly labeled water (DLW; Table 6.1). When comparing physical activity assessed by questionnaire against physical activity records or histories, correlation coefficients on the order of 0.5 to 0.6 have been obtained. Against physiologic measures, the magnitude of the coefficients have been lower (0.3 to 0.5), which is expected because other factors (besides physical activity, such as diet for HDL cholesterol or body fat) also influence these measures. With regard to comparisons against measured energy intake (when weight is constant), mechanical/electronic devices measuring movement, and DLW, correlation coefficients on the order of 0.4 to 0.5 have been reported. Notably, there is a good correlation coefficient of 0.67 observed between questionnaire-estimated energy expended on sports/recreational activities and DLW-estimated energy expenditure, considered a "gold standard" measure (Bonnefoy et al., 2001). On the whole, no large differences in validity have been noted between men and women; however, validity for high-intensity activities and sports generally has been noted to be superior to that for moderate- or light-intensity activities (Ainsworth et al., 1993b; Bonnefoy et al., 2001).

It is important to note that the correlation coefficients obtained from the validity studies in Table 6.1 assess *ranking* order, without regard to the absolute value of the parameter assessed. That is, when a high correlation coefficient is observed in Table 6.1, this indicates that the ranking of participants (e.g., from low to high), as assessed by the Harvard Alumni Health Study physical activity questionnaire, compares well with the ranking when using a validation standard (e.g., accelerometers). It does not necessarily indicate that the absolute value of the energy expended in physical activity, assessed by questionnaire, compares well with the absolute value as assessed by the validation standard. For example, if the questionnaire were to consistently overestimate energy expenditure by 500 kcal/week—a large amount—in every participant, the value of the correlation coefficient would still be a perfect 1.0.

The Harvard Alumni Health Study questionnaire appears to underestimate the actual amount of energy expended in *all* physical activity. This is not surprising, because the questionnaire was designed to assess only leisure-time physical activity and walking and stair-climbing rather than all energy expended (such as on activities of daily living, including grooming, self-care, etc.). In a study of 19 healthy, older men ages 66 to 82 years, investigators assessed total energy expenditure using DLW and resting energy expenditure using indirect calorimetry (Bonnefoy et al., 2001). Investigators then estimated the energy expended on *all* physical activity by subtracting resting energy expenditure from total energy expenditure. On average, this was 802 (standard deviation: 462) kcal/day, compared to the Harvard Alumni Health Study questionnaire estimate of 716 kcal/day expended on physical activity (this excluded three men who reported unusually high levels of activity during the period of DLW assessment). Again, this "underestimate" by the questionnaire is expected, because the questionnaire was not designed to assess *all* physical activity apart from resting energy expenditure. (As an aside, recent findings from the Harvard Alumni Health Study have been based on older men, in the age range of subjects in the study by Bonnefoy et al. The results from the study by Bonnefoy et al. suggest that the physical activity questionnaire used is a reasonable tool for assessing physical activity among older men.)

In summary, the physical activity questionnaire used in the Harvard Alumni Healthy Study has repeatedly been shown to be reasonably reliable and valid for large epidemiologic studies. Additionally, it has demonstrated face validity, as evidenced by expected associations between physical activity and several health outcomes described later.

Assessment of Health Outcomes

In the Harvard Alumni Health Study, men self-report physician-diagnosed, chronic diseases (e.g., CHD, site-specific cancers, diabetes, etc.) on health surveys that are mailed periodically. In validation studies, the self-reports of these educated subjects have compared well with information obtained from their physicians. For example, confirmation rates of 96% were observed for reported CHD (Lee et al., 2003b) and greater than 90% for various site-specific cancers (Lee et al., 1991; Lee et al., 1992). For mortality follow-up, information obtained from the alumni office regarding alumni who have died is used to request copies of death certificates from state agencies to ascertain the fact and cause(s) of death. In a validation study, we compared our method of ascertaining deaths to the National Death Index, a national compilation of decedents, and found the study method ascertained more than 99% of deceased alumni (Lee et al., 2000).

Early Investigations

When the Harvard Alumni Health Study was started in the early 1960s, investigators were concerned about the rates of CHD—which had been increasing since the beginning of the century (*see* additional discussion in Chapter 1)—but knew little about risk factors for the disease. Initial investigations from the study included assessments of early precursors (i.e., those ascertained during college time) associated with fatal CHD (Paffenbarger et al., 1966) as well as fatal stroke (Paffenbarger and Wing, 1967). Early in the course of the study, physical inactivity was very interesting as a risk factor, with investigators noting inverse associations between activity levels and risk of CHD or stroke death. Specific questions asked by investigators included how much physical activity was needed; 2,000 kcal/week was deemed necessary and associated with about a 40% reduction in risk (Paffenbarger et al., 1978; additionally, investigators did observe age-adjusted rates of heart attack declined steadily from <500 kcal/week to 2,000–2,999 kcal/week, beyond which rates stabilized). Also, investigators questioned what intensity of activity was needed, observing "strenuous" sports but not "light" sports to be associated with risk reduction (Paffenbarger et al., 1978). They also questioned what timing of physical activity was beneficial, noting that "alumni physical activity supplanted student athleticism assessed in college 16–50 years earlier" and that "ex-varsity athletes retained lower risk only if they maintained a high physical activity index as alumni" (Paffenbarger et al., 1978).

Although cardiovascular disease was a major focus of the study in the early years, investigators also examined physical activity in relation to other disease conditions, including suicide (Paffenbarger and Asnes, 1966), diabetes mellitus (Paffenbarger and Wing, 1973), peptic ulcer (Paffenbarger et al., 1974), and Parkinson's disease (Sasco et al., 1992).

Refinement of Early Investigations

By the early 1990s, there was a large body of epidemiologic literature showing that physical activity was associated with lower rates of cardiovascular disease and all-cause mortality. In 1992, the American Heart Association (AHA) formally recognized inactivity as a risk factor for CHD (Fletcher et al., 1992). Investigators in the Harvard Alumni Health Study then turned their attention to clarifying details of the association, including those discussed later.

Intensity of Physical Activity

One specific research question of interest related to the required intensity of physical activity, particularly because evolving public health recommendations in the mid-1990s had started to emphasize the value of moderate-intensity physical activity, in contrast to earlier recommendations that promoted vigorous activities only (Pate et al., 1995). Early investigations in the Harvard Alumni Health Study had noted that "strenuous," but not "light," sporting activity was associated with lower rates of heart attack (Paffenbarger et al., 1978). However, the interpretation of these early findings was limited because of potential confounding by total energy expenditure. That is, higher intensity activities cost more energy than lower intensity ones. Therefore, the observation that strenuous activity was needed to lower the risk of heart attack might simply be reflecting the need for higher *total* energy expenditure to lower risk, not necessarily that only higher intensity activities were associated with lower risk.

To clarify this issue further, investigators adapted analytic methods that had been developed for dietary studies to control for confounding by total energy expenditure, as well as confounding by different kinds of physical activity (for additional discussion, *see* Chapter 4). Subsequent analyses, using multivariate models to simultaneously adjust for activities of different intensity, continued to show that only vigorous (≥6 METs or ≥6 times the resting metabolic rate), but not light- or moderate-intensity (<6 METs), activities were associated with lower CHD rates (Sesso et al., 2000). Additionally, analyses using the "energy decomposition" method also supported the observation that only vigorous, but not non-vigorous, activities were associated with lower all-cause mortality rates during follow-up (Lee et al., 1995). Furthermore, when examining participants who engaged in only vigorous-intensity activities (thereby preventing confounding by non-vigorous activities; i.e., using "restriction" analysis), greater amounts of energy expended in vigorous activities were associated with lower rates of mortality during follow-up. However, when examining participants who engaged in only non-vigorous intensity activities (preventing confounding by vigorous activities), greater amounts of energy expended in non-vigorous activities were not associated with lower mortality rates (Lee et al., 1995).

These observations appear to support the need for higher intensity physical activity to decrease risks of CHD and all-cause mortality, at least in this group of subjects. However, as noted in the aforementioned validation studies, activities of higher intensity and sporting activities reported on the questionnaire show better validity than lower intensity activities. Therefore, the lack of association with lower intensity activities might be a reflection of the lower precision of assessment of these activities on questionnaire. Another explanation, as discussed in detail in Chapter 4, may be related to the nature of the study population—subjects in the Harvard Alumni Health Study represented individuals at the higher end of the physical activity spectrum, such that men in the reference group were those already at a high level of activity, and much larger increases in intensity of physical activity (e.g., vigorous-intensity) may have been needed for further risk reduction. (It is worth noting that other studies conducted among less active individuals, such as women in the Nurses' Health Study discussed later, have shown that moderate-intensity physical activity is associated with lower rates of cardiovascular disease among these individuals.)

Absolute Versus Relative Intensity of Physical Activity

Another research question of interest to the Harvard Alumni Health Study was more detail related to the intensity of physical activity required. Two scales used to define the intensity of physical activity are the absolute scale and the relative scale. On the absolute scale, vigorous physical activity is typically defined as any activity requiring 6 or more METs (≥6 times the resting metabolic rate), and moderate-intensity physical activity is any activity requiring 3 to <6 METs (Pate et al., 1995). For example, a slow jog requires 6 METs and is considered vigorous; brisk walking at 3–4 mph, which requires 4 METs, is typically regarded as a moderate-intensity activity (Ainsworth et al., 1993a). However, as the terminology suggests, the classification is "absolute," with no regard to the physical conditioning (cardiorespiratory fitness) of the individual. Under the absolute scale, a fit, 20-year-old male walking at 3–4 mph is classified as undertaking a moderate-intensity activity, even if this activity were to feel easy to him because of his conditioning. Additionally, on the absolute scale, a 90-year-old woman undertaking the same activity also is regarded as performing a moderate-intensity activity, even if this activity requires a high degree of effort on her part. In contrast, classifying the intensity of activities on the relative scale accounts for the cardiorespira-tory fitness of the individual (Howley, 2001). Thus, for poorly conditioned or older individuals, activities requiring less than 6 METs may indeed be considered vigorous on the relative scale.

In studies of physical activity, intervention studies typically use the relative scale for gaging the intensity of physical activity prescribed (e.g., Church et al., 2007). Subjects are assessed at baseline for their level of cardiorespiratory fitness in the laboratory, and moderate- or vigorous-intensity exercise is prescribed accordingly. However, observational epidemiologic studies almost always use the absolute intensity scale to classify intensity of physical activity. This is partly because of the impracticality of bringing thousands of subjects into the laboratory to assess cardiorespiratory fitness and define relative intensity for each individual.

As individuals age, cardiorespiratory fitness typically declines, such that in older individuals, the absolute scale for measuring intensity may not match well with the actual effort required for carrying out a particular activity (Howley, 2001). Therefore, in the Harvard Alumni Health Study, we were interested in the association between *relative intensity* of physical activity (as contrasted to the investigations described earlier, which examined *absolute intensity*) and risk of developing CHD among older men with mean age of 66 years (Lee et al., 2003b). Men were asked to report their usual perceived level of exertion when exercising using the Borg Scale (i.e., relative intensity). The Borg Scale is commonly used during exercise stress testing, and good correlation exists between ratings on this scale and heart rate, a measure of exertion required by an individual. In multivariate analyses, the relative risks RRs of CHD among men who perceived their exercise exertion as "moderate," "somewhat strong," and "strong" or more intense were 0.86 (95% confidence interval [CI], 0.66–1.13), 0.69 (0.51–0.94), and 0.72 (0.52–1.00), respectively (p-trend = 0.02) compared with those who perceived their exercise exertion as "weak" or less intense. More interesting was the observation that even among men who did not engage in activities requiring 3 METs or more, the inverse association persisted (p-trend = 0.007).

In the 1995 physical activity recommendation from the Centers for Disease Control and the American College of Sports Medicine (CDC/ACSM), moderate-intensity activities of 3 to 6 METs were recommended (Pate et al., 1995). The finding of an inverse relationship between relative intensity and CHD risk from the Harvard Alumni Health Study, even among men with no activities in the 3- to 6-MET range of absolute intensity, suggests that relative intensity is the preferred scale for classifying intensity among older individuals. This was recognized in an update to the 1995 recommendation by ACSM and AHA published in 2007 (Haskell et al., 2007; Nelson et al., 2007). Separate recommendations are now made for adults and for older adults (age ≥65 years), with moderate-intensity physical activity still recommended but accounting for the older adult's level of cardiorespiratory fitness.

Short Versus Long Bouts of Physical Activity

The 1995 CDC/ACSM recommendation allowed for the accumulation of physical activity in short bouts of at least 8 to 10 minutes each to count toward the goal of 30 minutes/day of moderate-intensity physical activity (Pate et al., 1995). Hardly any direct data were available to support the concept of accumulation (for additional discussion, *see* Chapter 4), and none related to the development of clinical outcomes (i.e., data were available only for risk factors). Therefore, to provide information we examined the question of short vs. long bouts of physical activity in relation to CHD risk in the Harvard Alumni Health Study (Lee et al., 2000).

Of particular concern in analyses was separating the *duration* of activity from the *volume* of energy expended—that is, a person who exercises for a longer duration will also expend more energy. The question of interest was not whether longer bouts of activity, which generate higher levels of total energy expenditure, predict lower CHD risk (because this association already had been established); rather, the pertinent research question was: For the same level of total energy expended, does it matter whether this occurs in shorter bouts (and, hence, greater frequency) or longer bouts (and lesser frequency, to result in the same total energy expended)?

Subjects were classified according to the longest duration reported per episode of activity, based on the different activities (and different durations) they declared. We assumed that if there were increased benefit with longer durations of activity, the longest duration would be most relevant. In age-adjusted analyses, we found a significant, inverse dose–response relationship between duration of activity and risk of developing CHD (p-trend = 0.04). However, the findings from the age-adjusted analyses did not differentiate between these alternate explanations that *(a)* longer durations are more beneficial than shorter ones or *(b)* longer durations simply expend more energy, which is more beneficial. We then proceeded to adjust for the volume of energy expended (i.e., making comparisons of different bout lengths among individuals with the same volume of energy expended), as well as other potential confounders (smoking, alcohol, diet, diabetes, hypertension, early parental mortality, and participation in vigorous activities). In these analyses, there was no longer an association with duration (p-trend = 0.25) once the volume of energy expenditure was controlled; however, volume of energy expended continued to show a significant, inverse association with CHD risk (p-trend = 0.046). These results suggest that it is the volume of energy expended that is important rather than the duration (i.e., shorter bouts can be accumulated).

Pattern of Physical Activity

A commonly cited barrier to being physically active is lack of time. Current physical activity guidelines require a non-inconsequential time commitment, asking for participation on at least 3 to 5 days a week (Haskell et al., 2007). Some individuals may choose to compress their exercise into fewer days, such as during weekends only ("weekend warriors"). Although exercising only once or twice a week, each activity session may have a long duration, resulting in a total energy expenditure that can be at least as much as that generated under current guidelines. However, U.S. national surveys do not count "weekend warriors" as achieving recommended levels of activity, because they do not satisfy the 3 to 5 days per week frequency. Little is known about whether health benefits are associated with such an activity pattern; thus, we investigated the association of this physical activity pattern with all-cause mortality in the Harvard Alumni Health Study.

In these analyses, we classified men into four groups: sedentary men, expending less than 500 kcal/week on physical activity; insufficiently active men, expending 500 to 999 kcal/week; weekend warriors, who expended 1,000 kcal/week or more by participating in sports and recreational activities only one to two times per week; and regularly active men, who expended 1,000 kcal/week or more by participating in sports and recreational activities at least three times/week (Lee et al., 2004). Overall, compared with sedentary men, the multivariate RRs for all-cause mortality among sedentary men, insufficiently active men, weekend warriors, and regularly active men were 1.00 (referent), 0.75 (95% CI, 0.62–0.91), 0.85 (0.65–1.11), and 0.64 (0.55–0.73), respectively. In stratified analysis, among men without major risk factors, weekend warriors had a lower risk of dying during follow-up compared with sedentary men (RR = 0.41; 95% CI, 0.21–0.81). This was not seen among men with at least one major risk factor (i.e., smoking, overweight, hypertension, or hypercholesterolemia; all men in the study were free of cardiovascular disease, cancer, and diabetes at study entry); the corresponding RR was 1.02 (0.75–1.38). We hypothesized that high-risk men may not benefit from sporadic frequency of physical activity, such as the weekend warrior pattern, because several beneficial effects of physical activity, such as improvements in blood pressure, lipid profile, and insulin sensitivity are short-lived (Haskell, 1994). We thus concluded that a pattern of regular physical activity, as recommended by current guidelines, is preferable to more sporadic patterns such as the weekend warrior pattern. However, if time is an issue and individuals cannot be active on a more regular basis, among individuals with no major risk factors, even one to two episodes per week of physical activity that generates 1,000 kcal/week or more (i.e., approximately equivalent to the energy expended over 3–5 days/week under current guidelines) may postpone mortality.

Physical Inactivity Versus Overweight/Obesity As Risk Factors for Chronic Disease

There continues to be debate regarding the importance of physical inactivity or lack of cardiorespiratory fitness vs. increased adiposity as risk factors for the development of chronic diseases (Blair and Church, 2004). Some investigators have suggested that physical activity or fitness can completely ameliorate the adverse effects of increased adiposity, whereas others disagree (for additional discussion, *see* Chapter 12). In the Harvard Alumni Health Study, several investigations, including those discussed earlier, clearly document associations between higher levels of physical activity and lower rates of cardiovascular disease and all-cause mortality, after accounting for differences in body mass index (BMI). Additionally, other investigations in the study have shown that higher levels of BMI are associated with increased mortality rates, independent of physical activity (Lee et al., 1993).

In observational epidemiologic studies, investigators commonly analyze physical activity and BMI (or other markers of adiposity) as independent variables. Higher levels of physical activity are compared against a reference level, which is set at a RR of 1.00 (or, lower levels of activity may be compared with the highest level, set as the referent). Simultaneously, different levels of BMI are categorized in similar fashion, with the referent again set at a RR of 1.00. In such an analysis, one cannot compare the risk factors with each other, because the comparison being made in this analysis is across levels of the same risk factor and not across the two risk factors. To be able to make cross-comparisons, subjects need to be cross-classified by *both* risk factors; for example, active and normal-weight persons can be compared against these three other groups: active but overweight, inactive and normal weight, and inactive and overweight.

In the Harvard Alumni Health Study, our findings suggest that the magnitude of physical inactivity as a risk factor vs. being overweight or obese depends on the outcome being studied. For all-cause mortality, each risk factor appears to be associated with increased risk of premature mortality, of about equal magnitude (Lee and Paffenbarger, 2000). Compared with inactive and overweight men, in multivariate analyses, those who were inactive but normal weight had a RR of 0.90 (0.79–1.02). Corresponding results were 0.80 (0.71–0.91) for active (satisfying the 1995 CDC/ACSM recommendation) but overweight men and 0.67 (0.60–0.75) for active and normal weight men.

However, for type 2 diabetes, adiposity appears to be more strongly related to risk than inactivity. In an analysis that included subjects from the Harvard Alumni Health Study, as well as alumni from the University of Pennsylvania, we observed the well-established association between higher BMI and increased risk of type 2 diabetes (Oguma et al., 2005). Additionally, we observed that weight gain between young adulthood and middle age

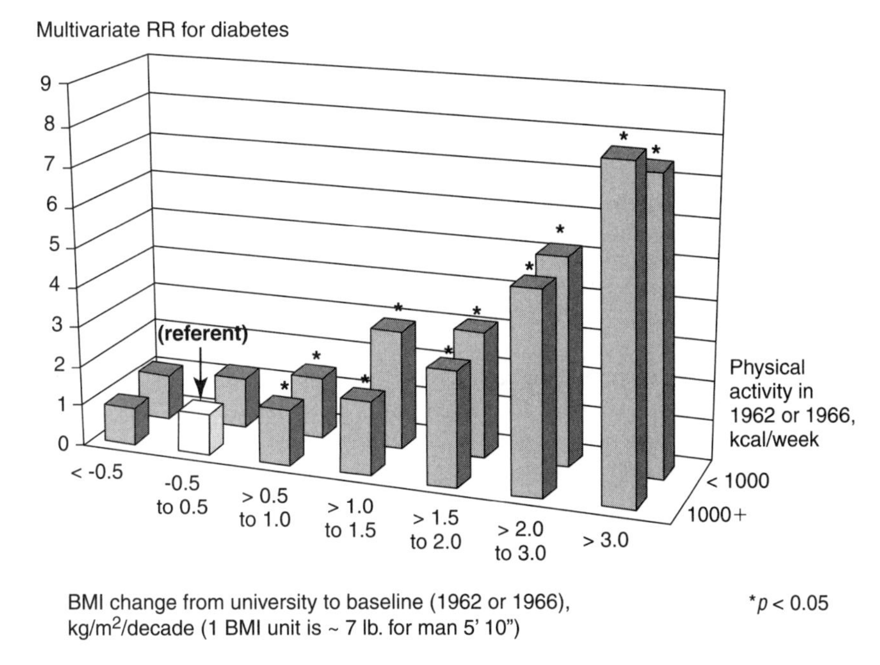

Figure 6.2 Physical Activity, Weight Change, and Risk of Type 2 Diabetes.
[A total of 20,187 men with mean age 46 years at baseline in 1962 or 1966. During follow-up through 1998, 1223 men developed type 2 diabetes. Multivariate relative risks (RRs) were adjusted for age, smoking, hypertension, parental history of diabetes, and body mass index (BMI) at university entry.]

increased risk, even among the leanest young adults with BMI less than 21 kg/^{2}. In examining the joint relationship between physical activity and weight gain with risk of type 2 diabetes (Figure 6.2), the strong, positive association between weight gain and risk of type 2 diabetes was observed both among inactive and active men who fulfilled the 1995 CDC/ACSM physical activity recommendation. The interaction between physical activity and weight gain was not significant ($p = 0.77$)—that is, inactive and active men experienced similar increases in risk with similar amounts of weight gain, and being active did not ameliorate the increase in risk of type 2 diabetes with weight gain. (Findings in women from the Women's Health Study, discussed later, support this observation in men that adiposity is a stronger risk factor for the development of type 2 diabetes than inactivity.)

Other Investigations of Physical Activity and Health Outcomes

In the Harvard Alumni Health Study, the techniques for addressing several methodologic issues pertinent to epidemiologic studies of physical activity (such as those discussed in the previous section) primarily were developed for investigations of all-cause mortality and cardiovascular disease. However, the relationship of physical activity to other health outcomes also has been of interest, with the appropriate methodologic techniques applied where needed. In addition to the diseases investigated in the early years of the study (described earlier), over the past decade, other health outcomes studied in relation to physical activity have included various cancers (e.g., Lee et al., 2003a), type 2 diabetes (Oguma et al., 2005), gallbladder disease (Sahi et al., 1998), and Parkinson's disease (Logroscino et al., 2006). Detailed discussion of their findings is beyond the scope of the chapter.

The Nurses' Health Study

Design and Rationale

The Nurses' Health Study was established in 1976 to study adverse health effects potentially associated with the use of oral contraceptive pills. At that time, use of oral contraceptives among U.S. women had been widespread for about a decade, but there was uncertainty regarding whether these drugs might increase the risk of diseases, such as cardiovascular disease and breast cancer (Colditz et al., 1997). The study was started to investigate this specific research question; since then, it has grown to encompass study of, and has provided important information on, many other questions related to lifestyle and women's health (Hankinson et al., 2002). Professor Frank Speizer was the founder of this study; several other investigators also were instrumental in helping with the scientific direction and conduct of the study since its initiation. With regard to interest in physical activity as a predictor of good health outcomes, Professor Walter Willett and other senior investigators were responsible for incorporating this into the study beginning in 1980, and Professor Willett also was responsible for including a detailed dietary component beginning the same year.

Similarly to the Harvard Alumni Health Study, the Nurses' Health Study is an ongoing prospective cohort study. Subjects are approximately 122,000 female, registered nurses, born between January 1, 1921 and December 31, 1946, who reside in 11 U.S. states with the largest number of registrants, based on data from the 1972 American Nurses Association. The choice of nurses as study participants reflected similar concerns that had arisen in the Harvard Alumni Health Study: investigators required that subjects would have a long-term commitment to the study, possess high rates of follow-up (by virtue of their being willing to provide prompt information on address changes), and be able to provide accurate health information in a cost-effective fashion through mailed health surveys. In addition to the health surveys mailed every 2 years, the Nurses' Health Study has requested biological samples from participants; these have included toenail clippings (to assess selenium consumption) obtained from approximately 68,000 nurses in 1982 and blood samples from approximately 33,000 women in 1988 (Hankinson et al., 2002).

Assessment of Physical Activity

In 1980, the first assessment of physical activity in the Nurses' Health Study was brief, asking women about the average number of hours per day during the past month that they had engaged in vigorous activity and, separately, in moderate activity. Separate estimates for each were requested for a weekday and a weekend day. On the next questionnaire in 1982, the number of hours per week in vigorous activity was queried.

In 1986, the physical activity questions were expanded (Figure 6.3). The format of the questions was then made similar to those used in the Harvard Alumni Health Study. Women were asked to report their usual walking pace outdoors and the number of flights of stairs climbed daily. In contrast to the Harvard Alumni Health Study, close-ended options were provided (rather than the "write-in" answers requested from the alumni). Additionally, the average time per week spent in each of several specified, leisure-time activities was requested, again with close-ended options. The activities selected (Wolf et al., 1994) were those most commonly reported by women in another study initiated by Professor Paffenbarger that enrolled male and female alumni from the University of Pennsylvania and included (e.g., in 1998) walking; jogging; running; bicycling; playing tennis, squash, or racquetball; lap swimming; other aerobic exercises; lower intensity exercises; and other vigorous activities. The data collected are used to derive a weekly physical activity score that is an estimate of

1. What is your normal walking pace outdoors?

☐ Slow (<2mph) ☐ Normal, average (2 to 2.9 mph) ☐ Brisk pace (3 to 3.9 mph) ☐ Very brisk, striding (4 mph or faster) ☐ Unable to walk

2. How many flights of stairs (not steps) do you climb daily?

☐ No flights ☐ 1–2 flights ☐ 3–4 flights ☐ 5–9 flights ☐ 10–14 flights ☐ 15 or more flights

3. During the past year, what was your average time **per week** spent at each of the following recreational activities?

	TIME PER WEEK									
	Zero	1–4 Min.	5–19 Min.	20–59 Min.	One Hr.	1–1.5 Hrs.	2–3 Hrs.	4–6 Hrs.	7–10 Hrs.	11+ Hrs.
Walking for exercise or walking to work	☐	☐	☐	☐	☐	☐	☐	☐	☐	☐
Jogging (slower than 10 minutes/mile)	☐	☐	☐	☐	☐	☐	☐	☐	☐	☐
Running (10 minutes/mile or faster)	☐	☐	☐	☐	☐	☐	☐	☐	☐	☐
Bicycling (including stationary machine)	☐	☐	☐	☐	☐	☐	☐	☐	☐	☐
Tennis, squash, racquetball	☐	☐	☐	☐	☐	☐	☐	☐	☐	☐
Lap swimming	☐	☐	☐	☐	☐	☐	☐	☐	☐	☐
Other aerobic exercise (aerobic dance, ski or stair machine, etc.)	☐	☐	☐	☐	☐	☐	☐	☐	☐	☐
Lower intensity exercise (yoga, stretching, toning)	☐	☐	☐	☐	☐	☐	☐	☐	☐	☐
Other vigorous activities (e.g., lawn mowing)	☐	☐	☐	☐	☐	☐	☐	☐	☐	☐

Figure 6.3 Nurses' Health Study Physical Activity Questionnaire.

the energy expended on all these activities, expressed in MET-hours/week. Nurses are typically asked to update the information on their physical activity every 2 years.

Reliability and Validity of Physical Activity Assessment

The reliability of the Nurses' Health Study physical activity questionnaire was investigated by comparing two questionnaires administered to a random sample of 151 nurses and 84 African-American nurses, randomly selected from African-American nurses (mean age in both groups: 39 years) in the Nurses' Health Study II, which enrolled a similar group of participants as the Nurses' Health Study (Wolf et al., 1994). Test-retest correlation coefficients of 0.59 and 0.39 were observed in the random and African-American samples, respectively. Because 2 years is a relatively long time-interval, some degree of change in physical activity was likely to have occurred; thus, the observed correlation coefficients likely underestimated the true reliability.

Validity was assessed by comparing questionnaire estimates of physical activity against four past-week physical activity recalls and four 7-day physical activity diaries, administered at 3-month intervals in the year prior to the administration of the physical activity questionnaire (Wolf et al., 1994). The correlation coefficient (corrected for within-person measurement error) for physical activity recalls was 0.79 in the random sample and 0.62 in the diaries. For African-American nurses, the correlation coefficients were similar: 0.83 and 0.59, respectively. As discussed previously for the Harvard Alumni Health Study, although the correlation coefficients may be high, indicating good agreement with regard to *ranking*, this does not necessarily mean that the absolute values agree on the different assessment tools. The mean physical activity level assessed via questionnaire was 19.5 MET-hours/week (95% CI, 16.4–22.9) compared with 23.8 MET-hours/week (20.8–27.1) from the recalls and 17.5 MET-hours/week (15.3–19.8) from the diaries, with scores from the recalls and diaries calculated only using the same activities that were queried on the questionnaire.

Thus, the questionnaire in the Nurses' Health Study is reasonably reliable and valid for use in large epidemiologic studies. Further evidence for its validity is shown in studies demonstrating expected associations between physical activity and several disease outcomes, including CHD (Manson et al., 1999), colon cancer (Martinez et al., 1997), and type 2 diabetes (Hu et al., 1999).

Assessment of Health Outcomes

On follow-up questionnaires sent every 2 years, women are asked about the occurrence of endpoints of interest. Investigators then request permission from the participant or next of kin for permission to obtain medical records and pathology reports pertaining to the diagnosis. Deaths in the study are reported by family members or the postal service, as well as through state registries or the National Heath Index. Where appropriate, death certificates and autopsy medical records are additionally reviewed to confirm the diagnoses of interest. Mortality follow-up in this population is more than 98% complete (Stampfer et al., 1984).

Select Investigations of Physical Activity

Walking Versus Vigorous-Intensity Physical Activity in Coronary Heart Disease Prevention

With the 1995 CDC/ACSM recommendation focused on moderate-intensity physical activity, the Nurses' Health Study became interested in examining whether walking, a common moderate-intensity activity undertaken by Americans, is associated with lower rates of CHD (Manson et al., 1999). To prevent confounding by vigorous activities, investigators examined only women who did not report participation in vigorous activities (47% of women). Among these women, the multivariate RRs associated with 0.5 or less, 0.6 to 2.0, 2.1 to 3.8, 3.9 to 9.9, and 10 or more MET-hours/week of walking were 1.00 (referent), 0.78 (95% CI, 0.57–1.06), 0.88 (0.65–1.21), 0.70 (0.51–0.95), and 0.65 (0.47–0.91), respectively (p-trend = 0.02). Therefore, as little walking as 3.9 to 9.9 MET-hour/week, the equivalent of 1 to 2.5 hours/week of brisk walking, was associated with a significantly lower risk of developing CHD. Additionally, investigators noted a significant inverse trend with walking pace; women whose usual pace was 3 mph or faster had a 36% lower risk than those whose usual pace was slower than 2 mph.

To compare walking with vigorous physical activity, investigators cross-classified women according to both the total energy expended on walking and the total energy expended on vigorous activities. The association of walking or vigorous activity with CHD risk appeared equivalent: compared with sedentary women (0–0.6 MET-hour/week of walking and 0 MET-hours/week of vigorous activity), women who walked 7 MET-hours/week or more, but who did no vigorous activity, had a multivariate relative risk for CHD of 0.74 (0.57–0.97). This reduction was comparable among women expending about an equal amount of energy but primarily in vigorous activities only (≥7 MET-hours/week in vigorous activities and 0–0.6 MET-hour/week in walking); the RR was 0.76 (0.49–1.17). (Seven MET-hours/week can be expended by approximately 2 hours of brisk walking or 1 hour of jogging.) These data do not necessarily indicate no added benefit associated with vigorous activities—because there were few women at very high levels of vigorous activity (only 26% participated in vigorous activities for at least 1 hr/wk), potentially added benefits may not have been observable.

Physical Inactivity Versus Obesity As Risk Factors for Chronic Disease

To provide information on the importance of each these factors toward the risk of developing CHD, investigators from the Nurses' Health Study examined groups of women classified according to both physical activity and BMI (Li et al., 2006). Women were classified according to their BMI in 1980; this was not updated over time to minimize the potential for bias (i.e., women who become unhealthy may lose weight). In contrast, all available information on physical activity over time was used because the present data (e.g., Paffenbarger et al., 1978) have indicated that recent, rather than remote, physical activity has been associated with decreased CHD risk. In the Nurses' Health Study, physical activity was assessed with different questionnaires early (prior to 1986; *see "Assessment of Physical Activity"* above) and later in the study. Therefore, investigators tried to use a measure that was common across the different questionnaires, hours per week spent in moderate-to-vigorous activities. To give greater weight to recent, rather than more distant, physical activity, investigators used the cumulative average of time in moderate-to-vigorous activities from all questionnaires at the start of each 2-year follow-up interval (e.g., hours of physical activity per week in 1980 were related to CHD events occurring between 1980 and 1982; the average of hours of physical activity per week between 1980 and 1982 was related to CHD events occurring between 1982 and 1986, the next year that physical activity was assessed; this last value and 1988 hours of physical activity were then averaged and related to CHD events occurring between 1986 and 1988, etc.).

In multivariate analyses, physical activity was significantly and inversely related to CHD risk (p-trend = 0.001) after adjustment for BMI. Additionally, BMI was significantly and directly related to CHD risk (p-trend = 0.001) after adjustment for physical activity. In joint analyses, higher levels of physical activity did not remove the increased risk associated with obesity. Compared with normal-weight, active (≥3.5 hours/week of moderate-to-vigorous activity) women, obese women with the same level of physical activity had a significantly elevated RR, 2.48 (96% CI, 1.84–3.34), for CHD. Normal-weight women who were inactive (<1 hour/week) also experienced a higher RR, 1.48 (1.24–1.77), whereas obese and inactive women had the highest RR, 3.44 (2.81–4.21).

Similar analyses were conducted with all-cause mortality as the outcome of interest (Hu et al., 2004). Again, using normal-weight, active women as referent, obese women with the same level of physical activity had a significantly elevated RR, 1.91 (96% CI, 1.60–2.30), for all-cause mortality, after adjusting for potential confounders. Normal-weight women who were inactive (<1 hour/week) also had a higher RR, 1.55 (1.42–1.70), whereas obese and inactive women again experienced the highest RR, 2.42 (2.14–2.73). These findings mirror those from the Harvard Alumni Health Study for men discussed earlier (Lee and Paffenbarger, 2000), in that either factor appears to be associated with increased risk of premature mortality, of very approximately equal magnitude, and that possessing both further increases risk.

Proportion of Coronary Heart Disease That Is Preventable Through a Healthy Lifestyle Including Physical Activity

Investigators in the Nurses' Health Study attempted to estimate the proportion of coronary events (non-fatal myocardial infarction or CHD death) in the study population that might be preventable by following a healthy lifestyle including physical activity (Stampfer et al., 2000). They defined a group of nurses considered to possess a healthy lifestyle, with the following characteristics: engaged in 30 min/day or more of moderate-to-vigorous physical activity (as recommended by the 1995 ACSM/CDC guidelines; Pate et al., 1995), did not smoke, possessed a BMI less than 25 kg/m^2, consumed a moderate amount of alcohol, and ate a healthy diet (low trans fat and glycemic load; high cereal fiber, marine *n*-3 fatty acids, and folate; and high ratio of polyunsaturated to saturated fat).

Only 3% of women fell into this low-risk group, which experienced substantially lower rates of CHD compared with the rest of the cohort. After adjusting for differences in age, parental history of myocardial infarction before age 60 years, menopausal status, use of postmenopausal hormones, hypertension and high cholesterol, the RR of developing a coronary event was only 0.17 (0.07–0.41) in this low-risk group, compared with other study subjects. Investigators estimated that 82% of coronary events—a very large proportion indeed—among the nurses might have been prevented if all women had followed the low-risk lifestyle.

Physical Activity and Transient Risk of Sudden Cardiac Death

As discussed in detail in Chapter 13, physical activity can be a two-edged sword: habitual physical activity can reduce the overall, long-term risk of CHD and sudden death, but it is also capable of causing a transient increase in the risk of acute cardiac events, especially in individuals who are not regularly active. There are few data from prospective cohort studies to examine the transient risk of acute cardiac events during exercise, with the Nurses' Health Study providing some of these data (Whang et al., 2006). In this study, the overall incidence of sudden cardiac death during moderate-to-vigorous exercise (requiring ≥5 METs) was very low (1 per 36.5 million hours of exertion) compared to activity of lesser exertion or during no exertion (1 per 59.4 million hours). Investigators calculated a RR of 2.38 (1.23–4.60) for sudden cardiac death associated with moderate-to-vigorous exercise. However, this was modified by habitual physical activity: women who usually engaged in moderate-to-vigorous physical activity 2 or more hours per week did not have a significantly elevated transient risk with these activities (RR = 1.49; 0.61–3.61), but women who reported less than 2 hours/week did have a substantial transient increase in risk (RR = 8.98; 3.32–24.3).

Other Investigations of Physical Activity and Health Outcomes

The Nurses' Health Study also has investigated the relationship between physical activity and numerous other health outcomes, such as type 2 diabetes (e.g., Hu et al., 1999), various cancers (e.g., Holmes et al., 2005), hip fractures (Feskanich et al., 2002), and cognitive function (Weuve et al., 2004); however, space constraints prevent discussion of their findings. Several of the methodologic issues discussed in this chapter that are relevant to studying physical activity, and the strategies to address them, have been included in these other investigations.

Other Studies

The Women's Health Study

The Women's Health Study is a completed, randomized, controlled trial testing low-dose aspirin and vitamin E in the prevention of heart disease and cancer in approximately 40,000 women. As part of the trial, data also were collected on physical activity (to evaluate, and ensure that randomization resulted in similar distribution of physical activity across randomized arms) using a very similar questionnaire to that used in the Nurses' Health Study (Figure 6.3). One contribution of this study has been to provide data on the relationship between walking and the risk of developing CHD (Lee et al., 2001). Women who reported walking also were more likely to participate in vigorous activities (Lee and Buchner, in press); thus, we restricted the analyses to women who did not participate in any vigorous activities to prevent confounding by such activities. The data showed that women who walked as little as 1 to 1.5 hours per week had significantly lower risk: compared with to women who did not usually walk, the multivariate relative risks for CHD associated with walking less than 1, 1 to 1.5 and 2 hours/week or more were 0.86 (0.57–1.29), 0.49 (0.28–0.86), and 0.48 (0.29–0.78), respectively (*p*-trend <0.001).

This study also has used the technique of a common reference group (discussed earlier) to compare physical inactivity and obesity as risk factors for developing type 2 diabetes (Weinstein et al., 2004). As in the Harvard Alumni Health Study (Figure 6.2), the Women's Health Study showed that obesity is more strongly related to risk of developing this disease than physical inactivity. Compared with normal-weight and active women, the multivariate relative risk for developing type 2 diabetes in normal-weight but inactive women was 1.15 (0.83–1.59). However, for obese and active women, this was 11.5 (8.34–11.9), and an elevated RR of similar magnitude was seen in women who were both obese and inactive, 11.8 (8.75–16.0), indicating a large effect on risk with obesity but only a small effect with inactivity.

The Women's Health Initiative Observational Study

The Women's Health Initiative is a study of approximately 162,000 ethnically diverse, postmenopausal women in four major study components: three randomized clinical trials (with these primary aims: low-fat eating pattern in the prevention of breast and colorectal cancer; postmenopausal hormone therapy in the prevention of CHD and other cardiovascular diseases, with increased breast cancer risk as a possible adverse outcome; calcium and vitamin D supplementation in the prevention of hip fractures) and a prospective cohort study, the Women's Health Initiative Observational Study, which comprises approximately 94,000 women (Women's Health Initiative Study Group [WHI], 1998). An important contribution of the observational study has been to provide data on the association of physical activity, comparing walking and vigorous activity, with the risk of developing cardiovascular disease. In this analysis (Manson et al., 2002), investigators classified women according to both the energy expended on walking and the energy expended on vigorous activities (Figure 6.4). In age-adjusted analysis, the data appeared to indicate that as long as the *total* energy expended was similar, whether this was derived from walking or from vigorous activities, the risk reduction for cardiovascular disease risk was similar. Compared with sedentary women (≤2.5 MET-hours/week in walking and no vigorous activities), women who spent more than 100 min/week in vigorous activities (this is equivalent to some 10 MET-hours/week) and 2.5 MET-hours/week or less in walking had an age-adjusted RR of 0.71. Women who did no vigorous activities but who walked for more than 10 MET-hours/week experienced a similar age-adjusted RR of 0.67. Thus, both groups of women expended similar amounts of energy—some 10 to 12.5 MET-hours/week—and the former group achieved this primarily through vigorous activities, and the latter group achieved this mainly by means of walking.

As in the Nurses' Heath Study discussed earlier, these data do not conclusively indicate no added benefit associated with vigorous activities. It is likely that few women in this study, just as among the nurses, participated in high levels of vigorous activity, so that potential, further risk reductions with vigorous activity could not be observed.

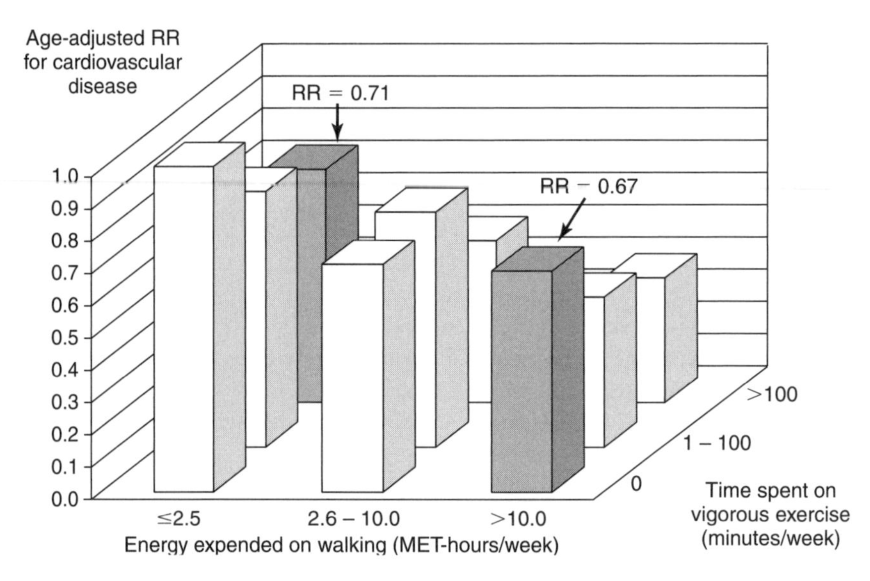

Figure 6.4 Moderate- (Walking) and Vigorous-Intensity Physical Activity and Risk of Cardiovascular Disease. [Data from the Women's Health Initiative Observational Study (Manson et al., 2002). Shaded bars represent women expending similar amounts of energy (approximately 10–12.5 MET-hours/week); the relative risks for cardiovascular disease are similar, regardless of whether the energy expended was derived primarily from walking or primarily from vigorous exercise.]

The Health, Aging, and Body Composition Study

Prospective cohort studies of physical activity and health primarily have used questionnaires to assess physical activity levels (although validation of the questionnaire may have used several other objective measures of physical activity, such as those listed in Table 6.1). The Health, Aging, and Body Composition Study (Manini et al., 2006) is unique because this study used DLW to estimate energy expenditure in approximately 300 high-functioning, community-dwelling adults ages 70 to 82 years. In multivariate analyses, higher levels of physical activity were associated with lower rates of mortality during follow-up (55 deaths over 6 years). Compared with individuals expending less than 521 kcal/day, those who expended 521 to 770 and more than 770 kcal/day (representing tertiles of study subjects) experienced RRs of 0.65 (0.33–1.28) and 0.33 (0.15–0.74), respectively (p-trend = 0.007).

A major advantage of this method of measuring physical activity is its precision, because DLW is considered a "gold standard" for determining energy expenditure. However, its limitation is that it does not inform regarding the activities that contributed to total energy expenditure (e.g., What intensity? Did activity occur in bouts of at least 10 minutes' duration?). This study also observed that self-reported high-intensity activities did not differ across tertiles of energy expenditure, as measured by DLW. However, the questionnaire asked subjects only to self-report the frequency of these activities, but not the duration; thus, this finding is not necessarily an indictment of self-reported physical activity data. Subjects self-reported the frequency and duration of other activities, and self-reported *total* activity (apart from high-intensity activities), whether duration or amount of energy expended, differed significantly across tertiles of energy expenditure measured using DLW.

Additional Studies

In addition to the studies described earlier, many other prospective cohort studies, although not initially designed to be studies of physical activity, have analyzed the data collected to address hypotheses related to physical activity and health. These studies—including the following selected examples: the Health Professionals' Follow-up Study (e.g., Tanasescu et al., 2002), the Iowa Women's Health Study (e.g., Kushi et al., 1997), the Framingham Heart Study (e.g., Franco et al., 2005), the Canada Fitness Survey (e.g., Katzmarzyk and Craig, 2006), the British Regional Heart Study (e.g., Shaper et al., 1991), the European Prospective Investigation into Cancer and Nutrition Cohort Study (e.g., Lahmann et al., 2007), the Finnish Twin Cohort Study (e.g., Kujala et al., 1998)—all have had to face the methodologic issues related to epidemiologic studies of physical activity that are discussed in this chapter.

Finally, the intent of this chapter is to focus on studies of physical activity, rather than physical fitness. Studies of physical fitness, a marker of recent physical activity, cannot provide the direct information needed to make public health recommendations with regard to the kinds of activity, their intensity, duration, and frequency that is needed for health. Nonetheless, prospective cohort studies of physical fitness in relation to health outcomes (e.g., the Aerobics Center Longitudinal Study; Blair et al., 1996), the St. James Women Take Heart Project (Gulati et al., 2005), a study by Myers et al. (2002) have contributed importantly to the body of knowledge showing an inverse relationship between levels of physical fitness and good health, in congruence with findings from the studies of physical activity discussed in this chapter.

Personal Perspective

In medical research, the randomized clinical trial often is considered the "gold standard" of study designs (and, by implication, the prospective cohort study, a "poor relative"). It is undoubtedly true that such trials, if well-designed and -conducted, are more likely to yield unbiased and unconfounded results compared to other study designs. However, it is not always appropriate to conduct randomized clinical trials. With regard to physical activity, this study design is impractical if long-term health outcomes (e.g., the development of coronary events or cancer in a healthy population) are the endpoints of interest. The costs of conducting such a trial would be prohibitive. More importantly, good compliance (particularly to the physical activity or intervention arms), which is crucial to obtaining valid results, would surely be impossible over a period of many years. Additionally, cost considerations make it impractical to plan multiple intervention arms that mimic the myriad activity patterns seen in real life. Another limitation of randomized clinical trials is the select nature of participants in these studies. Often, for safety reasons, investigators place selection criteria that exclude high-risk patients from participation; furthermore, subjects who choose to participate in clinical trials can be a very exclusive group. For example, in a recently completed randomized clinical trial examining different doses of physical activity on change in physical fitness among sedentary women, only 10% of women screened eventually were randomized into the trial (Church et al., 2007)

Therefore, prospective cohort studies play an important role in providing answers to research questions related to physical activity and long-term health outcomes in particular. There are, of course, limitations to the data provided by such studies (just as there are limitations to data derived from other study designs). In designing, conducting, and analyzing the data from prospective cohort studies, consideration of the methodologic issues discussed in this chapter (as well as in Chapter 4) can minimize some of the limitations. To provide a good, complete picture of the relationships between physical activity and health, the data from many different kinds of studies—including observational (e.g., cohort studies) and experimental (e.g., trials) designs—are needed to flesh out the hues.

References

Ainsworth BE, Haskell WL, Leon AS, et al. 1993a. Compendium of physical activities: classification of energy costs of human physical activities. *Med Sci Sports Exerc* 25: 71–80.

Ainsworth BE, Leon AS, Richardson MT, Jacobs DR, Paffenbarger RS, Jr. 1993b. Accuracy of the College Alumnus Physical Activity Questionnaire. *J Clin Epidemiol* 46: 1403–11.

Albanes D, Conway JM, Taylor PR, Moe PW, Judd J. 1990. Validation and comparison of eight physical activity questionnaires. *Epidemiology* 1: 65–71.

Bassett DR, Jr., Cureton AL, Ainsworth BE. 2000. Measurement of daily walking distance-questionnaire versus pedometer. *Med Sci Sports Exerc* 32: 1018–23.

Bassett DR, Vachon JA, Kirkland AO, Howley ET, Duncan GE, Johnson KR. 1997. Energy cost of stair climbing and descending on the college alumnus questionnaire. *Med Sci Sports Exerc* 29: 1250–4.

Blair SN, Church TS. 2004. The fitness, obesity, and health equation: is physical activity the common denominator? *JAMA* 292: 1232–4.

Blair SN, Kampert JB, Kohl HW, 3rd, et al. 1996. Influences of cardiorespiratory fitness and other precursors on cardiovascular disease and all-cause mortality in men and women. *JAMA* 276: 205–10.

Bonnefoy M, Normand S, Pachiaudi C, Lacour JR, Laville M, Kostka T. 2001. Simultaneous validation of ten physical activity questionnaires in older men: a doubly labeled water study. *J Am Geriatr Soc* 49: 28–35.

Cauley JA, LaPorte RE, Sandler RB, Schramm MM, Kriska AM. 1987. Comparison of methods to measure physical activity in postmenopausal women. *Am J Clin Nutr* 45: 14–22.

Church TS, Earnest CP, Skinner JS, Blair SN. 2007. Effects of different doses of physical activity on cardiorespiratory fitness among sedentary, overweight or obese postmenopausal women with elevated blood pressure: a randomized controlled trial. *JAMA* 297: 2081–91.

Colditz GA, Manson JE, Hankinson SE. 1997. The Nurses' Health Study: 20-year contribution to the understanding of health among women. *J Womens Health* 6: 49–62.

Feskanich D, Willett W, Colditz G. 2002. Walking and leisure-time activity and risk of hip fracture in postmenopausal women. *JAMA* 288: 2300–6.

Fletcher GF, Blair SN, Blumenthal J, et al. 1992. Statement on exercise. Benefits and recommendations for physical activity programs for all Americans. A statement for health professionals by the Committee on Exercise and Cardiac Rehabilitation of the Council on Clinical Cardiology, American Heart association. *Circulation* 86: 340–4.

Franco OH, de Laet C, Peeters A, Jonker J, Mackenbach J, Nusselder W. 2005. Effects of physical activity on life expectancy with cardiovascular disease. *Arch Intern Med* 165: 2355–60.

Gulati M, Black HR, Shaw LJ, et al. 2005. The prognostic value of a nomogram for exercise capacity in women. *N Engl J Med* 353: 468–75.

Hankinson SE, Colditz GA, Manson JE, Speizer FE (Eds.). 2002. *Healthy women, healthy lives: A guide to preventing disease, from the landmark Nurses' Health Study*. New York, NY: Fireside.

Haskell WL. 1994. J.B. Wolffe Memorial Lecture. Health consequences of physical activity: understanding and challenges regarding dose-response. *Med Sci Sports Exerc* 26: 649–60.

Haskell WL, Lee IM, Pate RR, et al. 2007. Physical Activity and Public Health: Updated Recommendation for Adults from the American College of Sports Medicine and the American Heart Association. *Med Sci Sports Exerc* 39: 1423–34.

Helmrich SP, Ragland DR, Leung RW, Paffenbarger RS, Jr. 1991. Physical activity and reduced occurrence of non-insulin-dependent diabetes mellitus. *N Engl J Med* 325: 147–52.

Holmes MD, Chen WY, Feskanich D, Kroenke CH, Colditz GA. 2005. Physical activity and survival after breast cancer diagnosis. *JAMA* 293: 2479–86.

Howley ET. 2001. Type of activity: resistance, aerobic and leisure versus occupational physical activity. *Med Sci Sports Exerc* 33: S364–9; discussion S419–20.

Hu FB, Sigal RJ, Rich-Edwards JW, et al. 1999. Walking compared with vigorous physical activity and risk of type 2 diabetes in women: a prospective study. *JAMA* 282: 1433–9.

Hu FB, Willett WC, Li T, Stampfer MJ, Colditz GA, Manson JE. 2004. Adiposity as compared with physical activity in predicting mortality among women. *N Engl J Med* 351: 2694–703.

Jacobs DR, Jr., Ainsworth BE, Hartman TJ, Leon AS. 1993. A simultaneous evaluation of 10 commonly used physical activity questionnaires. *Med Sci Sports Exerc* 25: 81–91.

Katzmarzyk PT, Craig CL. 2006. Independent effects of waist circumference and physical activity on all-cause mortality in Canadian women. *Appl Physiol Nutr Metab* 31: 271–6.

Kriska AM, Caspersen CJ (Eds.). 1997. *A collection of physical activity questionnaires for health-related research. Med Sci Sports Exerc*, Vols. 29(Suppl): S1–S205.

Kujala UM, Kaprio J, Sarna S, Koskenvuo M. 1998. Relationship of leisure-time physical activity and mortality: the Finnish twin cohort. *JAMA* 279: 440–4.

Kushi LH, Fee RM, Folsom AR, Mink PJ, Anderson KE, Sellers TA. 1997. Physical activity and mortality in postmenopausal women. *JAMA* 277: 1287–92.

Lahmann PH, Friedenreich C, Schuit AJ, et al. 2007. Physical activity and breast cancer risk: the European Prospective Investigation into Cancer and Nutrition. *Cancer Epidemiol Biomarkers Prev* 16: 36–42.

LaPorte RE, Black-Sandler R, Cauley JA, Link M, Bayles C, Marks B. 1983. The assessment of physical activity in older women: analysis of the interrelationship and reliability of activity monitoring, activity surveys, and caloric intake. *J Gerontol* 38: 394–7.

Lee I-M, Buchner DM. The importance of walking to public health. *Med Sci Sports Exerc* (In press.)

Lee IM, Hsieh CC, Paffenbarger RS, Jr. 1995. Exercise intensity and longevity in men. The Harvard Alumni Health Study. *JAMA* 273: 1179–84.

Lee IM, Manson JE, Hennekens CH, Paffenbarger RS, Jr. 1993. Body weight and mortality. A 27-year follow-up of middle-aged men. *JAMA* 270: 2823–8.

Lee IM, Paffenbarger RS, Jr. 2000. Associations of light, moderate, and vigorous intensity physical activity with longevity. The Harvard Alumni Health Study. *Am J Epidemiol* 151: 293–9.

Lee IM, Paffenbarger RS, Jr., Hsieh C. 1991. Physical activity and risk of developing colorectal cancer among college alumni. *J Natl Cancer Inst* 83: 1324–9.

Lee IM, Paffenbarger RS, Jr., Hsieh CC. 1992. Physical activity and risk of prostatic cancer among college alumni. *Am J Epidemiol* 135: 169–79.

Lee IM, Rexrode KM, Cook NR, Manson JE, Buring JE. 2001. Physical activity and coronary heart disease in women: is "no pain, no gain" passe? *JAMA* 285: 1447–54.

Lee IM, Sesso HD, Oguma Y, Paffenbarger RS, Jr. 2003a. Physical activity, body weight, and pancreatic cancer mortality. *Br J Cancer* 88: 679–83.

Lee IM, Sesso HD, Oguma Y, Paffenbarger RS, Jr. 2003b. Relative intensity of physical activity and risk of coronary heart disease. *Circulation* 107: 1110–6.

Lee IM, Sesso HD, Oguma Y, Paffenbarger RS, Jr. 2004. The "weekend warrior" and risk of mortality. *Am J Epidemiol* 160: 636–41.

Lee IM, Sesso HD, Paffenbarger RS, Jr. 2000. Physical activity and coronary heart disease risk in men: does the duration of exercise episodes predict risk? *Circulation* 102: 981–6.

Li TY, Rana JS, Manson JE, et al. 2006. Obesity as compared with physical activity in predicting risk of coronary heart disease in women. *Circulation* 113: 499–506.

Logroscino G, Sesso HD, Paffenbarger RS, Jr., Lee IM. 2006. Physical activity and risk of Parkinson's disease: a prospective cohort study. *J Neurol Neurosurg Psychiatry* 77: 1318–22.

Manini TM, Everhart JE, Patel KV, et al. 2006. Daily activity energy expenditure and mortality among older adults. *JAMA* 296: 171–9.

Manson JE, Greenland P, LaCroix AZ, et al. 2002. Walking compared with vigorous exercise for the prevention of cardiovascular events in women. *N Engl J Med* 347: 716–25.

Manson JE, Hu FB, Rich-Edwards JW, et al. 1999. A prospective study of walking as compared with vigorous exercise in the prevention of coronary heart disease in women. *N Engl J Med* 341: 650–8.

Martinez ME, Giovannucci E, Spiegelman D, Hunter DJ, Willett WC, Colditz GA. 1997. Leisure-time physical activity, body size, and colon cancer in women. Nurses' Health Study Research Group. *J Natl Cancer Inst* 89: 948–55.

Morris JN, Heady JA, Raffle PA, Roberts CG, Parks JW. 1953. Coronary heart-disease and physical activity of work. *Lancet* 265: 1053–7.

Myers J, Prakash M, Froelicher V, Do D, Partington S, Atwood JE. 2002. Exercise capacity and mortality among men referred for exercise testing. *N Engl J Med* 346: 793–801.

Nelson ME, Rejeski WJ, Blair SN, et al. 2007. Physical activity and public health in older adults: recommendation from the American College of Sports Medicine and the American Heart Association. *Med Sci Sports Exerc* 39: 1435–45.

Oguma Y, Sesso HD, Paffenbarger RS, Jr., Lee IM. 2005. Weight change and risk of developing type 2 diabetes. *Obes Res* 13: 945–51.

Paffenbarger RS, Jr., Asnes DP. 1966. Chronic disease in former college students. 3. Precursors of suicide in early and middle life. *Am J Public Health Nations Health* 56: 1026–36.

Paffenbarger RS, Jr., Wing AL. 1967. Characteristics in youth predisposing to fatal stroke in later years. *Lancet* 1: 753–4.

Paffenbarger RS, Jr., Wing AL. 1973. Chronic disease in former college students. XII. Early precursors of adult-onset diabetes mellitus. *Am J Epidemiol* 97: 314–23.

Paffenbarger RS, Jr., Wing AL, Hyde RT. 1974. Chronic disease in former college students; 13. Early precursors of peptic ulcer. *Am J Epidemiol* 100: 307–15.

Paffenbarger RS, Jr., Wing AL, Hyde RT. 1978. Physical activity as an index of heart attack risk in college alumni. *Am J Epidemiol* 108: 161–75.

Paffenbarger RS, Jr., Wolf PA, Notkin J, Thorne MC. 1966. Chronic disease in former college students. I. Early precursors of fatal coronary heart disease. *Am J Epidemiol* 83: 314–28.

Pate RR, Pratt M, Blair SN, et al. 1995. Physical activity and public health. A recommendation from the Centers for Disease Control and Prevention and the American College of Sports Medicine. *JAMA* 273: 402–7.

Rauh MJ, Hovell MF, Hofstetter CR, Sallis JF, Gleghorn A. 1992. Reliability and validity of self-reported physical activity in Latinos. *Int J Epidemiol* 21: 966–71.

Sahi T, Paffenbarger RS, Jr., Hsieh CC, Lee IM. 1998. Body mass index, cigarette smoking, and other characteristics as predictors of self-reported, physician-diagnosed gallbladder disease in male college alumni. *Am J Epidemiol* 147: 644–51.

Sasco AJ, Paffenbarger RS, Jr., Gendre I, Wing AL. 1992. The role of physical exercise in the occurrence of Parkinson's disease. *Arch Neurol* 49: 360–5.

Sesso HD, Paffenbarger RS, Jr., Lee IM. 1998. Physical activity and breast cancer risk in the College Alumni Health Study (United States). *Cancer Causes Control* 9: 433–9.

Sesso HD, Paffenbarger RS, Jr., Lee IM. 2000. Physical activity and coronary heart disease in men: The Harvard Alumni Health Study. *Circulation* 102: 975–80.

Shaper AG, Wannamethee G, Weatherall R. 1991. Physical activity and ischaemic heart disease in middle-aged British men. *Br Heart J* 66: 384–94.

Siconolfi SF, Lasater TM, Snow RC, Carleton RA. 1985. Self-reported physical activity compared with maximal oxygen uptake. *Am J Epidemiol* 122: 101–5.

Stampfer MJ, Hu FB, Manson JE, Rimm EB, Willett WC. 2000. Primary prevention of coronary heart disease in women through diet and lifestyle. *N Engl J Med* 343: 16–22.

Stampfer MJ, Willett WC, Speizer FE, et al. 1984. Test of the National Death Index. *Am J Epidemiol* 119: 837–9.

Strath SJ, Bassett DR, Jr., Swartz AM. 2004. Comparison of the college alumnus questionnaire physical activity index with objective monitoring. *Ann Epidemiol* 14: 409–15.

Tanasescu M, Leitzmann MF, Rimm EB, Willett WC, Stampfer MJ, Hu FB. 2002. Exercise type and intensity in relation to coronary heart disease in men. *JAMA* 288: 1994–2000.

Washburn RA, Smith KW, Goldfield SR, McKinlay JB. 1991. Reliability and physiologic correlates of the Harvard Alumni Activity Survey in a general population. *J Clin Epidemiol* 44: 1319–26.

Weinstein AR, Sesso HD, Lee IM, et al. 2004. Relationship of physical activity vs body mass index with type 2 diabetes in women. *JAMA* 292: 1188–94.

Weuve J, Kang JH, Manson JE, Breteler MM, Ware JH, Grodstein F. 2004. Physical activity, including walking, and cognitive function in older women. *JAMA* 292: 1454–61.
Wolf AM, Hunter DJ, Colditz GA, et al. 1994. Reproducibility and validity of a self-administered physical activity questionnaire. *Int J Epidemiol* 23: 991–9.
Women's Health Initiative Study Group. 1998. Design of the Women's Health Initiative clinical trial and observational study. The Women's Health Initiative Study Group. *Control Clin Trials* 19: 61–109.

7 Physical Activity Surveillance

Harold W. Kohl III
and C. Dexter Kimsey Jr.

Physical activity surveillance has become an integral and necessary part of physical activity epidemiology, primarily by enabling an understanding of prevalence and trends in participation. Uses of surveillance data are varied and broad, but perhaps most importantly, such data provide useful guidance for physical activity program planning and policy development. The purposes of this chapter are to review key components of physical activity surveillance, describe the main physical activity surveillance tools in the United States, illustrate (through case example) issues in physical activity surveillance, and discuss future needs in physical activity surveillance.

Data Collected in Physical Activity Surveillance

Public health surveillance has been defined as "the ongoing systematic collection, analysis, and interpretation of outcome-specific data for use in the planning, implementation, and evaluation of public health practice" (Thacker and Berkelman, 1988). As a central component of public health practice, surveillance is used for planning and to assess the magnitude of a public health problem; to detect and document the distribution and spread of health events; and to help define public health priorities, monitor changes, evaluate public health programs, identify research needs, and facilitate research (Teutsch and Churchill, 2000). The collection, analysis, and dissemination of data are the foundation of any surveillance system. Surveillance was initially used in public health to monitor development of specific infectious diseases, but today public health surveillance is "often applied to almost *any* effort to monitor, observe, or determine health status, diseases or risk factors within a population" (Teutsch and Churchill, 2000).

A survey, as defined by Merriam-Webster, is "to query (someone) in order to collect data for the analysis of some aspect of a group or area" (Merriam-Webster Online Dictionary: http://www.merriam-webster.com/dictionary/survey). A survey does not become surveillance unless it is repeated over time at determined intervals (Teutsch and Churchill, 2000). Numerous methods are used in population-based surveys, and to be able to compare data from surveys (for surveillance purposes), they must use a common methodology. Surveillance is usually conducted to better understand the extent of diseases or behaviors, to monitor the progress of prevention efforts, and to help public health professionals make more timely and effective decisions regarding control efforts.

To understand the national patterns and trends in physical activity, surveillance systems attempt to collect information on the components of physical activity in individuals, then aggregate this information by group (e.g., by age or race/ethnicity). Current Centers for Disease Control and Prevention (CDC)–American College of Sports Medicine (ACSM) physical activity guidelines recommend that adults perform 30 minutes or more of moderate-intensity physical activity on most, preferably all, days—either in a single session or accumulated in multiple bouts of at least 10 minutes (Pate et al., 1995). This level of physical activity is considered the minimum amount required for the achievement of health benefits.

Information about physical activity is usually obtained in one of three ways: questionnaire, observation and direct measurement, or diary/log. Questionnaires ask a respondent to recall and report recent or usual participation in activities or in sedentary behavior, usually for an identified period of time. The observation and direct measurement method may include use of devices such as pedometers, motion detectors, or heart rate monitors to record movements or physiological responses to movement. Another method in this category is direct observation, such as watching and recording playground use during school recess. In the diary method of obtaining physical activity information, an individual records all activity for a defined period of time (usually a day or a week). Once data using any of these methods are gathered, estimates or indicators of energy expenditure (e.g., metabolic equivalents [METs]) or indices of physical activity are obtained. (Additional discussion of methods for measuring physical activity is provided in Chapters 2 and 3.)

Currently in surveillance, physical activity is measured through questionnaires (self-report surveys) that attempt to capture the frequency, duration, and intensity of activity and, at times, also the mode and domain of the activity. Frequency is often described as the number of days per (usual) week that activity occurs. For example, the frequency of regular physical activity is activity performed on most days of the week (defined as 5 days or more), preferably daily (again, according to the CDC–ACSM guidelines).

Duration is the length of time that the physical activity is performed (usually in a day). Duration may be continuous (e.g., a 40-minute run) or accumulated (in bouts of activity; e.g., three 10-minute periods of walking the dog).

Intensity refers to the level of effort or amount of energy expended in performing the activity and is often categorized as light, moderate, or vigorous. Under one classification scheme (relative intensity), these intensity levels are related to perceived exertion (Borg scale) or METs and are defined relative to a person's capacity for a specific type of activity (U.S. Department of Health and Human Services, 1996). This relativity to an individual's capacity is important, as capacity typically changes as someone ages, so that what was once light-intensity physical activity may become moderate- or vigorous-intensity activity at different ages (additional discussion is provided in Chapter 6).

The mode of physical activity refers to the type of activity, such as walking, swimming, or gardening. Data on mode of activity have been and still are collected by some surveillance systems, but this component of physical activity is being replaced by intensity and duration of activity because these aspects of physical activity (i.e., intensity and duration) are specified in CDC–ACSM guidelines (Pate et al., 1995) and Healthy People 2010 objectives (U.S. Department of Health and Human Services, 2000; Healthy People 2010 website: http://www.healthypeople.gov/).

Physical activities are classified into domains that represent the situation or environment in which the activity occurs. The four most common domains are leisure-time, occupational, household, and transportation activities. Most surveillance systems that collect physical activity information concern themselves mainly with leisure-time activities.

Physical Activity Goals in the United States

As mentioned earlier, current CDC–ACSM physical activity guidelines recommend that adults perform 30 minutes or more of moderate-intensity physical activity on most, preferable all, days—either in a single session or accumulated in multiple bouts of at least 10 minutes (Pate et al., 1995). This level of activity is considered the minimum amount required for the achievement of health benefits.

Achieving the recommended level of physical activity is one of the goals of Healthy People 2010, a comprehensive set of disease prevention and health promotion objectives for the nation. Healthy People 2010 presents health objectives in a format that enables diverse groups to combine their efforts and work as a team. Healthy People 2010 has two overarching goals: *(1)* increase quality and years of healthy life and *(2)* eliminate health disparities. Healthy People 2010 has 28 focus areas, each of which is addressed by a chapter. Chapter 22 of Healthy People 2010, "Physical Activity and Fitness," has 15 objectives. These objectives are tracked using national surveillance systems such as the National Health Interview Survey (NHIS), Youth Risk Behavior Surveillance System (YRBSS), School Health Policies and Programs Study (SHPPS), and the National Personal Transportation Survey (NPTS) (U.S. Department of Health and Human Services, 2000).

For the first time, there are 10 leading health indicators that reflect the major health concerns in the United States at the beginning of the twenty-first century and that are used to measure the health of the nation. Each leading health indicator (physical activity being one of them) has one or more focus areas from Healthy People 2010 associated with it. The leading health indicators were selected on the basis of their ability to motivate action (in individuals and communities), the availability of data to measure progress, and their importance as public health issues (U.S. Department of Health and Human Services, 2000).

Physical Activity Surveillance in the United States

Several different national surveys are used to track physical activity among many age groups for Healthy People 2010 objectives and public health trends. This section provides a background for understanding and comparing these surveys and their methods.

Existing physical activity assessment (surveillance) questionnaires measure different domains, with some assessing multiple domains. In the past, strategies to promote physical activity emphasized increasing leisure-time physical activity, and consequently, many questionnaires previously focused only on this domain. More recently, strategies to promote physical activity have emphasized the health benefits of all kinds of physical activity. As a result, more physical activity assessment questionnaires are being designed to measure more than one, if not all four, domains of activity.

The CDC–ACSM recommendations for physical activity and public health are considered to be attained when survey respondents report participating in moderate-intensity activity (at least 30 minutes on 5 days or more per week), vigorous-intensity physical activity (at least 20 minutes on 3 days or more per week), or both. Historically, the health benefits of vigorous physical activity were emphasized, leading to the recommendations that adults should be physically active 3 days or more per week for 20 or more minutes on each occasion (U.S. Department of Health and Human Services, 1996). The public health benefits of moderate physical activity first became prominent in the mid 1990s with the publication of the physical activity and public health recommendations from the CDC and the ACSM (Pate et al., 1995) and the U.S. Surgeon General's Report on *Physical Activity and Health* (U.S. Department of Health and Human Services, 1996). Both reports indicate that adults can be classified as meeting the moderate physical activity recommendation if they participate in moderate activity for at least 30 minutes per day on most days of the week.

U.S. national health surveys that assess and track physical activity in individuals typically include questions on physical activity as just one of many health-related topics. Most current national surveys no longer use a more detailed physical activity questionnaire like those typically used in research studies. Furthermore, no national physical activity or health surveys have yet employed observational methods of physical activity assessment, except National Health and Nutrition Examination Survey (NHANES), which in 2003 to 2004 began requiring respondents 6 years and older to wear a physical activity monitor for 7 days. In addition to asking questions about cardiovascular-related physical activities, some national health surveys also query muscle-strengthening and flexibility activities. Travel and transportation surveys, designed to track individual transportation and movement habits, rely on diaries for information on daily walking and bicycling habits.

Once assessment is completed, responses must be summarized for analysis and reporting purposes. Methods to create summary scores from physical activity questionnaires can result in either continuous scores (e.g., total kilocalories expended in physical activity over a given time period) or categorical scores (e.g., low, medium, or high levels of physical activity). A frequently used scoring algorithm in U.S. national surveys relies on an external standard (a pre-established physical activity recommendation or recommendations such as those established by the CDC and ACSM). Individual survey respondents are classified into three categories: sufficiently active (meeting recommendations for either moderate- and/or vigorous-intensity physical activity); insufficiently active (some reported physical activity but not enough to meet existing recommendations); and inactive (no reported physical activity). All public health indicators used for tracking progress toward meeting the Healthy People 2010 objectives, including objectives for physical activity, are categorical summary measures (meets/does not meet the objective).

General Health Surveys

Five national health surveillance systems provide information on physical activity levels of the U.S. population (Table 7.1) and one survey (the SHPPS, discussed in the Policy Surveys Subheading) contains relevant data on policies for physical activity promotion. Each survey uses a different set of questions because the purposes of each survey differ. Compiling and evaluating data from all of these surveys allows a more complete picture of the physical activity levels and trends among Americans than can be obtained from a single survey alone.

Results from these surveys paint a similar picture—most adults and youth are not physically active at recommended levels. Each survey, however, shows slightly different results, and these differences have the potential for confusion. To reduce confusion when citing results, it is recommended that authors provide specific details about the name of the survey, the year of the results, and the domains of physical activity that were assessed. Each of the surveys is described in detail in the following paragraphs.

The Behavioral Risk Factor Surveillance System (BRFSS) began in 1984. The BRFSS is a cross-sectional, random-digit, dialed telephone survey and is the world's largest telephone survey. Information that is collected monthly provides ongoing prevalence data on major behavioral risk factors among adults (18 years and older) who live in households in the United States and its territories, with an emphasis on state-level surveillance and comparisons across states. The BRFSS collects data from approximately 304,000 people (in 2004) in 50 states, the District of Columbia, Puerto Rico, the U.S. Virgin Islands, and Guam. The BRFSS consists of a core set of questions (fixed and rotating cores) and optional modules. The main purpose of the physical activity portion of BRFSS is to track the proportion of

Table 7.1 U.S. National Surveys for Physical Activity

*Survey**	*Target population*	*Data collection mode*	*Data collection frequency*	*Physical activity domains*	*Healthy People 2010 tracking*
BRFSS	Adults (age ≥18 years) in U.S. states, territories, and the District of Columbia. ~304,000 respondents in 2004	Telephone interview (one adult per household)	Annual (fixed core questions asked every year; rotating core questions asked every other year)	Leisure-time domestic transportation	Used for tracking state progress toward some HP2010 objectives
NHIS	Adults and children in U.S. states and the District of Columbia. ~100,000 respondents in 2004; 31,000 adults sampled about physical activity	Personal interview (household interview survey)	Annual	Leisure-time	Objectives 22-1 through 22-5
NHANES	Children and adults in United States ~10,000 respondents in 2001–2002	Personal interview; health examination	Ongoing, 2-year cycle	Leisure-time domestic transportation	—
YRBSS	High school students in United States (grades 9–12). >15,200 respondents in 2003	School-based student self-administered paper survey	Every 2 years	Leisure-time domestic transportation	Objectives 22-6 through 22-11
NHTS	U.S. households. >25,000 respondents	Household survey using Computer-Assisted Telephone Interviewing (CATI) technology	Every 5–7 years	Transportation	Objectives 22-14 and 22-15
SHPPS	U.S. school districts, state education organizations, and classrooms	Self-administered mail survey (state, district levels); computer-assisted personal interviews (school, classroom levels)	Periodic (1994, 2000, 2006)	Physical activity policies and curricula	Objectives 22-8 and 22-12

*Abbreviations: BRFSS: Behavioral Risk Factor Surveillance System; NHIS: National Health Interview Survey; NHANES: National Health and Nutrition Examination Survey; YRBSS: Youth Risk Factor Behavior Surveillance System; NHTS: National Household Transportation Survey; SHPPS: School Health Policies and Programs Study.

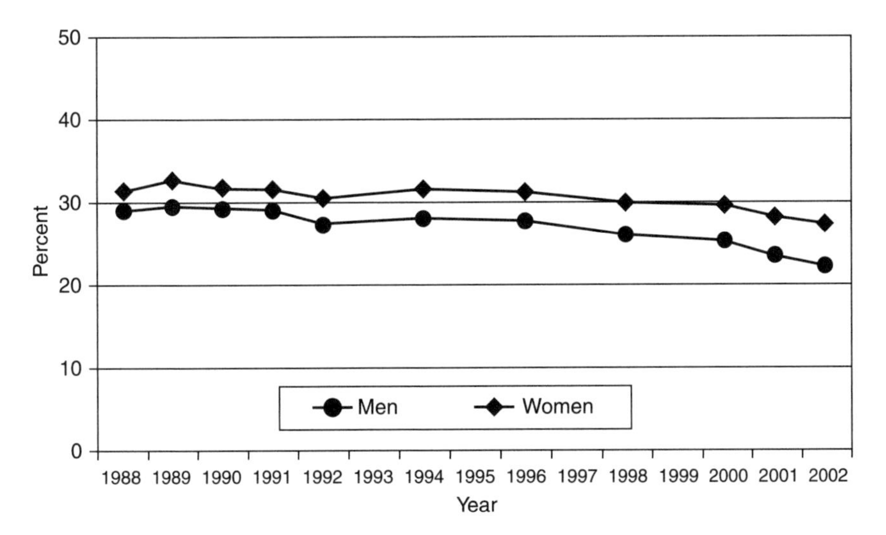

Figure 7.1 Trends in physical inactivity during leisure time among U.S. adults in 35 states, Behavioral Risk Factor Surveillance System 1986–2003 (Ham et al., 2004).

respondents who meet or exceed the public health recommendations for physical activity (e.g., CDC–ACSM recommendations). The main results from the survey are the proportions of American adults that are sufficiently active, insufficiently active, and inactive (BRFSS and CDC–Physical Activity Resources websites). The data in Figure 7.1 show the trend in physical inactivity during leisure-time among U.S. adults in 35 states from BRFSS (Ham et al., 2004).

The NHIS provides statistics about the health of the civilian, non-institutionalized population of the United States and is used to track progress toward national health objectives (currently those of Healthy People 2010). The NHIS is a large cross-sectional (epidemiologic study design), household personal interview survey (approximately 40,000 households and 100,000 respondents) conducted by the National Center for Health Statistics (NCHS), part of the CDC. The ongoing, annual NHIS consists of a core component, which remains the same from year to year (Family, Sample Adult, and Sample Child questionnaires), and a supplement component that changes with changing data needs and funding. Its strength is its capability to look at health characteristics by many demographic and socioeconomic characteristics. The leisure-time physical activity questions are included in the Sample Adult core questionnaire and asked of one randomly selected adult age 18 years and over per family (approximately 30,000 adults annually). The physical activity questions in NHIS provide information about progress in meeting Healthy People 2010 objectives 22-1 through 22-5. The NHIS periodically assesses physical activity using closed-ended questions that ask about physical activity only in the leisure-time domain. The questions used from 1985 to 1996 were revised in 1997 to keep pace with changing data needs. The older surveys asked about 24 types of leisure-time activities, whereas and the newer surveys query about light- to moderate-intensity physical activity, vigorous activity, and strengthening activity, rather than specific modes of activity. Notably, the current NHIS physical activity questions include an assessment of light-to-moderate-intensity physical activities, an approach that differs from that of other questionnaires, which focus only on moderate- and vigorous-intensity activities (NHIS and CDC–Physical Activity Resources websites).

Specialized Health Surveys

The NHANES gathers statistics about the health of Americans using methods of personal interviews and direct physical examination. The NHANES is an NCHS population-based survey designed to collect information on the health and nutrition of the U.S. household population and is substantially smaller (approximately 10,000 persons in 2001–2002) than either the BRFSS or the NHIS, but it provides much more specialized information than can be collected in the other surveys. The NHANES became a continuous survey in 1999, with data released in 2-year cycles (e.g., 1999–2000, 2001–2002, etc.). Although the NHANES collects information on many aspects of health of U.S. children and adults, it has traditionally emphasized relationships among dietary intake, nutrition, and measured health outcomes. The first NHANES (NHANES I) in the 1970s included physical activity questions; however, these have changed over the years, with the current physical activity questions first being used in 1999. For adults, the survey measures three domains (leisure-time, domestic, and transport activities) using separate questions in closed-ended format. For children, only leisure-time physical activity is assessed. Sedentary behavior is also assessed for both children and adults. Notably, the NHANES physical examination of adults currently includes a cardiovascular fitness evaluation (submaximal treadmill test) for persons ages 12 to 49 years and a musculoskeletal fitness test (strength testing; although discontinued after 2003 for those adults age 50 years and older), and, in 1999, a 20-feet timed walk was added for adults age 50 years and older. These evaluations provide the only national data available on physical fitness measures in adults (NHANES and CDC–Physical Activity Resources websites).

The YRBSS is a school-based survey of U.S. high school students (grades 9–12) that monitors six categories of health-risk behavior. YRBSS is a large CDC survey with more than 15,000 respondents from public and private schools in the 50 U.S. states and the District of Columbia. The purpose of the survey is to help determine national prevalence and age-at-initiation of key health-risk behaviors. Physical activity data from the YRBSS are used to monitor progress toward Healthy People 2010 objectives 22-6 through 22-11. Current YRBSS physical activity questions use a closed-ended format and measure factors related to physical activity participation (including moderate- and vigorous-intensity activity, muscle strengthening, and flexibility), physical education class attendance and availability, and television viewing habits. Three domains of activity (leisure-time, transport, and domestic) are measured in the YRBSS. Occupational activity is not believed to be a major source of physical activity in this age group (YRBSS and CDC–Physical Activity Resources websites: http://www.cdc.gov/HealthyYouth/yrbs/; http://www.cdc.gov/nccdphp/dnpa/physical/stats/index.htm).

The NHTS is an integration of two national travel surveys previously conducted: the Nationwide Personal Transportation Survey and the American Travel Survey. It is conducted by the U.S. Department of Transportation and consists of a random-digit, dialed telephone survey and diaries of travel modes, commuting habits, and long-distance trips. The NHTS provides national estimates of daily trip frequency, trip distance, means of transportation, and trip time for persons age 5 years and older. The unit of analysis in this survey is the trip, rather than the individual respondent. For 2001, there were approximately 66,000 households in the final NHTS data set: about 26,000 households in the national sample and 40,000 households from nine add-on areas. The NHTS provides information solely in the transport domain of physical activity. This survey is periodic (currently approximately every 5 years), with survey data available for 1969, 1977, 1983, 1990, 1995, and 2001–2002. Estimates from this survey are used to track progress toward Healthy People 2010 objectives 22-14 and 22-15 regarding walking and bicycling habits in general, and to school in particular. Notably, dozens of regional counterparts to the NHTS are conducted by regional transportation authorities, a federal requirement for those regions to receive federal highway funds. Unlike the BRFSS (with its state-based estimates), these regional surveys are not coordinated by a federal agency to ensure consistent implementation protocols and quality. Therefore, comparisons of results among regions and with national estimates are not advised (NHTS and CDC–Physical Activity Resources websites).

Policy Surveys

The SHPPS is a periodic, national mail survey designed to assess school health policies and programs at the state, school district, and classroom levels. Policies and programs in elementary, middle, and high schools are included. State education agencies, district level representatives, and classroom teachers at designated schools provide the respondent base for this survey. Physical activity questions on the SHPPS are designed to assess physical education curriculum offerings, availability of recess and intramural sports programs, and state and district curricular requirements for physical education. Physical activity data from the SHPPS are used to measure progress toward Healthy People 2010 objectives 22-8 and 22-12 (SHPPS and CDC–Physical Activity Resources websites).

Behavioral Risk Factor Surveillance System—Physical Activity: A Case Study

As noted earlier, the BRFSS is an ongoing health behavior surveillance system that relies on telephone interviews and is designed to allow state health departments to gather representative data for their states. Because national data from other surveillance systems (such as the NHANES and the NHIS) may not be appropriate for extrapolation at the state level, the BRFSS draws samples to allow for state-level estimates and, in some cases, estimates for areas within states. State health authorities use this tool to collect data for surveillance and health planning and policy. A core set of BRFSS questions used for all states allows for comparisons of health behaviors across states.

Since its inception, the BRFSS has revised its physical activity questions one time. Between 1984 and 2000, the questions focused on measurement of only one domain of physical activity, leisure-time, using mainly open-ended questions (Table 7.2). These questions asked respondents to name two primary leisure-time physical activities. For each named activity, respondents were asked to provide frequency and duration of participation. One question regarding physical inactivity in leisure time has remained as part of the core BRFSS questions since 1984, thus allowing for a consistent way to measure trends in physical inactivity.

With the publication of the CDC–ACSM Recommendations for Physical Activity and Public Health (Pate et al., 1995) and the U.S. Surgeon General's Report on *Physical Activity and Health* (U.S. Department of Health and Human Services, 1996), it became clear that a revision of the BRFSS physical activity surveillance questions was necessary for states to better track physical activity behavior that more closely represented those in the new recommendations—specifically including moderate-intensity activities that were performed for at least 10 minutes and that contributed to the 30-minute daily minimum. These recommendations also reflected Healthy People 2000 objectives for physical activity. Importantly, the new recommendations allowed for non-leisure-time physical activity (e.g., walking for transportation, housework) to contribute toward the 30-minute goal, in contrast to the earlier BRFSS questions, which could not adequately assess these non-sport or leisure activities.

Table 7.2 BRFSS Physical Activity Questions, 1984–2000

The next few questions are about exercise, recreation, or physical activities other than your regular job duties.

1. During the past month, did you participate in any physical activities or exercises such as running, calisthenics, golf, gardening, or walking for exercise?
2. What type of physical activity or exercise did you spend the most time doing during the past month?
3. How far did you usually walk/run/jog/swim?
4. How many times per week or per month did you take part in this activity during the past month?
5. And when you took part in this activity, for how many minutes or hours did you usually keep at it?
6. Was there another physical activity or exercise that you participated in during the last month?
7. What other type of physical activity gave you the next most exercise during the past month?
8. How far did you usually walk/run/jog/swim?
9. How many times per week or per month did you take part in this activity?
10. And when you took part in this activity, for how many minutes or hours did you usually keep at it?

Below is the activity-coding list from which the telephone surveyor could choose according to the respondent's answers:

1. Aerobics class
2. Back packing
3. Badminton
4. Basketball
5. Bicycling for pleasure
6. Boating or canoeing, rowing, sailing for pleasure, or camping
7. Bowling
8. Boxing
9. Calisthenics
10. Canoeing/rowing in competition
11. Carpentry
12. Dancing-Aerobics/Ballet
13. Fishing from river bank or boat
14. Gardening(spading, weeding, digging, filling)
15. Golf
16. Handball
17. Healthclub exercise
18. Hiking cross-country
19. Home exercise
20. Horseback riding
21. Hunting large game (deer, elk)
22. Jogging
23. Judo/Karate
24. Mountain climbing
25. Mowing lawn
26. Paddleball
27. Painting/papering house
28. Racquetball
29. Raking lawn
30. Running
31. Rope skipping
32. Scuba diving
33. Skating (ice or roller)
34. Sledding, tobogganing
35. Snorkeling
36. Snow shoeing
37. Snow shoveling
38. Snow blowing
39. Snow skiing
40. Soccer
41. Softball
42. Squash
43. Stair climbing
44. Stream fishing in waders
45. Surfing
46. Swimming laps
47. Table tennis
48. Tennis
49. Touch football
50. Volley ball
51. Walking
52. Water skiing
53. Weight lifting
54. Other
55. Bicycling machine exercise
56. Rowing machine exercise

Table 7.3 BRFSS Physical Activity Questions, 2001 to present

1. During the past month, other than your regular job, did you participate in any physical activities or exercises such as running, calisthenics, golf, gardening, or walking for exercise?
2. When you are at work, which of the following best describes what you do?
   Mostly sitting or standing
   Mostly walking
   Mostly heavy labor or physically demanding work
3. We are interested in two types of physical activity: moderate and vigorous. Vigorous activities cause large increases in breathing or heart rate, whereas moderate activities cause small increases in breathing or heart rate.
4. Now thinking about the moderate activities you do, in a usual week, do you do moderate activities for at least 10 minutes at a time, such as brisk walking, bicycling, vacuuming, gardening, or anything else that causes some increase in breathing or heart rate?
5. How many days per week do you do these moderate activities for at least 10 minutes at a time?
6. On days when you do moderate activities for at least 10 minutes at a time, how much total time per day do you spend doing these activities?
7. Now thinking about the vigorous activities you do, in a usual week, do you do vigorous activities for at least 10 minutes at a time, such as running, aerobics, heavy yard work, or anything else that causes large increases in breathing or heart rate?
8. How many days per week do you do these vigorous activities for at least 10 minutes at a time?
9. On days when you do vigorous activities for at least 10 minutes at a time, how much total time do you spend doing these activities?

Optional BRFSS Physical Activity Questions for State Use

10. In a usual week, do you walk for at least 10 minutes at a time for recreation, exercise, to get to and from places, or for any other reason?
11. How many days per week do you walk for at least 10 minutes at a time?
12. On days when you walk for at least 10 minutes at a time, how much total time do you spend walking?
13. In a usual week, do you do any activities designed to increase muscle strength or tone, such as lifting weights, pull-ups, push-ups, or sit-ups?
14. How many days per week do you do these activities?

Thus, in 2001, the BRFSS implemented a new set of questions to capture data on three key physical activity domains: leisure-time, domestic, and transportation (Table 7.3). These questions were designed to assess frequency and duration of both moderate and vigorous activities in these domains. With the new questions, the BRFSS no longer assessed specific types of physical activities in which people participate. Currently, the BRFSS also queries occupational physical activity, but because of technical reasons, such activity does not contribute to a physical activity summary score. That is, the occupational activity question asks respondents to classify their activity as mostly sitting or standing, mostly walking, or mostly heavy lifting or physically demanding work; these data cannot be easily translated for their contribution toward meeting current recommendations for physical activity.

Methodological Issues in Physical Activity Surveillance

The aforementioned case study illustrates several methodological issues in physical activity surveillance. First, questionnaires, with their attendant limitations (for additional discussion, *see* Chapters 2 and 3), are most feasible when surveying large numbers of individuals (>300,000 in the 2004 BRFSS), although subgroups can be targeted for additional, more precise assessments (e.g., submaximal treadmill testing and 20-feet timed walk in smaller samples in the NHANES). Additionally, physical activity surveillance is typically part of a larger surveillance that includes other health parameters; therefore, time constraints during the interview process limits the number of physical activity questions that can be asked. The questions used also may not have been extensively tested for reliability and validity; rather, they may have been developed based on expert opinion and have face validity. Tests of reliability and validity may be conducted after the questions have already been implemented. For example, the BRFSS occupational activity questions have been routinely quantified in health surveys for state use since 2001; however, findings on its reliability were published in 2005 (Yore et al., 2005).

As mentioned previously, surveillance can capture physical activity in one or more domains: leisure-time, occupational, household, and transportation activities. Thus, data from different studies may not be comparable if they assess different domains of physical activity. Data at different time-points from the same survey also may not be comparable. In the case study mentioned earlier, prior to 2001, the BRFSS assessed only leisure-time physical activity but, subsequently, assessed moderate- and vigorous-intensity physical activity in non-leisure activities as well (Table 7.2). This was to keep pace with research studies showing that such activities can contribute to health benefits (Pate et al., 1995). Therefore, the prevalence of individuals meeting physical activity recommendations prior to and after 2001 cannot be directly compared, because of the change of questions. To have a consistent measure of physical activity patterns over the long term, the BRFSS did maintain a single question on physical inactivity that did not change in 2001, allowing long-term trends in physical inactivity to be directly compared (Figure 7.1).

It is interesting to compare physical activity patterns across different countries in the world. However, as discussed in the previous paragraph, comparability across surveys in the United States and even across time within the same survey can be difficult; cross-country comparisons are likely to be even more complex. Efforts have begun to address physical activity surveillance across countries. In 1996, an international group of physical activity assessment experts formed a working group to develop a reliable, valid questionnaire for measuring physical activity that was suitable for both surveillance, as well as research, in different countries. This resulted in the development of the International Physical Activity Questionnaire (IPAQ; International Physical Activity Questionnaire website: http://www.ipaq.ki.se/ipaq.htm), which has been tested in 12 countries and shows reasonable reliability and validity for physical activity surveillance in adults (Craig et al., 2003).

Personal Perspective

Physical activity surveillance will continue to grow in prominence and importance in the foreseeable future. Policy development and research progress depend on consistent, understandable assessments of prevalence and trends in physical activity and inactivity behavior.

Although the level of physical activity surveillance and the complexity of the surveillance systems in the United States are at a historical apex, advances must be made in several key areas. First, an instrument, or preferably a system, that is internationally accepted and implemented is needed to allow country-level comparisons of physical activity prevalence and trends. The cultural and sociodemographic differences among countries are among the factors that can affect instrument compatibility. Initial attempts to develop an internationally standardized instrument, the IPAQ, have begun (Craig et al., 2003) and have provided a base on which the next generation of instruments can be built. Such international tools must at a minimum provide data on physical activity that coincide with health-related recommendations.

Surveillance indicators can and do change. As new scientific knowledge becomes available, existing indicators and systems must be reassessed and, if appropriate, changed to match the current science. The 2001 shift in the BRFSS physical activity surveillance instrument is an example of this point. Importantly, a balance must be struck between making changes in existing tools to match emerging science and maintaining constancy to be able to effectively assess trends. Too many changes or changes that are too substantial can result in a loss of continuing information that would show trends. Conversely, not making changes can result in the omission of important indicators or the use of indicators that do not match the needs of policymakers and health authorities.

Another important future need in physical activity surveillance is the development of indicators for surveillance of the environment and policy. Existing systems have allowed for effective surveillance of physical activity participation by individuals. The environmental level factors that may support or inhibit the physical activity behaviors of individuals are also interesting. The recommendations on increasing physical activity from the Task Force on Community Preventive Services (Kahn et al., 2001) reflect the importance of the environment in influencing physical activity. The strategies recommended for promoting physical activity include environmental interventions such as access to places for physical activity along with an emphasis on neighborhood factors (e.g., street lighting, sidewalks) that have been shown to affect physical activity behaviors. Without validated surveillance systems designed to monitor the prevalence of, and trends in, such environmental interventions, there is no way to monitor progress in this critical area. With the growing understanding that environmental factors affect physical activity behavior, surveillance systems designed to address environmental supports and barriers should be developed, tested, and implemented.

References

Behavioral Risk Factor Surveillance System: http://www.cdc.gov/brfss/ (accessed August 15 2007).

Centers for Disease Control and Prevention, Physical Activity Resources for Health Professionals: http://www.cdc.gov/nccdphp/dnpa/physical/health_professionals/index.htm. (accessed August 15 2007).

Craig CL, Marshall AL, Sjostrom M, et alP. 2003. International physical activity questionnaire: 12-country reliability and validity. *Med Sci Sports Exerc* 35(8):1381–95.

Ham SA, Yore MM, Fulton JE, Kohl HW. 2004. Trends in physical inactivity during leisure time, 35 states and District of Columbia, United States – 1988–2002. *MMWR* 53:76–81.

Healthy People 2010: www.healthypeople.gov/About (accessed August 15 2007).

International Physical Activity Questionnaire: http://www.ipaq.ki.se/ (accessed August 15 2007).

Kahn EB, Ramsey LT, Brownson RC, et al. 2002. The effectiveness of interventions to increase physical activity. *Am J Prev Med* 22: 73–107.

Kahn EB, Ramsey LT, Heath GW, et al. 2001. Increasing Physical Activity: A Report on Recommendations of the Task Force on Community Preventive Services. *MMWR* 50(RR-18): 1–16.

Merriam-Webster Online Dictionary: www.m-w.com/ (accessed August 15 2007).

National Health and Nutrition Examination Survey: www.cdc.gov/nchs/nhanes.htm (accessed August 15 2007).

National Health Interview Survey: www.cdc.gov/nchs/nhis.htm (accessed May 22 2005).

National Household Travel Survey: http://nhts.ornl.gov/index.shtml (accessed August 15 2007).

Pate RR, Pratt M, Blair SN, et al. 1995 Physical activity and public health: a recommendation from the Centers for Disease Control and Prevention and the American College of Sports Medicine. *JAMA* 273:402–407.

School Health Policies and Programs Study: www.cdc.gov/HealthyYouth/shpps (accessed August 15 2007).

Teutsh SM, Churchill RE (Eds.). 2000. *Principles and Practice of Public Health Surveillance.* New York, NY: Oxford University Press.

Thacker SB, Berkelman RL. 1988. Public health surveillance in the United States. *Epidemiol Rev* 10:164–90.

U.S. Department of Health and Human Services. 1996. *Physical Activity and Health: A Report of the Surgeon General.* Atlanta, GA: U.S. Department of Health and Human Services, Centers for Disease Control and Prevention, National Center for Chronic Disease Prevention and Health Promotion.

U.S. Department of Health and Human Services. 2000. *Healthy People 2010: Understanding and Improving Health.* 2nd ed. Washington, DC: U.S. Government Printing Office.

Yore MM, Ham SA, Ainsworth BE, Macera CA, Jones DA, Kohl HW III. 2005. Occupational physical activity: reliability and comparison of activity levels. *JPAH.* 3: 358–65.Youth Risk Behavior Surveillance System: www.cdc.gov/HealthyYouth/yrbs/index.htm (accessed August 15 2007).

II

Epidemiologic Data

8

Physical Activity, Fitness, and Delayed Mortality

Michael J. Lamonte
and Steven N. Blair

"Few of us will approach these [Olympic athlete] levels of performance in our own physical endeavors. The good news is that we do not have to scale Olympian heights to achieve significant health benefits. We can improve the quality of our lives through a lifelong practice of moderate amounts [and intensities] of regular physical activity."

—David Satcher, M.D., Ph.D.; Philip R. Lee, M.D.; Florence Griffith Joyner, Atlanta, GA (U.S. Department of Health and Human Services, 1996)

As noted by Satcher and colleagues in the Forward of the seminal report on Physical Activity and Health by the U.S. Surgeon General, few individuals will ever achieve the level of athletic performance displayed by participants competing in the Olympic games, but everyone can benefit from an active way of living (U.S. Department of Health and Human Services, 1996). In fact, human evolution has depended on a physically active lifestyle (Eaton et al., 1988), and our genetic constitution has not changed significantly in the past 10,000 years (Macaulay, Richards et al., 1999). Thus, existence in a modern world where physical activity has largely been engineered out of daily living habits is an unnatural aberration from our evolutionary constitution. Therefore, a sedentary way of life should logically be unhealthy to our species, and considerable evidence indicates that sedentary habits and low cardiorespiratory fitness (CRF) are among the strongest predictors of premature mortality (U.S. Department of Health and Human Services, 1996). Indeed, Hahn et al. (1990) estimated that more than 250,000 deaths annually could be attributed to physical inactivity, a number comparable to the deaths attributed to other established predictors of mortality such as hypertension, hypercholesterolemia, obesity, and smoking.

A large amount of evidence amassed from observational studies indicates that low levels of physical activity and CRF are associated with increased mortality risk, and these data have thoroughly been reviewed elsewhere (U.S. Department of Health and Human Services, 1996; Lee and Skerrett, 2001). In this chapter, we draw from selected epidemiological studies to broadly illustrate this line of research and to discuss specific issues that must be considered when interpreting and generalizing existing study findings. We also summarize available data on physical activity, CRF, and mortality risk in several population subgroups according to their demographic and health status. Because other chapters review the evidence for an association between physical activity or CRF and the major causes of mortality, we further delimit our focus to only investigations of all-cause mortality as the study outcome.

When possible, we comment on the characteristics of the exposure–response gradient. Potential biological mechanisms that may explain the lower death rates from specific chronic diseases observed among active and fit individuals, compared to their sedentary and unfit counterparts, are covered in detail in other chapters of this book.

An important distinction to make is that physical activity refers to a behavior—specifically, body movement that occurs from skeletal muscle contraction and results in increased energy expenditure above resting metabolic rate (U.S. Department of Health and Human Services, 1996). It is now accepted that activity-related energy expenditure, or the total dose of physical activity, appears to be more important for overall health benefits than the specific type of physical activity performed (e.g., walking, running, cycling; *see* Chapter 4 for additional discussion of this issue) (LaMonte and Ainsworth, 2001). Physical fitness is a set of physiological attributes that may be enhanced through participation in regular physical activity (U.S. Department of Health and Human Services, 1996). The major component of physical fitness that has been related to mortality risk is CRF or "aerobic power." Several factors influence CRF, including age, sex, health status, genetics, and habitual physical activity level. In fact, in one study, more than 70% of the variation in maximal treadmill exercise duration was accounted for by detailed records of habitual physical activity (Paffenbarger et al., 1993). Thus, CRF can be used as an objective, surrogate measure of recent physical activity patterns, with the understanding that other factors also underlie the expression of CRF. Additionally, it is possible that other components of physical fitness—such as muscular strength or endurance—may predict mortality risk; however, few data from large prospective studies currently exist to support these relationships. Therefore, only data relating levels of physical activity or CRF with mortality risk are presented here.

Physical Activity and Mortality Risk in Men

Research on physical activity and mortality did not begin in earnest until the second half of the twentieth century with the seminal studies by Professor Jeremy Morris on male British Civil Servants (Morris and Heady, 1953), by Professor Henry Taylor on male U.S. railroad employees (Taylor et al., 1962), and by Professor Ralph Paffenbarger, Jr., on male San Francisco longshoremen (Paffenbarger et al., 1987). Physical activity exposures were based on job classification and were categorized according to the level of effort involved in the work performed—for example, light effort (clerks), intermediate effort (masons, bricklayers, railroad switchmen), and heavy effort (iron miners, boilermakers, railroad section men, dockworkers). In each study, men who performed intermediate and heavy effort job activities had a 48% to 49% and a 63% to 69% lower risk of mortality, respectively, than men whose jobs required light effort. The influence of confounding factors such as smoking and blood pressure was considered only in the study of longshoreman; the inverse association between occupational physical activity and mortality persisted thereafter ($p < 0.001$). The inverse gradient of mortality risk across job categories requiring incremental physical effort that was seen in these early studies of British and U.S. men generally has been consistent with subsequent observations by later investigations on occupational physical activity and mortality in which a variety of confounding factors were also considered (U.S. Department of Health and Human Services, 1996; Lee and Skerrett, 2001).

Classifying occupational physical activity levels according to job title provides only a crude physical activity exposure because this approach assumes that all persons expend a similar amount of energy to perform a given job task, and it does not account for non-occupational forms of physical activity-related energy expenditure that may contribute to lower mortality risk. As the nature of occupational work changed with the industrialization movement throughout the twentieth century, fewer people performed hard physical labor at work, and more workers spent the majority of their day sitting or standing and doing light work. Thus, it seemed logical to expand physical activity epidemiology studies to include leisure-time activity exposures. As such, Professor Ralph Paffenbarger, Jr., initiated in the early 1960s a prospective investigation of lifestyle characteristics and health in men who entered Harvard College during the period from 1916 to 1950. In either 1962 or 1966, these men completed an extensive baseline health and lifestyle questionnaire that included several questions aimed at quantifying energy expended in walking, sports, and other leisure-time activities (Pereira et al., 1997). From 1962 to 1978, Paffenbarger recorded 1,413 deaths in a cohort of 16,936 Harvard alumni who were ages 35 to 74 years and healthy at baseline (Paffenbarger et al., 1986). When the men were grouped on their baseline total leisure-time physical activity-related energy expenditure (from <500 to ≥3500 kcal/week, by ≈500 kcal/week increments), a significant steep inverse gradient in age-adjusted mortality risk was observed across incremental categories of energy expenditure. Compared to men who expended less than 500 kcal/week, relative risk (RR) estimates decreased from 0.78 in men who expended 500 to 999 kcal/week to 0.46 in men who expended 3,000 to 3499 kcal/week, and were 0.62 in men who expended 3500 kcal/week or more. After further adjusting for potential confounding factors such as baseline differences in blood pressure, smoking status, body weight, and premature parental death, men who reported expending 2000 kcal/week or more in leisure-time physical activity had a 23% (95% confidence intervals [CI], 13%–32%) lower mortality risk during follow-up than men whose activity level was less than 2000 kcal/week. Based on the observed exposure prevalence and associated mortality risk in the population sample of male Harvard alumni, Paffenbarger computed attributable fractions for each exposure to estimate the number of deaths that would have been avoided if no men were exposed to the adverse condition. Sedentary lifestyle (<2000 kcal/week) accounted for 16% of deaths, second only to being a current smoker, which accounted for 23% of deaths. Data from the Harvard Alumni Health Study, along with the studies on occupational physical activity, established the foundation of epidemiological evidence supporting physical activity as an important determinant of mortality. The extent of the quantitative approach to assessing physical activity used in the Harvard Alumni Health Study was novel, and this further allowed for characterizing the dose–response between activity-related energy expenditure and mortality risk, for identifying a potential threshold of physical activity for informing public health recommendations, and for estimation of the population mortality burden conferred by sedentary living habits, based on the study definition. An important issue to consider when interpreting dose–response relationships between physical activity and mortality is the summary units for the physical activity exposure (LaMonte and Ainsworth, 2001). We illustrate this point using physical activity and mortality data among men in the Harvard Alumni Health Study (Paffenbarger et al., 1986) and the British Regional Heart Study (Wannamethee et al., 1998). Both studies generally supported a strong inverse gradient of mortality risk across incremental categories of physical activity. The Harvard study showed about a 40% lower age-adjusted mortality risk at an energy expenditure of about 1500 kcal/week, whereas the British study showed a similar reduction in age-adjusted mortality risk at a physical activity level defined as "occasional." The unitless index that was used to categorize physical activity in the British study prevents comparison of the dose–response between the two studies and illustrates some of the difficulty in combining data from different studies regarding the dose of physical activity required to reduce mortality risk in middle-age men (*see also* Chapters 2 and 4 for additional discussion of this issue).

Physical Activity and Mortality Risk in Women

Although early epidemiological studies on physical activity and mortality were conducted almost exclusively in men, more recent investigations have examined this issue in women. One of the largest and most influential studies on women's health has been the Nurses' Health Study I, a prospective follow-up of more than 120,000 U.S. female registered nurses who were ages 30 to 55 years at the time of completing an extensive baseline health questionnaire in 1976 (Rockhill et al., 2001). Post-baseline questionnaires were administered every 2 years, and physical activity was first assessed in 1980 with questions similar to those used in the Harvard Alumni Health Study. Rockhill et al. (2001) examined the association between physical activity and mortality risk in 80,348 women followed for mortality between 1982 and 1996, during which 4,746 deaths occurred. Physical activity information was updated every 2 years between 1980 and 1992 and was categorized as the average number of hours per week in moderate- to vigorous-intensity activities (<1, 1–1.9, 2–3.9, 4–6.9, ≥7 hr/week). Physical activity was significantly and inversely associated with mortality, with age-adjusted risk estimates starting at 1.0 (referent) in the group with less than 1 hr/week and ranged from 0.76 in the group with 1 to 1.9 hr/week to 0.62 in the group with 7 hr/week or more. Further adjustment for smoking, alcohol intake, body size, and postmenopausal hormone therapy slightly attenuated the risk estimates but did not eliminate the significant inverse association between physical activity and mortality (p-trend <0.001). Other large prospective studies of women (Kaplan et al., 1996; Kushi et al., 1997; Barengo et al., 2004) have reported findings that are consistent with the observations in the Nurses' Health Study.

Some studies have not shown an association between physical activity and mortality risk in women. For example, in the Framingham Heart Study, (Kannel and Sorlie, 1979) 2,311 women ages 35 to 64 years completed a physical activity questionnaire in 1955 to 1956 and were then followed for 14 years, during which 269 deaths occurred. No association was noted between reported levels of physical activity and mortality risk. In this study, physical activity was quantified as the sum of time (hours per day) spent sleeping and in occupational and sport activities, which was weighted for the estimated energy cost of the specific activities. Interestingly, the questionnaire items and associated energy costs had originally been developed and validated in men (Reiff et al., 1967). Thus, one possible explanation for the null finding may have been misclassification of energy costs in women. However, in a later follow-up of these women, from 1969 to 1973 until 1985 to 1989, physical activity was now found to be significantly related to lower mortality during follow-up (Sherman et al., 1994). The authors attributed the difference in findings to greater statistical power in their later analyses.

In another study, 6,620 Canadian women age 30 years or older completed an extensive baseline questionnaire to quantify usual daily physical activity-related energy expenditure during the past year (Weller and Corey, 1998). Follow-up was for 7 years, during which 449 women died. Age-adjusted odds ratios (95% CI) were 1.0 (referent), 0.86 (0.66–1.13), 0.68 (0.51–0.91), and 0.73 (0.54–1.00) across incremental fourths of total energy expenditure. However, further investigation revealed that of the 8.2 kcal/kg/day average daily total energy expenditure, only 1.2 kcal/kg/day (15%) was spent in sport and leisure activities, whereas 7.0 kcal/kg/day (85%) was spent in non-leisure activities (e.g., house and family care). Figure 8.1 shows age-adjusted estimates of mortality risk according to fourths of leisure and non-leisure physical activity. There was no association between mortality and leisure activity; however, a significant inverse association was observed between non-leisure activity and mortality risk. Similarly to the Framingham study, the physical activity questionnaire used in the Canadian study was based on an instrument originally developed and

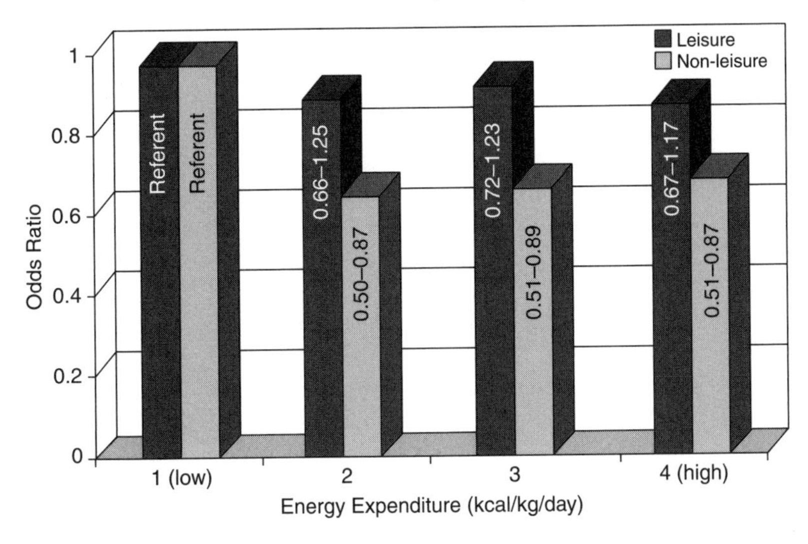

Figure 8.1 Age-adjusted odds ratios of all-cause mortality by physical activity (PA) levels (leisure and non-leisure) in 6620 initially healthy women (449 deaths) followed for 7 years—Canadian Fitness Survey, 1981–1988. (Numbers on bars are 95% confidence interval [CI].)

validated in men (Taylor et al., 1978). Because computing energy expended in leisure activity can lead to an underestimation of physical activity-related energy expenditure in those women whose primary daily physical activity was house and family care, the true association between physical activity and mortality in these women may have been missed when examining only leisure activity. The data from the Framingham and Canadian studies illustrate an important methodological issue: the influence that physical activity assessment methods can have in studies of mortality risk in women (*see also* Chapter 2 for additional discussion of this issue) (LaMonte and Ainsworth, 2001). The use of assessment methods that are less ideal for measuring physical activity in women may partly explain why a significant inverse association between physical activity and mortality is less consistently observed in women than men and, when observed, why the effect sizes tend to be smaller in women than in men (U.S. Department of Health and Human Services, 1996; Lee and Skerrett, 2001).

Cardiorespiratory Fitness and Mortality Risk

As discussed in Chapters 2 and 3, and as illustrated earlier, questionnaire-based physical activity assessment can result in misclassification on exposure and dilution of the exposure–outcome relationship, particularly in women. CRF can be assessed more objectively than physical activity and, thus, may more accurately reflect the consequences of a sedentary lifestyle. One of the first large-scale epidemiological studies to examine the relationship between CRF expsoures and mortality risk has been the Aerobics Center Longitudinal Study (ACLS), which is a prospective follow-up of individuals who have had a preventive health examination at the Cooper Clinic in Dallas, Texas (Blair et al., 1989). Our initial report was based on 10,244 men and 3,120 women who were apparently healthy at baseline, at which time they completed detailed health and lifestyle questionnaires and had clinical measures, including fasting blood chemistry, resting blood pressure, and a maximal treadmill exercise test (Blair et al., 1989). CRF was categorized as fifths of the age- and sex-specific distribution of maximal exercise duration. During an average follow-up of 8 years, we recorded 240 deaths in men and 43 deaths in women. Figure 8.2 shows a significant steep inverse gradient in age-adjusted mortality rates across incremental categories of CRF in women and men. The inverse pattern of association between CRF and mortality risk persisted in both sexes after accounting for differences in baseline clinical characteristics and for early mortality. In multivariable analyses that adjusted for differences in age, smoking habits, fasting levels of serum total cholesterol and glucose, systolic blood pressure, and family history of CHD, women and men in the upper four-fifths of CRF had a 52% (95% CI, 35%–77%) and 63% (95% CI, 35%–77%) lower mortality risk, respectively, than their peers in the lowest fifth of CRF. Following the methods used by Professor Paffenbarger, we also computed attributable fractions for mortality based on the observed exposure prevalence and associated RRs for mortality. Approximately 9% of the deaths in men and 15% of the deaths in women could have been avoided if no study participant had been exposed to low fitness (i.e., lowest fifth of treadmill performance).

The ACLS has strengths that minimize two sources of potential bias that are common concerns in prospective observational studies: confounding and reverse causation. By design, a prospective study aims to assess the exposure variable(s) before the occurrence of the study outcome. Confounding occurs when a potential source of extraneous variation in the exposure–response relationship is not adequately accounted for in the analysis. Control for confounding may not be complete when information on potential confounding factors is obtained by questionnaire and thus is subject to recall error, or when additional but unmeasured factors influence the exposure–outcome relationship. Reverse causation occurs when subclinical disease is undetected at baseline and affects the exposure by limiting a

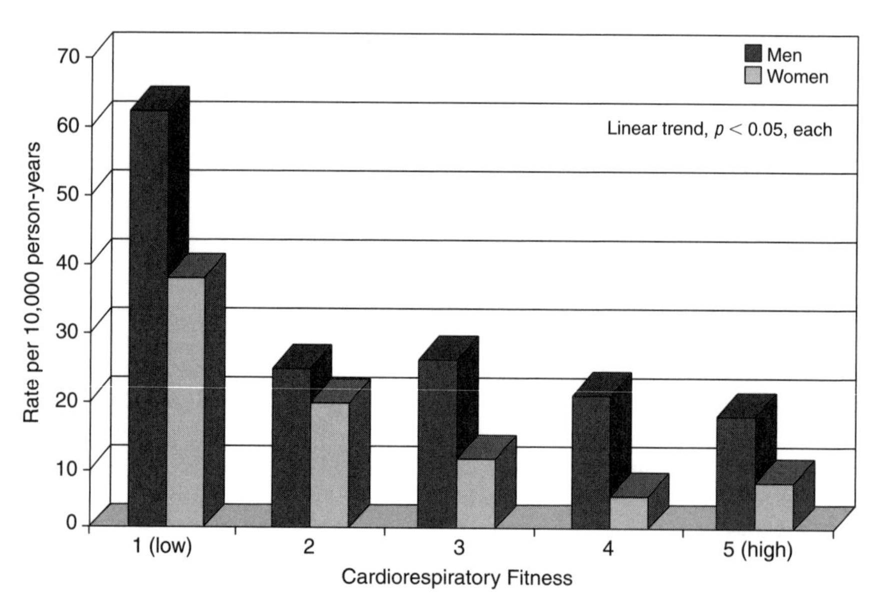

Figure 8.2 Age-adjusted rates of all-cause mortality by cardiorespiratory fitness (CRF) levels in 13,344 initially healthy men (240 deaths) and women (43 deaths) followed for an average of 8 years—Aerobics Center Longitudinal Study, 1970–1985.

participant's habitual physical activity level or exercise test performance. This could selectively increase the death rates among those with low physical activity or CRF levels and, therefore, result in a spuriously high inverse association between the exposure and outcome. Reverse causation can be difficult to address in large-population epidemiological studies when the exposure assessment is performed exclusively by questionnaire. However, in the ACLS, each participant completed a comprehensive baseline history and thorough physical examination with a physician and had several clinical measures, including fasting blood chemistries, resting and exercise electrocardiograms, and blood pressures. In the analysis summarized earlier, to minimize bias from reverse causation, individuals were excluded if they did not achieve at least 85% of age-predicted maximal heart rate during the exercise test, if they had an abnormal resting or exercise electrocardiogram, or if they had a history of physician-diagnosed disease at baseline. These objective assessments increase our confidence that subclinical disease was not a major issue in our analysis. Furthermore, we found nearly identical estimates and patterns of association when analyses were repeated in subgroups of participants who died early in follow-up and who died later in the follow-up. Additionally, we were able to account for the potential confounding influence of blood pressure, glucose, lipids, and body size by using measured clinical phenotypes rather than self-reported information. There is some debate, however, whether blood pressure, glucose, lipids, and body size represent true confounders or whether they represent intermediate mechanisms through which CRF decreases mortality risk. If the latter is true, adjustment for these factors would dilute the true exposure-outcome relationship, and thus result in a conservative estimate of the association between physical activity or CRF and mortality. Thus, we believe that confounding and reverse causation are unlikely explanations for the strong inverse mortality gradient observed across levels of CRF in the ACLS.

Additional confidence in the initial observations on CRF and mortality in the ACLS has been found in recent investigations in other population samples that have been consistent in showing an inverse pattern of association between CRF and mortality risk in women as well as in men (Laukkanen et al., 2001; Myers et al., 2002; Gulati et al., 2003; Mora et al., 2003). For example, Laukkanen et al. (2001) examined the association between CRF and mortality risk in 1,294 Finnish men ages 42 to 61 years who were followed an average of 11 years, during which 124 men died. Whereas in essentially all other prospective studies CRF is estimated from submaximal heart rate responses, maximal exercise duration, or the maximal work rate achieved during the exercise test, a unique aspect of this study was that CRF was quantified as metabolic equivalent (MET) levels of maximal oxygen uptake (1 MET = 3.5 mL O_2 uptake/kg/minute) measured with indirect calorimetry. Age- and examination year-adjusted RRs (95% CI) for mortality were 1.0 (referent), 1.47 (0.71–3.01), 2.79 (1.44–5.39), and 3.85 (2.02–7.32), (p-trend < 0.001) across CRF categories of more than 10.6, 9.3 to 10.6, 7.9 to 9.2, and less than 7.9 METs. Two recent studies have confirmed observations in the ACLS of significantly lower mortality rates in women with higher levels of CRF. In one of the longest mortality follow-up studies to date, Mora et al. (2003) related CRF levels with 20-year death rates in 2,994 women (427 deaths) who had participated in the Lipid Research Clinics Prevalence Study. CRF was quantified as METs estimated from the duration of a treadmill exercise test to 90% or more of age- and physical activity-standardized heart rate response. On average, each 1-MET increment in treadmill performance was associated with a 10% (95% CI, 6%–15%) lower multivariable adjusted mortality risk. Similarly, after accounting for conventional risk predictors, Gulati et al. (2003) observed an average of 17% (95% CI, 11%–22%) lower mortality risk for each 1-MET increment in maximal treadmill exercise performance in 5,721 women older than age 35 years who were followed an average of 8 years (180 deaths).

Physical Activity, Cardiorespiratory Fitness, and Mortality: Influence of Age and Ethnicity

Studies of physical activity or CRF and mortality risk generally have included only middle-age, non-Hispanic white individuals, with few data on older individuals or those from different ethnic subgroups. The few data do support that higher levels of physical activity are associated with delayed mortality in older adults. Paffenbarger and associates (Paffenbarger et al., 1986) reported that within age groups of 35 to 49, 50 to 59, 60 to 69, and 70 to 84 years, mortality risk was 21% to 49% lower in men whose weekly energy expenditure was 2000 kcal/week or more compared to less than 500 kcal/week. Fried et al. (1998) showed a significant inverse mortality gradient across incremental levels of physical activity-related energy expenditure in 5,201 women and men age 65 years or older who were followed for 5 years in the Cardiovascular Health Study. After adjusting for age, race, and other measured clinical risk factors, mortality risk was 44% (95% CI, 26%–57%) lower in participants who were in the highest (≥1890 kcal/week) compared to the lowest (≤67.5 kcal/week) physical activity category. In a 17-year follow-up of women and men age 60 years or older at baseline who were living in Alameda County, California, mortality risk was 28% (95% CI, 8%–43%) and 27% (95% CI, 8%–42%) lower in active compared to inactive participants ages 60 to 69 years and 70 years or older, respectively (Kaplan et al., 1987).

The prognostic value of CRF assessed by maximal exercise testing also has been examined in older individuals. In a recent study of 7,354 medically stable adults age 65 years or older who completed a symptom-limited maximal exercise treadmill test at the Cleveland Clinic and were then followed an average of 3.7 years (842 deaths), those whose CRF (based on peak exercise work rate) was in the upper four-fifths of the age- and sex-standardized sample distribution had a 63% lower risk (95% CI, 55%–68%) of mortality than participants in the lowest fifth of CRF (Messinger-Rapport et al., 2003). We recently extended mortality surveillance in the ACLS up to 2003, which has allowed us to conduct a preliminary analysis of CRF and mortality in adults ages 60 to 99 years. A total of 3,046 men and 997 women who were ages 60 to 99 years at baseline were followed for an average of 14 years. Those participants who were in the lowest fifth of maximal treadmill exercise performance were classified as unfit, and the other participants were classified as fit. Age-adjusted mortality rates were significantly lower in fit compared to unfit men grouped into age categories of 60 to 69 years (693 deaths) and 70 to 99 years (151 deaths) (Figure 8.3). Death rates also were significantly lower in fit than unfit women ages 60 to 69 years (112 deaths) but did not differ by CRF level in women ages 70 to 99 years, among whom the number of deaths was small ($n = 32$). Adjustment for smoking and prevalent disease at baseline did not materially change the associations observed in men or in women. Based on available data, it appears that higher levels of physical activity and CRF also are associated with significantly lower mortality risk in older adult population samples, consistent with the findings from younger and middle-age cohorts.

It is plausible that cultural differences in physical activity patterns or in the interaction of physical activity and other risk predictors may result in race/ethnic differences in associations between physical activity and mortality. A prospective study comparing race or ethnicity-specific associations between physical activity or CRF and mortality among race/ethnic subgroups within a large diverse population sample does not exist. However, in the Cardiovascular Health Study (Fried et al., 1998), the Alameda County Study (Kaplan et al., 1987), the Corpus Christi Heart Project (Steffen-Batey et al., 2000), and in NHANES I (Fang et al., 2005), inverse associations between physical activity and mortality were observed after statistical adjustment for differences in race/ethnicity. Furthermore, significant

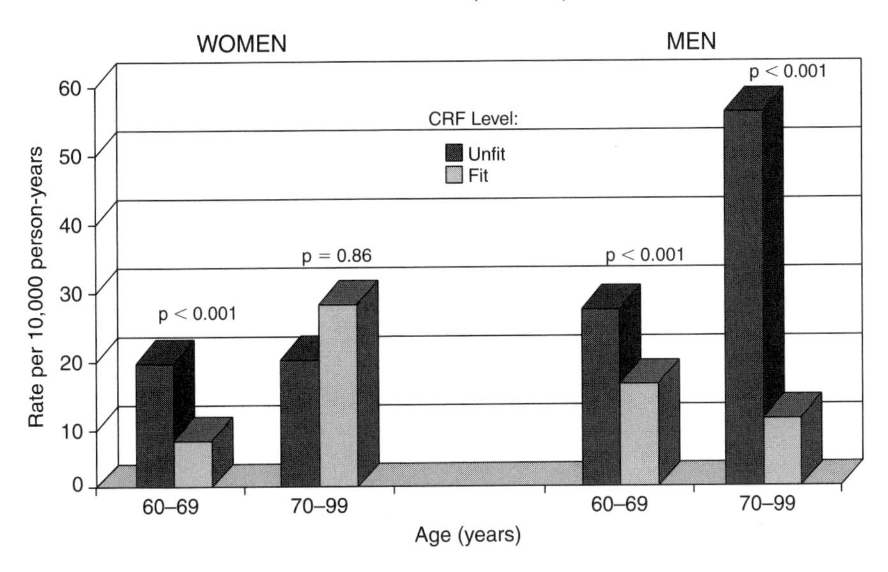

Figure 8.3 Age-adjusted rates of all-cause mortality by CRF levels in 3046 men (844 deaths) and 997 women (144 deaths), ages 60 to 69 and 70 to 99 years, who were initially healthy and were followed an average of 14 years—Aerobics Center Longitudinal Study, 1970–2003.

inverse associations between physical activity and mortality have been reported in population samples of Japanese men living in Hawaii (Hakim et al., 1998), women and men living in Barcelona, Spain (Ruigomez et al., 1995), black women and men in the Adventist Health Study (Fraser et al., 1997), and women and men living in Eastern Finland (Laukkanen et al., 2001; Barengo et al., 2004). The hypothesis that race/ethnicity does not modify the association between physical activity and mortality has yet to be definitively tested. To do so would require a prospective study with a large ethnically diverse population and adequate statistical power to examine race-specific associations between physical activity and mortality. This should be a focus of future research aimed at improving public health physical activity recommendations. Notwithstanding, the consistency of available data showing an inverse association between physical activity and mortality among individuals from different race/ethnic population subgroups increases our confidence that differences in race/ethnicity are not a major source of variation in this relationship.

Physical Activity, Cardiorespiratory Fitness, and Mortality: Low-Risk Versus High-Risk Populations

Evidence of the inverse relationship between physical activity or CRF on mortality risk has been observed in population subgroups that could be considered low-risk on the basis of healthy lifestyle practices or high-risk because of the presence of adverse risk factor profiles or clinically manifest disease. Lindsted et al. (1991) reported findings from a 26-year follow-up of 9,484 male Seventh-Day Adventists who, because of adherence to religion-based lifestyle practices, have substantially lower rates of total and cause-specific mortality than the overall U.S. population. Baseline physical activity was assessed by questionnaire in 1960, and mortality follow-up lasted through the end of 1985, during which 3,799 men died. In each 10-year age stratum from 50 to 99 years, significant inverse associations were seen between physical activity categories (inactive and moderate and high activity) and mortality risk, even after accounting for reported levels of risk factors and prevalent disease. Similarly, in the Lipid Research Clinics Prevalence Study cohort of women and men, a high proportion of whom had hypercholesterolemia and thus elevated risk for mortality, CRF remained significantly inversely associated with mortality risk after adjustment for differences in age and clinical risk factors (Ekelund et al., 1988; Mora et al., 2003).

Although data from the Lipid Research Clinics Prevalence study suggest that higher physical activity or CRF may protect against premature mortality in high-risk individuals, more convincing evidence has been found in population samples of adults who have manifest clinical disease. Table 8.1 summarizes findings from several recent prospective observational studies that related physical activity or CRF exposures with mortality risk in adults with clinically diagnosed diabetes, hypertension, metabolic syndrome, cardiovascular disease, and obesity (Wei et al., 1999; Wannamethee et al., 2000; Church et al., 2001; Myers et al., 2002; Kavanagh et al., 2002; Kavanagh et al., 2003; Church et al., 2004; Katzmarzyk et al., 2004; Hu et al., 2004; Hu et al., 2005; Fang et al., 2005). In each study, after adjustment for potential confounders such as smoking habits and alcohol intake, family history of disease, as well as other factors, mortality risk was significantly lower in individuals with manifest clinical disease who had higher levels of physical activity or CRF compared to inactive or low fit peers. In several of the studies, confounding and reverse causation were addressed by adjusting for medication or diet therapy and by subgroup analyses that eliminated early deaths. In support of a causal association, several of the exposure–response relationships also demonstrated an inverse, dose–response gradient.

Changes in Physical Activity or Cardiorespiratory Fitness and Subsequent Mortality

The vast majority of studies, including those reviewed earlier, have related a single baseline physical activity or CRF exposure with mortality risk. Misclassification, because of changes in physical activity or CRF during follow-up, can lead to biased estimates of the exposure–response association with this study design, although this bias is likely to be toward the null for prospective studies. An additional test for a causal relationship is to examine the association between a change in exposure and the subsequent risk of death. In other words, do individuals who are initially sedentary or unfit but who subsequently become physically active and fit have a lower mortality risk than do individuals who remain sedentary and unfit across two separate assessments? The first large-scale epidemiological investigation of this issue was conducted by Professor Paffenbarger in the Harvard Alumni Health Study (Paffenbarger et al., 1993). Physical activity questionnaires were completed in 1962 or 1966 and again in 1977 by 10,269 men, of whom 476 died during the subsequent 11-year follow-up. After accounting for differences in several health characteristics, initially sedentary men who took up physical activity of moderate or higher intensity had a 23% (95% CI, 4%–42%) lower mortality risk than their peers who were sedentary across both physical activity assessments.

We examined mortality risk in 9,777 men in the ACLS who had their CRF assessed by maximal treadmill exercise testing at two examinations separated by an average of 5 years who were then followed, on average, for an additional 5 years (Blair et al., 1995). After adjusting for age and changes in several clinical risk predictors, including body mass index, initially unfit men (lowest fifth of age-standardized treadmill performance) who were classified as being fit on the second treadmill test had a 64% lower mortality risk than men who were unfit at both examinations ($p < 0.05$). This observation persisted when analyses were performed on subgroups of the cohort who died within 3 years of follow-up and in those

Table 8.1 Prospective Studies of the Association Between Physical Activity or Cardiorespiratory Fitness and Mortality in Individuals with Clinically Manifest Disease

Reference	*Population*	*Follow-up (deaths)*	*Exposure*	*Main findings for PA or CRF RR (95% CI)**
Diabetes				
Hu et al., 2005	3708 Finnish men and women, ages 25–74 years, diabetes by physician diagnosis, FPG >126 mg/dL and OGTT criteria	18.7 years (1423)	Self-reported PA	Low: RR = 1.00 (referent) Mod: RR = 0.61 (0.51–0.73) High: RR = 0.52 (0.45–0.60)
Church et al., 2004	2196 ACLS men, ages 23–79 years, diabetes by physician diagnosis or FPG >126 mg/dL	14.6 years (275)	CRF from a maximal exercise test	METs >11.71: RR = 1.00 (referent) 10.09–11.71: RR = 1.60 (0.93–2.76) 8.83–10.08: RR = 2.77 (1.65–4.66) ≤8.82: RR = 4.99 (2.64–7.64)
Hypertension				
Fang et al., 2005	4857 U.S. men and women in NHANES I, ages 25–74 years, hypertension by physician diagnosis and measured BP ≥140/90 mmHg	17.0 years (2244)	Self-reported PA	Least: RR = 1.00 (referent) Mod: RR = 0.88 (0.80–0.98) Most: RR = 0.83 (0.72–0.95)
Church et al., 2001	3184 ACLS men, ages 20–85 years, hypertension by physician diagnosis	10.3 years (151)	CRF from a maximal exercise test	Physician diagnosed hypertension: Quintile (Q) 1: RR = 1.00 (referent) Q2–Q3: RR = 0.56 (0.38–0.82) Q4–Q5: RR = 0.57 (0.35–0.95)
	3257 ACLS men, ages 20–85 years, hypertension by measured BP ≥140/90 mmHg	10.3 years (152)		Measured BP ≥140/90 mmHg: Q1: RR = 1.00 (referent) Q2–Q3: RR = 0.49 (0.40–0.98) Q4–Q5: RR = 0.49 (0.36–0.96)

Continued

Table 8.1 Prospective Studies of the Association Between Physical Activity or Cardiorespiratory Fitness and Mortality in Individuals with Clinically Manifest Disease *(Continued)*

Reference	*Population*	*Follow-up (deaths)*	*Exposure*	*Main findings for PA or CRF RR (95% CI)**
Metabolic Syndrome				
Katzmarzyk et al., 2004	3757 ACLS men, ages 20–83 years, metabolic syndrome by ATP-III criteria	9.5 years (132)	CRF from a maximal exercise test	Q1: RR = 1.00 (referent) Q2–Q5: RR = 0.49 (0.34–0.72)
Cardiovascular Disease				
Wannamethee et al., 2000	772 British men, ages 52–73 years, physician-diagnosed myocardial infarction or angina	5.0 years (131)	Self-reported PA	Inactive/ Occasional: RR = 1.00 (referent) Light: RR = 0.42 (0.25–0.71) Moderate: RR = 0.47 (0.24–0.92) Vigorous: RR = 0.63 (0.39-1.03) Walking, minutes/day None: RR = 1.00 (referent) 1 to 40: RR = 0.73 (0.49–1.09) >40: RR = 0.48 (0.30–0.77)
Myers et al. 2002	3679 men, average age 61 years, physician-diagnosed cardiovascular disease	6.2 years (968)	CRF from a maximal exercise test	Each 1-MET increment in exercise performance: RR = 0.91 (0.88–0.94)
Kavanagh et al. 2003	2380 medically stable women, average age 59.7 years, ≈14 weeks postmyocardial infarction or CABG	6.1 years (209)	CRF from a maximal exercise test	Peak METs <3.7: RR = 1.00 (referent) ≥3.7: RR = 0.71 (0.53–0.95)

Kavanagh et al. 2002	12,169 men, average age 55 years, ≈14 weeks postmyocardial infarction or CABG	8.9 years (2352)	CRF from a maximal exercise test	Peak METs <4.3: RR = 1.00 (referent) 4.3 to 6.3: RR = 0.66 (0.59–0.73) >6.3: RR = 0.48 (0.42–0.55)
Overweight/obese				
Wei et al., 1999	25,714 ACLS men, ages 20–83 years	8.8 years (158)	CRF from a maximal exercise test BMI from measured height and weight	Fitness quintiles Q1 (low) to Q5 (high) Q1(in men with BMI = 18.5–24.9): RR = 1.00 (referent) Q2-Q5 (in men with BMI = 18.5–24.9): RR = 0.63 (0.48–0.78) Q2-Q5 (in men with BMI = 25.0–29.9): RR = 0.59 (0.50–0.71) Q2-Q5 (in men with BMI ≥30): RR = 0.44 (0.29–0.67)
Hu et al., 2004	116,564 women, ages 30–55 years	24 years (10,282)	Self-reported PA BMI from self-reported height and weight	BMI <25.0 kg/m^2 ≥3.5 hours/week: RR = 1.00 (referent) 1.0-3.4 hours/week: RR = 1.18 (1.09–1.29) <1.0 hours/week: RR = 1.55 (1.42–1.70) BMI 25.0-29.9 kg/m^2 ≥3.5 hours/week: RR = 1.28 (1.12–1.46) 1.0–3.4 hours/week: RR = 1.33 (1.20–1.47) <1.0 hours/week: RR = 1.64 (1.46–1.83) BMI ≥30.0 kg/m^2 ≥3.5 hours/week: RR = 1.91 (1.60–2.30) 1.0–3.4 hours/week: RR = 2.05 (1.82–2.30) <1.0 hours/week: RR = 2.42 (2.14–2.73)

Continued

Table 8.1 Prospective Studies of the Association Between Physical Activity or Cardiorespiratory Fitness and Mortality in Individuals with Clinically Manifest Disease *(Continued)*

Reference	*Population*	*Follow-up (deaths)*	*Exposure*	*Main findings for PA or CRF RR (95% CI)**
Hu et al., 2005	≈3081 men and ≈4287 women, ages 25–64 years, obesity defined as BMI ≥30 kg/m²	17.7 years (4563 men, 2831 women)	Self-reported PA BMI from measured height and weight	Men Active/non-obese: RR = 1.00 (referent) Active/obese: RR = 1.21 ($p < 0.05$) Inactive/non-obese: RR = 1.53 ($p < 0.05$) Inactive/obese: RR = 1.78 ($p < 0.05$) Women Active/non-obese: RR = 1.00 (referent) Active/obese: RR = 1.12 ($p < 0.05$) Inactive/non-obese: RR = 1.59 ($p < 0.05$) Inactive/obese: RR = 2.10 ($p < 0.05$)

*In each study, the point and interval estimates of association were adjusted for age, sex (where applicable), and a variety of risk predictors (space precludes listing each of the covariables used in the respective studies; interested readers can refer to the original manuscripts for greater details). For each study, we show estimates for the most fully adjusted model reported in the original work. For consistency with our approach in the text of the chapter, when possible, we show the data with low PA or CRF as the referent category, in some instances taking the reciprocal of the published estimates.

Abbreviations: ACLS: Aerobics Center Longitudinal Study; ATP: Adult Treatment Panel; BMI: body mass index; BP: resting blood pressure; CABG: coronary artery bypass graft surgery; CI: confidence interval; FPG: fasting plasma glucose; METs: metabolic equivalents (1 MET = 3.5 mL O_2 uptake/kg/minute); Mod: moderate; NHANES: National Health and Nutrition Examination Survey; OGTT: oral glucose tolerance test; RR: relative risk.

who died more than 3 years after the second clinic examination. Consistent with our findings in the ACLS and with those from the Harvard Alumni Health Study, other investigators subsequently have observed favorable associations between improvements in physical activity and mortality risk in women (Lissner et al., 1996; Gregg et al., 2003) as well as in men (Wannamethee et al., 1998; Johansson and Sundquist, 1999).

Summary and Future Directions

Over the past 50 years or so, the association of occupational and leisure-time physical activity or CRF with mortality risk has been examined in numerous prospective observational studies. Nearly all studies have found an inverse association, and many have also found a significant dose–response gradient between exposure categories and mortality risk (U.S. Department of Health and Human Services, 1996; Lee and Skerrett, 2001). Patterns of association are similar for women and men, although inadequate physical activity assessment may result in attenuated associations with mortality, particularly in women. Higher levels of physical activity and CRF confer protection against premature mortality across a wide age range and among population subgroups with clinically diagnosed disease. A small number of studies also have examined the influence of changes in physical activity or CRF exposures on subsequent mortality and have observed significantly lower mortality risk in initially sedentary or unfit individuals who become physically active and fit. The effect of delayed mortality by higher physical activity or CRF, or improvements therein, persists after accounting for potential confounding factors and in analyses that eliminate early deaths during follow-up. The majority of the studies on physical activity or CRF and mortality that were reviewed here and elsewhere (U.S. Department of Health and Human Services, 1996; Lee and Skerrett, 2001) meet all or most of the epidemiological criteria for causality (e.g., strength of association, temporality, biological gradient, consistency of findings; U.S. Department of Health and Human Services, 1996). Evidence for the criteria of biological plausibility is discussed in other chapters of this book that focus on potential mechanisms through which physical activity or CRF confers health benefits on specific diseases. Experimental evidence of a true association between physical activity or CRF and mortality does not exist, because there have not been controlled randomized trials of physical activity exposures and mortality outcomes. Clinical trial data, however, have demonstrated that increases in physical activity or CRF are associated with improved levels of biological factors (e.g., blood pressure, glucose, lipids, catecholamine and stress hormone levels, endothelial cell and autonomic function) that are intermediate in the causal pathway with mortality. Future studies should include a mixture of individuals of different race/ethnicity and should utilize objective, direct physical activity monitoring to quantify activity-related energy expenditure and its component dimensions of frequency, duration, and intensity. Investigators should examine physical activity–mortality relationships using physical activity exposures that are defined specific to current recommendations (e.g., at least 150 minutes/week in moderate-intensity or at least 60 minutes/week in vigorous-intensity activity; or 7.5–15.0 MET-hours/week of energy expenditure; U.S. Department of Health and Human Services, 1996; Haskell et al, 2007; Nelson et al, 2007).

In April 2006, an international congress on physical activity and health was held in Atlanta, Georgia (Kohl et al, 2006), commemorating the tenth anniversary of the U.S. Surgeon General's Report of Physical Activity and Health (U.S. Department of Health and Human Services, 1996). The Surgeon General's physical activity recommendation, similarly to the consensus recommendation first published in 1995 (Pate et al., 1995) was heavily influenced by a review of observational data on physical activity and mortality risk.

Since that writing, new prospective data have emerged, expanding on those studies that were reviewed in 1995. Available information from observational studies has suggested that a physical activity volume of at least 1,000 kcal/week in activities of at least moderate intensity (absolute intensity ≥3 METs) is associated with a 20% to 30% lower risk of all-cause mortality (Lee and Skerrett, 2001). Whether significantly lower mortality risk occurs at a physical activity volume less than 1,000 kcal/week, whether there is a physical activity volume above which benefits no longer occur and/or mortality risk increases, whether mortality risk varies according to differences in physical activity durations, frequencies, and intensities while holding physical activity volume constant, and whether a there is a threshold of CRF required for delayed mortality, each remain unresolved issues for future research (Lee and Skerrett, 2001).

Personal Perspective

Until the middle of the twentieth century, there was little systematic data published on the relationship of physical activity patterns and health outcomes. Professor Jeremy Morris of London set the stage for research on this topic with his observations on mortality risk among workers in sedentary or active occupations and later followed with studies that related leisure-time physical with CHD risk. Professor Ralph Paffenbarger soon contributed similar observations in the United States in his studies on San Francisco longshoremen and college alumni. In some ways it is remarkable that Professors Morris and Paffenbarger were able to find associations between physical activity and health outcomes given the complexity of physical activity behavior and the potential for misclassification on the exposure variable, both for job classifications and self-reporting of leisure and sporting activity habits. During the latest third of the twentieth century, numerous other investigators reported on inverse associations between physical activity and morbidity and mortality in a variety of populations. The consistency of the observations, the strength and independence of the associations, and the discovery of plausible biological mechanisms through controlled experiments has led to a conclusion that physical inactivity is causally associated with higher risk for numerous fatal and non-fatal health outcomes. The work on physical activity and health has been supported by studies in which the exposure was an objective measure of cardiorespiratory fitness, and more recently, it appears that muscular fitness also is related inversely to chronic disease and early mortality. In the first part of the twenty-first century, advances in technology led to improved objective methods of monitoring physical activity habits. These new devices can store data for many days and are capable of providing relatively precise estimates of not only the amount of physical activity but also information on its intensity, duration, and pattern. We believe that these methods will open a new era of investigation on topics of physical activity and health, and we welcome the advances in knowledge that will come from this work.

Although it now is more than 10 years later, the public health message conveyed in the Forward of the U.S. Surgeon General's Report of Physical Activity and Health as well as in the first consensus recommendation of physical activity and health remains the same: Everyone benefits from an active and fit way of living, and a primary benefit of regular physical activity and adequate CRF that can be enjoyed by many if not all individuals is delayed mortality.

Finally, we dedicate this chapter to two remarkable epidemiologists, Professors Ralph S. Paffenbarger, Jr and Jeremy Morris. They have provided direction, inspiration, counsel, and leadership to us and all others who work in physical activity epidemiology. We lost Professor Paffenbarger in 2007, and he is sorely missed. Professor Morris is actively engaged in research and continues to publish reports in peer-reviewed journal, at the age of 97 years. They are marvelous examples to all of us, not only for their scientific accomplishments, but also for their kindness and warm human spirit.

References

Barengo NC, Hu G, Lakka TA, Pekkarinen H, Nissinen A, Tuomilehto J. 2004. Low physical activity as a predictor for total and cardiovascular disease mortality in middle-aged men and women in Finland. *Eur Heart J* 25: 2204–11.

Blair SN, Kohl HW, III, Barlow CE, Paffenbarger RS, Jr., Gibbons LW, Macera CA, 1995. Changes in physical fitness and all-cause mortality: a prospective study of healthy and unhealthy men. *JAMA* 273: 1093–8.

Blair SN, Kohl HW, III, Paffenbarger RS, Jr., Clark DG, Cooper KH, Gibbons LW. 1989. Physical fitness and all-cause mortality: a prospective study of healthy men and women. *JAMA* 262: 2395–401.

Church TS, Cheng YJ, Earnest CP, et al. 2004. Exercise capacity and body composition as predictors of mortality among men with diabetes. *Diabetes Care* 27: 83–8.

Church TS, Kampert JB, Gibbons LW, Barlow CE, Blair SN. 2001. Usefulness of cardiorespiratory fitness as a predictor of all-cause and cardiovascular disease mortality in men with systemic hypertension. *Am J Cardiol* 88: 651–6.

Eaton SB, Konner M, Shostak M. 1988. Stone agers in the fast lane: chronic degenerative diseases in evolutionary perspective. *Am J Med* 84: 739–49.

Ekelund LG, Haskell WL, Johnson JL, Whaley FS, Criqui MH, Sheps DS. 1988. Physical fitness as a predictor of cardiovascular mortality in asymptomatic North American men: The Lipid Research Clinic's mortality follow-up study. *N Engl J Med* 319: 1379–84.

Fang J, Wylie-Rosett J, Alderman MH. 2005. Exercise and cardiovascular outcomes by hypertensive status: NHANES I epidemiological follow-up study, 1971–1992. *Am J Hypertens* 18: 751–8.

Fraser GE, Sumbureru D, Pribis P, Neil RL, Frankson MA. 1997. Association among health habits, risk factors, and all-cause mortality in a black California population. *Epidemiology* 8: 168–74.

Fried LP, Kronmal RA, Newman AB, et al. 1998. Risk factors for 5-year mortality in older adults: The Cardiovascular Health Study. *JAMA* 279: 585–92.

Gregg EW, Cauley JA, Stone K, et al. 2003. Relationship of changes in physical activity and mortality among older women. *JAMA* 289: 2379–86.

Gulati M, Pandey DK, Arnsdorf MF, et al. 2003. Exercise capacity and the risk of death in women: the St James Women Take Heart Project. *Circulation* 108: 1554–9.

Hahn RA, Teutsch SM, Rothenberg RB, Marks JS. 1990. Excess deaths from nine chronic diseases in the United States, 1986. *JAMA* 264: 2654–59.

Hakim AA, Petrovitch H, Burchfiel CM, et al. 1998. Effects of walking on mortality among nonsmoking retired men. *N Engl J Med* 338: 94–9.

Haskell WL, Lee I-M, Pate RR, et al 2007. Physical activity and public health. Updated recommendation for adults from the American College of Sports Medicine and the American Heart Association. *Circulation* 116:1081–93

Hu G, Eriksson J, Barengo NC, et al. 2004. Occupational, commuting, and leisure-time physical activity in relation to total and cardiovascular mortality among Finnish subjects with type 2 diabetes. *Circulation* 110: 666–73.

Hu G, Tuomilehto J, Silventoinen K, Barengo NC, Peltonen M, Jousilahti P. 2005. The effects of physical activity and body mass index on cardiovascular, cancer and all-cause mortality among 47 212 middle-aged Finnish men and women. *Int J Obes Relat. Metab Disord* 29: 894–902.

Johansson SE, Sundquist J. 1999. Change in lifestyle factors and their influence on health status and all-cause mortality. *Int J Epidemiol* 28: 1073–80.

Kannel WB, Sorlie P. 1979. Some health benefits of physical activity. The Framingham Study. *Arch Intern Med* 139: 857–61.

Kaplan GA, Seeman TE, Cohen RD, Knudsen LP, Guralnik J. 1987. Mortality among the elderly in the Alameda county study: behavioral and demographic risk factors. *Am J Pub Health* 77: 307–12.

Kaplan GA, Strawbridge WJ, Cohen RD, Hungerford LR. 1996. Natural history of leisure-time physical activity and its correlates: Associations with mortality from all causes and cardiovascular disease over 28 years. *Am J Epidemiol* 144: 793–7.

Katzmarzyk PT, Church TS, Blair SN. 2004. Cardiorespiratory fitness attenuates the effects of the metabolic syndrome on all-cause and cardiovascular disease mortality in men. *Arch Intern Med* 164: 1092–7.

Kavanagh T, Mertens DJ, Hamm LF, et al. 2002. Prediction of long-term prognosis in 12 169 men referred for cardiac rehabilitation. *Circulation* 106: 666–71.

Kavanagh T, Mertens DJ, Hamm LF, et al. 2003. Peak oxygen intake and cardiac mortality in women referred for cardiac rehabilitation. *J Am Coll Cardiol* 42: 2139–43.

Kohl HW, Lee IM, Vuori IM, et al. 2006. Physical activity and public health: the emergence of a subdiscipline. Report from the International Congress on Physical Activity and Public Health, April 17-21, 2006, Atlanta, Georgia. *J Phys Act Health* 3: 344–364.

Kushi LH, Fee RM, Folsom AR, Mink PJ, Anderson KE, Sellers TA. 1997. Physical activity and mortality in postmenopausal women. *JAMA* 277: 1287–92.

LaMonte MJ, Ainsworth BE. 2001. Quantifying energy expenditure and physical activity in the context of dose response. *Med Sci Sports Exerc* 33: S370-8.

Laukkanen JA, Lakka TA, Rauramaa R, et al. 2001. Cardiovascular fitness as a predictor of mortality in men. *Arch Intern Med* 161: 825–31.

Lee IM, Skerrett PJ. 2001. Physical activity and all-cause mortality: what is the dose-response relation? *Med Sci Sports Exerc* 33: S459-71.

Lindsted KD, Tonstad S, Kuzma JW. 1991. Self-report of physical activity and patterns of mortality in Seventh-Day Adventist men. *J Clin Epidemiol* 44: 355–64.

Lissner L, Bengtsson C, Bjorkelund C, Wedel H. 1996. Physical activity levels and changes in relation to longevity: A prospective study of Swedish women. *Am J Epidemiol* 143: 54–62.

Macaulay V, Richards M, Hickey E, et al. 1999. The emerging tree of West Eurasian mtDNAs: a synthesis of control-region sequences and RFLPs. *Am J Hum Genet* 64: 232–49.

Messinger-Rapport B, Pothier Snader CE, Blackstone EH, Yu D, Lauer MS. 2003. Value of exercise capacity and heart rate recovery in older people. *J Am Geriatr Soc* 51: 63–8.

Mora S, Redberg RF, Cui Y, et al. 2003. Ability of exercise testing to predict cardiovascular and all-cause death in asymptomatic women: a 20-year follow-up of the lipid research clinics prevalence study. *JAMA* 290: 1600–7.

Morris JN, Heady JA. 1953. Mortality in relation to the physical activity of work: a preliminary note on experience in middle age. *Br J Ind Med* 10: 245–54.

Myers J, Prakash M, Froelicher V, Do D, Partington S, Atwood JE. 2002. Exercise capacity and mortality among men referred for exercise testing. *N Engl J Med* 346: 793–801.

Nelson ME, Rejeski WJ, Blair SN, et al. 2007. Physical activity and public health in older adults. Recommendation from the American College of Sports Medicine and the American Heart Association. *Circulation* 116:1094–1105.

Paffenbarger RS, Jr., Blair SN, Lee I-M, Hyde RT. 1993. Measurement of physical activity to assess health effects in free-living populations. *Med Sci Sports Exerc* 25: 60–70.

Paffenbarger RS, Jr., Hyde RT, Wing AL. 1987. Physical activity and incidence of cancer in diverse populations: a preliminary report. *Am J Clin Nutr*, 45: 312–7.

Paffenbarger RS, Jr., Hyde RT, Wing AL, Hsieh C-C, 1986. Physical activity, all-cause mortality, and longevity of college alumni. *N Engl J Med* 314: 605–13.

Paffenbarger RS, Jr., Hyde RT, Wing AL, Lee I-M, Jung DL, Kampert JB. 1993. The association of changes in physical-activity level and other lifestyle characteristics with mortality among men. *N Engl J Med*, 328: 538–45.

Pate RR, Pratt M, Blair SN, et al. 1995. Physical activity and public health: a recommendation from the Centers for Disease Control and Prevention and the American College of Sports Medicine. *JAMA* 273: 402–7.

Pereira MA, FitzGerald SJ, Gregg EW, et al. 1997. A collection of physical activity questionnaires for health-related research. *Med Sci Sports Exerc* 29: S1-205.

Reiff GG, Montoye HJ, Remington RD, Napier JA, Metzner HL, Epstein FH. 1967. Assessment of physical activity by questionnaire and interview. *J Sports Med Phys Fitness* 7: 135–42.

Rockhill B, Willett WC, Manson JE, et al. 2001. Physical activity and mortality: a prospective study among women. *Am J Public Health* 91: 578–83.

Ruigomez A, Alonso J, Anto JM. 1995. Relationship of health behaviours to five-year mortality in an elderly cohort. *Age Ageing* 24: 113–9.

Sherman SE, D'Agostino RB, Cobb JL, Kannel WB. 1994. Physical activity and mortality in women in the Framingham Heart Study. *Am Heart J* 128: 879–84.

Steffen-Batey L, Nichaman MZ, Goff DC, et al. 2000. Change in level of physical activity and risk of all-cause mortality or reinfarction: The Corpus Christi Heart Project. *Circulation* 102: 2204–9.

Taylor HL, Jacobs DR, Jr., Schucker B, Knudsen J, Leon AS, Debacker G. 1978. A quesionnaire for the assessment of leisure time physical activities. *J Chronic Dis* 31: 741–55.

Taylor HL, Klepetar E, Keys A, Parlin W, Blackburn H, Puchner T. 1962. Death rates among physically active and sedentary employees of the railroad industry. *Am J Public Health* 52: 1697–707.

U.S. Department of Health and Human Services. 1996. Physical activity and health: A report of the Surgeon General. U.S. Department of Health and Human Services, Centers for Disease Control and Prevention, National Center for Chronic Disease Prevention and Health Promotion, Atlanta, GA.

Wannamethee SG, Shaper AG, Walker M. 1998. Changes in physical activity, mortality, and incidence of coronary heart disease in older men. *Lancet* 351: 1603–8.

Wannamethee SG, Shaper AG, Walker M. 2000. Physical activity and mortality in older men with diagnosed coronary heart disease. *Circulation* 102: 1358–63.

Wei M, Kampert JB, Barlow CE, et al. 1999. Relationship between low cardiorespiratory fitness and mortality in normal-weight, overweight, and obese men. *JAMA* 282: 1547–53.

Weller I, Corey P. 1998. The impact of excluding non-leisure energy expenditure on the relation between physical activity and mortality in women. *Epidemiology* 9: 632–5.

9

Physical Activity, Fitness, and the Prevention of Cardiovascular Disease

Shari S. Bassuk and
JoAnn E. Manson

Cardiovascular disease (CVD) is a major cause of morbidity and the leading killer of U.S. men and women (Rosamond et al., 2007). Coronary heart disease (CHD) and stroke account for an estimated 52% and 17% of cardiovascular deaths, respectively. The economic cost of CVD in this country has been estimated at $431.8 billion per year (Rosamond et al., 2007). This amount includes both direct health-care costs and indirect costs from lost productivity caused by illness or death.

A sedentary lifestyle should be considered an important modifiable risk factor for CVD in the general population. Researchers agree that physical activity provides cardiovascular benefits, although the volume or "dose"—a function of intensity, frequency, and duration—of activity required for optimal health remains controversial (*see* Chapter 4 for additional discussion). A review of prospective studies published between 1990 and 2000 concluded that the reduction in the risk of CHD associated with a physically active lifestyle, compared with a sedentary lifestyle, is 35% to 55% (Skerrett and Manson, 2002). Physical activity may slow the initiation and progression of atherosclerotic disease via favorable effects on body weight, blood pressure, insulin sensitivity, glycemic control, lipid profile, fibrinolysis, endothelial function, and inflammatory defense systems. This chapter reviews recent observational and clinical trial findings regarding the role of physical activity and fitness in preventing clinical and asymptomatic vascular disease. Dose–response issues and public health implications are highlighted.

Exercise intensity is typically measured in kilocalories (kcal) burned per minute of activity or in metabolic equivalents (METs), defined as the ratio of the metabolic rate during exercise to the metabolic rate at rest (*see* Chapter 2). Moderate-intensity activities, such brisk walking, are those that burn 3.5 to 7 kcal per minute or, equivalently, those that expend 3 to 6 METs. Vigorous activities, such as running, are those that burn more than 7 kcal per minute or expend more than 6 METs. The traditional view that physical activity must be vigorous to reduce the risk of CHD and other chronic diseases has been challenged by epidemiologic studies showing otherwise. Earlier recommendations promoting vigorous exercise for at least 20 minutes three times per week (American College of Sports Medicine, 1978) have been supplemented by guidelines issued by the Centers for Disease Control and the American College of Sports Medicine in 1995 (Pate et al., 1995) and the U.S. Surgeon General in 1996 (U.S. Department of Health and Human Services, 1996) advocating 30 minutes of moderate-intensity physical activity on most, and preferably all, days of the week. In 2002, the Institute of Medicine (IOM) doubled the daily moderate-intensity activity goal to 60 minutes, stating that one half-hour is not sufficient to maintain a healthy weight nor to achieve maximal health benefits (Institute of Medicine, 2002).

Although the IOM has been praised for portraying physical activity as an integral part of a healthy lifestyle, its recommendation has also been criticized for not balancing the issue of efficacy with that of feasibility, both of which are needed to achieve a public health goal. National data indicate that two of three U.S. adults do not meet the 30-minute guideline, and nearly two of five adults perform no leisure-time physical activity at all (Rosamond et al., 2007). Setting the benchmark even higher may weaken any motivation that the public, which already largely views the less stringent standard as too onerous, might muster to become more active. Based on this concern and on our review of recent epidemiologic findings, we believe that the primary public health message should continue to be that moderately intense exercise for one half-hour per day confers significant cardiovascular benefits. Indeed, physical activity guidelines issued in 2004 by the American Heart Association in a joint statement with the American Diabetes Association and the American Cancer Society reaffirm the 30-minute goal for the prevention of CVD, type 2 diabetes, and some types of cancer (Eyre et al., 2004). The World Health Organization included the 30-minute guideline in its 2004 blueprint for fighting these and other chronic diseases (World Health Organization, 2004). In 2005, the U.S. Department of Health and Human Services and the U.S. Department of Agriculture also espoused the 30-minute goal for disease risk reduction, although they concurred with the IOM that 60 minutes (or more) of physical activity may be required for weight control (U.S. Department of Health and Human Services and U.S. Department of Agriculture, 2005) (*see* Chapter 15 for additional discussion on the evolution of physical activity recommendations). The 30-minute recommendation does not imply the absence of a dose–response relationship between physical activity and cardiovascular outcomes; another half-hour of activity per day would, on average, be expected to confer additional protection against the development of CVD and would assist with weight control and prevention of obesity in persons with low baseline activity levels.

Clinical Cardiovascular Disease

Cohort studies consistently show a marked reduction in the incidence of CVD among physically active individuals compared with their inactive peers, and recent investigations provide empirical support for the prescription of 30 minutes per day of moderate-intensity physical activity in sedentary populations. In these studies, exposure data are derived from self-reported physical activity questionnaires. Among 73,743 postmenopausal women aged 50 to 79 years who participated in the Women's Health Initiative, walking briskly for at least 2.5 hours per week (e.g., a half-hour five times per week) was associated with a 30% reduction in cardiovascular events over 3.2 years of follow-up, after adjustment for age, body mass index (BMI), and other risk factors for CVD (Manson et al., 2002). Given equivalent total exercise energy expenditures, brisk walking and more vigorous exercise were associated with similar magnitudes of risk reductions, and the results did not vary substantially according to race, age, or baseline BMI (Fig. 9.1).

Effect of Gender and Age

Cardiovascular benefits of moderate-intensity exercise have been consistently observed in studies of women and older men. In the Nurses' Health Study, which followed 72,488 healthy female nurses aged 40 to 65 years for 8 years, women who walked briskly for 3 hours per week or, alternatively, performed more vigorous exercise for 1.5 hours per week

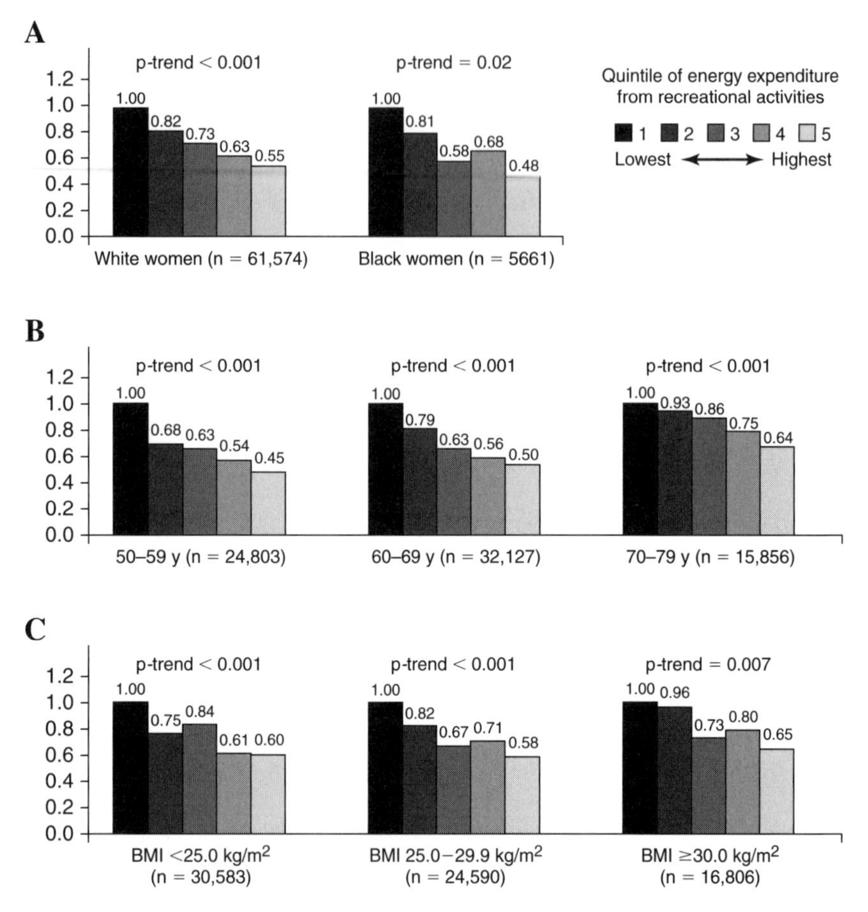

Figure 9.1 Age-adjusted relative risks of cardiovascular disease according to quintile of energy expenditure from recreational activities in subgroups defined by race (panel A), age (panel B), and body mass index (panel C). Quintile medians (ranges), in MET-hours per week, are as follows: quintile 1, 0 (0–2.4); quintile 2, 4.2 (2.5–7.2); quintile 3, 10.0 (7.3–13.4); quintile 4, 17.5 (13.5–23.3); quintile 5, 32.8 (≥23.4). Quintile 1 is the reference category. (From Manson et al., 2002, with permission.)

had a 30% to 40% lower rate of myocardial infarction than did their inactive counterparts (Manson et al., 1999). Among 39,372 healthy female health professionals aged 45 years and older who were followed for 7 years in the Women's Health Study, walking 1 hour or more per week was associated with a 50% reduction in CHD risk in respondents who reported no vigorous physical activity (Lee et al., 2001). In a 30-year study of 1,564 middle-aged University of Pennsylvania alumnae, women who walked at least 10 blocks per day experienced a 33% reduction in CVD incidence compared with women who walked less than 4 blocks per day (Sesso et al., 1999). Among 1,645 women and men aged 65 years and older in a large health maintenance organization, walking more than 4 hours per week, compared with walking less than 1 hour per week, significantly reduced the risk of hospitalization for cardiovascular reasons (LaCroix et al., 1996). In the Zutphen Elderly Study, men aged 64 to 84 years who walked or cycled at least three times per week for 20 minutes had a 31% reduction in CHD mortality over 10 years compared with their counterparts who were less active (Bijnen et al., 1998). In the Honolulu Heart Program, men aged 71 to 93 years who walked 1.5 miles per day had half the risk of CHD of those who walked less than one-quarter mile per day (Hakim et al., 1999). With the exception of the latter two estimates, these risk reductions reflect adjustment for the effects of BMI and other potential confounders.

Cardiovascular benefits of moderate-intensity exercise have also been observed in middle-aged men, although the associations are weaker and less consistent than those for women and older men, perhaps because of generally higher physical activity levels for middle-aged men (Lee, 2004). In the Health Professionals Follow-up Study, which followed 44,452 male health professionals aged 40 to 75 years for 12 years, 30 minutes or more per day of brisk walking was associated with an 18% reduction in CHD incidence among men who engaged in less than 1 hour of weekly vigorous exercise (Fig. 9.2; Tanasescu et al., 2002). Most studies of men have found that vigorous exercise leads to even greater risk reductions than does moderate-intensity exercise. In the Health Professionals

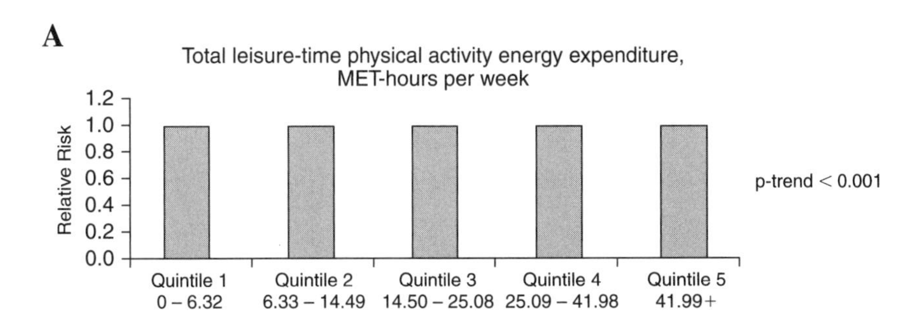

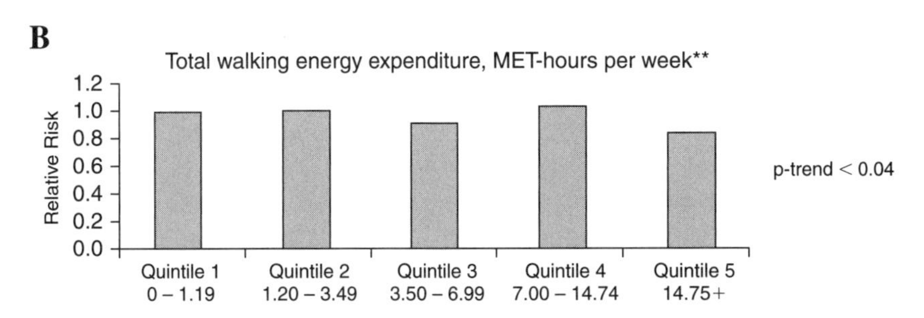

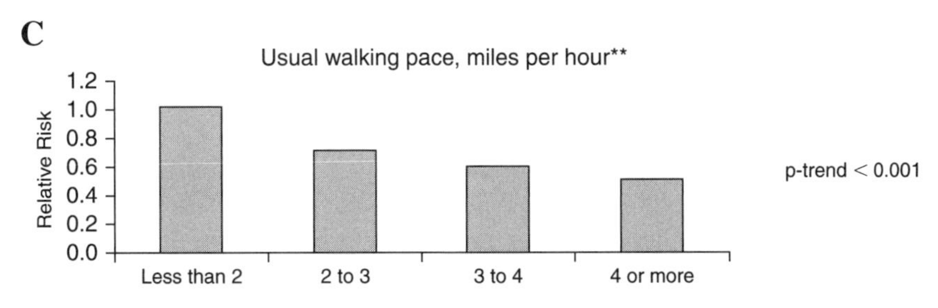

Figure 9.2 Relative risk* of coronary heart disease, according to physical activity, among men followed for 12 years in the Health Professionals Follow-up Study. (Data from Tanasescu et al., 2002.)
* Adjusted for alcohol use; smoking; family history of myocardial infarction; nutrient intake; presence of diabetes; high cholesterol level, and hypertension at baseline; and, for model C, total walking energy expenditure
** Among men who did not perform vigorous exercise regularly (i.e., <1 hr/week)

Follow-up Study, each 1-MET increase in exercise intensity was associated with a significant 4% reduction in CHD risk independently of total energy expenditure. Even variation in walking pace was strongly predictive of cardiovascular risk; compared with walking at an easy pace, the relative risks of CHD corresponding to normal pace (2–3 mph), brisk pace (3–4 mph), and very brisk pace (≥4 mph) were 0.72, 0.61, and 0.51, respectively (*p* for trend <0.001), after adjustment for walking energy expenditure. Data from this cohort also suggest that resistance exercise may be important in reducing CHD incidence; men who trained with weights for at least 30 minutes per week were 23% less likely to develop CHD over an 8-year follow-up period than men who did not train with weights. To date, comparable studies of resistance training and risk of CHD in women are lacking.

Although these investigations did not study physical activity patterns across the lifespan, other research indicates that previously sedentary individuals who become physically active in middle or late life derive cardiovascular benefit. A 10-year follow-up of two groups of initially inactive healthy men and women aged 55 to 75 years, one comprised of individuals who chose to participate in a supervised exercise program (30–45 minutes of walking three times per week) and the other of community controls, found that the exercise group experienced more favorable changes in systolic blood pressure, high-density lipoprotein (HDL) and total cholesterol, triglycerides, insulin, waist circumference, and percent body fat, as well as fewer abnormal electrocardiogram findings on exercise treadmill testing (Petrella et al., 2005). Among initially sedentary participants in the Nurses' Health Study, 6-year changes in activity level were associated in dose–response fashion with CHD incidence during the subsequent 8 years (Manson et al., 1999). Compared with the risk among women who remained sedentary, the relative risks of coronary events for women in increasing quintiles of total physical activity energy expenditure were 0.85, 0.79. 0.67, and 0.71 (*p* for trend = 0.03). The Study of Osteoporotic Fractures, which assessed changes in physical activity over 6 years among 7,553 women aged 65 years and older at baseline, found that women who increased their physical activity level were 36% less likely to die of cardiovascular causes during the subsequent 7 years than were women who remained inactive (Gregg et al., 2003a). The British Regional Heart Study, which examined physical activity changes over 14 years among 5,934 men aged 40 to 59 years at baseline, reported that participants who initiated even light activity in later life experienced a 34% reduction in cardiovascular mortality over the subsequent 4 years, as compared with those who stayed sedentary (Wannamethee et al., 1998). The latter two studies indicate that exercise must be current and habitual to confer cardiovascular protection; persons who became inactive in later life had a similar risk of cardiovascular death to those who had remained inactive over the course of follow-up.

Effect of Race

There are sparse data on the relationship between physical activity or fitness and CVD in non-white populations. Results from the Women's Health Initiative, one of the few studies to include a sufficient number of black participants to permit an examination of the association between physical activity and CHD in this group, indicate that black women derive comparable cardiovascular benefits from exercise to white women (Manson et al., 2002). As shown in Figure 9.1, the magnitude of the risk reduction across increasing quintiles of total recreational energy expenditure was nearly identical for black and white respondents. In both racial groups, 30 minutes per day of brisk walking was associated with an approximate 30% reduction in CHD risk. Such evidence regarding the applicability of national activity guidelines to U.S. blacks is important because of the high prevalence of physical inactivity, obesity, hypertension, type 2 diabetes, and CVD in this group. Although the reasons for racial disparities in health are not completely understood, with differing physical activity patterns being only one piece of a complex puzzle, targeted initiatives to increase physical activity among U.S. blacks may help ameliorate their disadvantaged cardiovascular status compared with U.S. whites.

Cardiorespiratory Fitness

Studies that use self-reported physical activity patterns as the exposure variable offer direct support for current public health guidelines for CVD prevention, which are framed in terms of physical activity, which is a behavior, rather than physical fitness, which is an attained physiologic state. However, cardiorespiratory fitness as assessed by maximal exercise testing is also inversely correlated with cardiovascular outcomes. For example, in a 20-year follow-up of 2,994 initially healthy women aged 30 to 80 years in the Lipid Research Clinics Prevalence Study, the risk of cardiovascular mortality and of all-cause mortality decreased by 17% and 11%, respectively, for every 1-MET increase in exercise capacity, after adjustment for multiple cardiovascular risk factors (Mora et al., 2003).

Although regular aerobic physical activity improves physical fitness, the degree to which being inactive and being unfit represent distinct cardiovascular risk factors is unclear. The volume of exercise necessary for CHD risk reduction likely varies according to age and baseline fitness level. This observation may explain the aforementioned gender and age differences in epidemiologic findings regarding the level of exercise intensity needed to reduce coronary risk. In general, studies that have shown an association between moderate-intensity activity and decreased CHD incidence or mortality have been conducted in women or older men, who tend to be less fit, whereas studies suggesting that vigorous activity is required to reduce cardiovascular risk have been conducted in young or middle-aged men, who tend to be more fit (Lee, 2004).

Short Versus Long Bouts of Exercise

Bouts of activity lasting as little as 10 minutes have been shown to improve the cardiovascular risk profile of otherwise sedentary individuals (Murphy et al., 2002). One prospective study has examined the relationship between short bouts of exercise and CVD itself. In a 5-year follow-up of 7,307 middle-aged and elderly male Harvard alumni, exercise sessions lasting 15, 30, or 45 minutes all provided equal protection against CVD after adjustment for total energy expenditure (Lee et al., 2000). From a public health perspective, this finding should encourage busy adults to view exercise as a manageable part of their daily routine rather than as a time-consuming activity to be reserved for rare occasions.

Prolonged Sitting and Other Sedentary Behaviors

Recent studies demonstrate the health benefits not only of obtaining adequate aerobic and resistance exercise but also avoiding sedentary behaviors such as prolonged sitting. Highlighting this distinction in future public health messages would seem to be warranted given that the typical U.S. adult spends 4 to 5 hours per day watching television, and many individuals sit for an additional 8 or more hours at work. Prolonged sitting predicts an increased risk for CVD, even after accounting for time spent in recreational exercise. In the Women's Health Initiative, women who spent 16 or more hours per day sitting were 68% more likely to develop CVD than those who spent less than 4 hours per day sitting (Manson et al., 2002).

Stroke

Most epidemiologic investigations of physical activity and clinical cardiovascular outcomes have focused on CHD or total CVD. However, prospective data also suggest that physical activity reduces the risk of stroke, although findings are less consistent than for CHD. In a quantitative analysis of 18 cohort studies with follow-up periods from 2 to 32 years, moderately active and highly active persons were 17% and 25% less likely, respectively, to have a stroke or die of stroke-related causes than were persons with low activity (Lee et al., 2003). On the basis of six studies of ischemic and three of hemorrhagic stroke in the analysis, physical activity appears to offer protection against both types of stroke. Compared with low-activity individuals, moderately active and highly active persons had a 9% and 21% lower risk, respectively, of ischemic stroke; the corresponding figures for hemorrhagic stroke were 15% and 34% (Lee et al., 2003). Unfortunately, variation in the measurement and classification of physical activity in the original studies did not allow for a precise definition of the "high," "moderate," and "low" activity categories. Also, gender-specific results were not provided, although both women and men were well-represented in the included studies. In the Nurses' Health Study, there was a strong dose–response relationship between the volume of physical activity and total stroke that primarily resulted from the association with ischemic rather than hemorrhagic stroke (Hu et al., 2000). Women in the highest activity category experienced only half the risk of ischemic stroke as the least active women after adjustment for BMI and other vascular risk factors. However, the Physicians' Health Study, which followed 21,823 men aged 40 to 84 years for 11 years, found an inverse gradient of risk for hemorrhagic, but not ischemic stroke, incidence (Lee et al., 1999). The Aerobics Center Longitudinal Study, a 10-year follow-up of 16,878 men aged 40 to 87 years, reported a strong inverse association between cardiorespiratory fitness and total stroke mortality, which persisted after adjustment for potential confounding variables. Compared with men in the bottom quintile of fitness, participants in the top two quintiles of fitness and those in the middle two quintiles had similar reductions in stroke mortality—68% and 63%, respectively (Lee and Blair, 2002). Data on stroke subtypes were not examined. More recently, the Kuipio Ischemic Heart Disease Risk Factor Study observed a strong inverse relationship between cardiorespiratory fitness and the 11-year incidence of both total and ischemic stroke among 2,011 middle-aged men (Kurl et al., 2003).

Coronary and Peripheral Artery Atherosclerosis

Data from cohort studies and clinical trials in Scandinavia and the United States provide some support for the hypothesis that physical activity retards the initiation or progression of coronary and peripheral artery atherosclerosis in asymptomatic individuals.

In the Tromsø Study, which followed 3,128 middle-aged Norwegians for 15 years, leisure-time physical activity was classified as a three-level ordinal variable, with levels roughly corresponding to no activity, moderate-intensity activity for at least 4 hours per week, and vigorous activity for at least 2 hours per week (Stensland-Bugge et al., 2000). Intensity of physical activity was inversely related to carotid intima-media thickness (IMT) in men but not women. The researchers offered several plausible explanations for the apparent effect modification by gender. First, the activity level among women, who as a group were more sedentary than the men, may have been too low to show a benefit. Second, because women may have been more likely than men to engage in housekeeping or caregiving activities requiring physical exertion, leisure-time activity may be less indicative of overall activity in women than in men. Finally, the benefit of exercise may occur via improvements in physiologic variables in which women have a comparative advantage over men, such as blood pressure or HDL cholesterol level.

Using a physical activity classification scheme similar to that of the Tromsø investigators, Swedish researchers examined whether intensity of activity was associated with asymptomatic leg atherosclerosis in a cohort of 363 male residents of Malmö followed for 13 years (Engström et al., 2001). After adjustment for potential confounders, intensity of physical activity at age 55 years and increases in activity intensity between ages 55 and 68 years were predictive of higher ankle-brachial blood pressure index at age 68 years, suggesting that exercise may retard atherosclerotic lesions even in those who become active late in life.

Among 854 middle-aged Finnish men in the Kuopio Ischemic Heart Disease Risk Factor Study, a high cardiorespiratory fitness level was predictive of a significant slowing in the progression of early atherosclerosis (Lakka et al., 2001). Strong, inverse, and graded associations between maximal oxygen uptake during baseline exercise and 4-year increases in maximal or mean carotid IMT, plaque height, and surface roughness were observed. However, there was no relationship between self-reported physical activity (total energy expenditure, duration, frequency, or mean intensity level) and 4-year changes in these parameters.

The Los Angeles Atherosclerosis Study investigated the relationship between leisure-time physical activity and early atherosclerotic progression in 500 middle-aged employees of a utility company (Nordstrom et al., 2003). Physical activity, classified as an ordinal three-level variable reflecting the intensity and frequency of activity, was strongly and inversely related to changes in mean carotid IMT over a 3-year period in both men and women.

Two randomized trials have tested whether physical activity slows the progression of atherosclerosis. The 6-year DNA Polymorphism and Carotid Atherosclerosis Study enrolled 140 healthy middle-aged Finnish men and assigned them to an exercise or control group (Rauramaa et al., 2004). For the first 3 months of the intervention, men in the exercise group were advised to perform exercise three times per week for 30 to 45 minutes per session; thereafter, they were asked to exercise five times per week for 45 to 60 minutes per session. Prescribed exercises included walking, jogging, cross-country skiing, swimming, and cycling. Exercise intensity was determined individually and modified when necessary to correspond to 40% to 60% of maximal oxygen uptake. Treatment assignment was not related to change in mean carotid IMT in the cohort as a whole. However, among men not taking statins, the exercise intervention was associated with a 40% reduction in the progression of atherosclerosis. The Women's Health Lifestyle Project assigned healthy women aged 44 to 50 years to a lifestyle intervention consisting of a low-fat, low-calorie diet and an increase in weekly leisure-time physical activity to 1000 to 1500 kcal of energy expenditure (Wildman et al., 2004). The intervention significantly slowed progression of atherosclerosis, measured by change in mean carotid IMT during 4 years of follow-up, among peri- and postmenopausal women but not among premenopausal women.

Methodologic Considerations

When interpreting the inverse associations between physical activity and clinical or subclinical atherosclerotic disease reported in observational studies, one must consider the possibility that unmeasured or unknown factors may influence the selection and participation of study participants (selection bias); the possibility that correlated factors, including unmeasured or unknown variables, account for the association (confounding); and the possibility that imperfectly measured exposure or disease status could influence the results (misclassification). For example, comparisons of questionnaire estimates with physical activity diaries or measures of cardiorespiratory fitness suggest that questionnaires more accurately capture vigorous activity than light or moderate activity, a finding that may account in part for the lack of association between the latter type of activities and risk of CVD noted in some studies of middle-aged men (Lee, 2004). However, the general consistency of the results across studies—including those that relied on exercise testing rather than physical activity questionnaires to assess exposure—supports a causal association, as does the biologic plausibility (the known beneficial effects of increased physical activity on the vascular risk factor profile).

Protective Mechanisms

Observational and experimental data indicate that habitual physical activity has beneficial effects on both atherosclerotic and thrombotic risk factors. These effects include reducing adiposity, blood pressure, diabetes incidence, atherogenic dyslipidemia (i.e., elevated triglycerides, low HDL cholesterol, and other lipoprotein abnormalities), and inflammation, as well as enhancing insulin sensitivity, glycemic control, fibrinolysis, and endothelial function.

Body Weight

The rationale for the aforementioned recommendation of 1 hour of moderate-intensity physical activity per day is that lesser amounts of activity have not been consistently shown to ensure weight maintenance within the healthy BMI range of 18.5 to 24.9 kg/m^2 or to promote weight loss in the absence of curtailing food intake. Exercising for weight control may be particularly important for females, because national data indicate that caloric intakes of U.S. women increased by a higher percentage than those of U.S. men in recent decades. From 1971 to 2000, the daily caloric intake of the average woman rose 22% (from 1542 to 1877 kcal), whereas the average man's intake increased by 7% (from 2450 to 2618 kcal) (Centers for Disease Control and Prevention, 2004). During this time, the prevalence of obesity soared in both genders. In the early 1960s, an estimated 32% of U.S. adults were overweight (BMI 25–29.9 kg/m^2) and 13% were obese (BMI $\geq$ 30 kg/m^2). By 2002, the proportion of overweight adults had increased slightly to 35%, while the proportion of obese adults more than doubled, to 30% (Hedley et al., 2004). An estimated 33.2% of U.S. women and 27.6% of U.S. men are obese. Although comparable data on national trends in physical activity during this period do not exist, activity levels among U.S. adults appeared to be stable during the 1990s (Centers for Disease Control and Prevention, 2001), suggesting that poor dietary habits are at least as responsible as sedentary lifestyle for Americans' expanding waistlines.

Data differ as to whether an hour of activity per day is necessary for weight control. In the National Weight Control Registry, a volunteer sample of 629 women and 155 men who lost an average of 30 kg and maintained a minimum weight loss of 13.6 kg for 5 years, the self-reported median weekly leisure-time exercise energy expenditure was 2800 kcal, or 1.5 hours per day of brisk walking for a 65-kg woman (Klem et al., 1997). In a database compiled by the IOM of some 400 healthy stable-weight men and women aged 19 to 70 years whose energy expenditures had been estimated with the doubly labeled water method, which is considered the gold standard of energy expenditure measurement, persons with BMI between 18.5 and 25.0 kg/m^2 expended a daily energy equivalent of substantially more than 1 hour of moderate activity. However, their age- and gender-matched overweight and obese counterparts also expended roughly the same amount of energy, a finding that undercuts the contention that at least 1 hour of daily activity is necessary to maintain a healthy weight (Blair et al., 2004). Moreover, findings from randomized trials of exercise

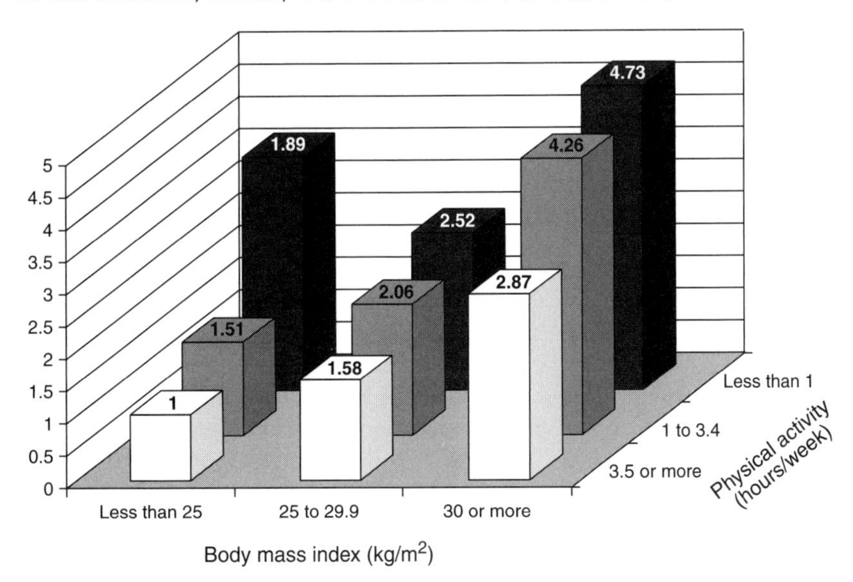

Figure 9.3 Relative risks of cardiovascular disease mortality according to body mass index and physical activity,* during 24 years of follow-up among 116,564 women in the Nurses' Health Study. (Data from Hu et al., 2004a.)
* Physical activity was defined as moderate to vigorous activity, including brisk walking. Relative risks were adjusted for age, smoking status, parental history of coronary heart disease, menopausal status and hormone use, and alcohol consumption.

in overweight, sedentary individuals who were asked to adhere to their usual diet indicate that lesser amounts of activity can also have a beneficial effect on weight regulation (Irwin et al., 2003; Slentz et al., 2004).

Although the exact shape of the dose–response curve between physical activity and body weight remains unclear, focusing on weight control as the main reason for engaging in physical activity yields an incomplete picture of exercise's impact on cardiovascular health. With few exceptions, prospective observational studies and clinical trials find that inverse relationships between physical activity—even at doses of 30 minutes per day of moderate-intensity exercise—and risk of CVD persist even after factoring out the effects of BMI, suggesting that the cardiovascular benefits derived from physical activity are not solely a function of weight regulation. Of course, this observation does not negate the strong deleterious impact of overweight and obesity; epidemiologic studies indicate that an estimated 25% of CHD cases are attributable to excess weight, and that each kg of weight gained during midlife increases CHD risk by 3% (Willett et al., 1995). Indeed, most studies of the "fit vs. fat" issue conclude that both physical activity and weight control are important and independent predictors of CVD incidence and mortality (Fig. 9.3; Hu et al., 2004a).

Blood Pressure

Prospective observational studies in men indicate that increased physical activity or fitness may protect against the development of hypertension (Pescatello et al., 2004). Three cohort studies have conducted gender-specific analyses of the association between physical activity and incident hypertension. The Atherosclerosis Risk In Communities (ARIC) investigators (Pereira et al., 1999), who followed 7,459 men and women aged 45 to 64 years for 6 years, and Haapenen and colleagues (1997), who followed 2,840 men and women aged 35 to 63 years for 10 years, reported an inverse association between physical activity and incident hypertension only in men. However, the largest study, a 10-year follow-up of 17,441 men and women aged 25 to 64 years, found that increased physical activity (a composite of amount and intensity of recreational, occupational, and commuting activity) predicted a lower risk of hypertension in both genders (Hu et al., 2004b). After adjustment for baseline blood pressure, BMI, and other covariates, the relative risks of hypertension associated with light, moderate, and high physical activity were 1.00, 0.60, and 0.59 (*p* for trend <0.001), respectively, in men and 1.0, 0.80, and 0.72 (*p* for trend = 0.006), respectively, in women.

Non-sport leisure activities such as walking or cycling were more strongly associated with reduced hypertension risk than were higher-intensity sport and exercise activities among men in the ARIC study, and only the association between the leisure index and incident hypertension was significant in a predictive model that included both the leisure and sport indices. Intensity of activity was not an important predictor of hypertension risk after adjustment for total physical activity among the men studied by Haapanen and colleagues.

Data from randomized trials also indicate that habitual moderate-intensity exercise is as effective as high-intensity exercise in lowering blood pressure. This pattern has been found in normotensive and hypertensive individuals, in women and men, and appears to be independent of weight change. In a meta-analysis of 54 randomized trials with a total of 2,419 participants, aerobic exercise was associated with a mean reduction in blood pressure of 3.9/2.6 mm Hg across all initial blood pressure levels and mean reduction of 4.9/3.7 mm Hg in hypertensive patients; the degree of blood pressure reduction did not differ by frequency or intensity of exercise (Whelton et al., 2002). Another meta-analysis of 47 aerobic exercise trials (2,543 participants) reported mean blood pressure decreases of 2/1 mm Hg (2%/1%) in normotensive persons and decreases of 6/5 mm Hg (4%/5%) in hypertensive persons (Kelley et al., 2001a). In a meta-analysis of 16 trials (650 participants) that employed walking as the sole intervention, decreases of 3/2 mm Hg occurred in both normotensive and hypertensive persons after a mean of 25 weeks of treatment (Kelley et al., 2001b). Resistance exercise may also reduce blood pressure. In a meta-analysis of 11 trials (320 participants) of strength training (an average of three 38-minute sessions per week over 14 weeks, with one to four sets ranging from 4 to 50 repetitions at 35% of participants' repetition maximum), the intervention produced blood pressure decreases of 3/3 mm Hg (2%/4%) (Kelley and Kelley, 2000).

Insulin Sensitivity and Glycemic Control

Observational and clinical trial data suggest that regular physical activity, either alone or combined with dietary therapy, improves insulin sensitivity, glycemic control, and the metabolic profile among both non-diabetic and diabetic populations. Moderate- and high-intensity exercise may confer comparable benefits. The Insulin Resistance Atherosclerosis Study reported significant cross-sectional relationships of similar magnitude between both moderate- and vigorous-intensity physical activity and insulin sensitivity among middle-aged men and women with and without type 2 diabetes (Mayer-Davis et al., 1998). Increases in moderate-intensity and vigorous physical activity of 200 kcal per day were associated with increases in insulin sensitivity of 2.9% and 2.6%, respectively. After adjustment for BMI and waist-to-hip ratio, the increases were somewhat attenuated—1.7% and 1.9%, respectively—but remained statistically significant.

Intervention studies have found a similar pattern of results. For example, a 6-month trial that randomly assigned middle-aged, overweight women and men with dyslipidemia to various exercise regimens or to a non-exercising control group found that equivalent durations of moderate-intensity and vigorous exercise were associated with nearly identical improvements in insulin sensitivity (Houmard et al., 2004). Compared with sedentary controls, participants who performed 170 minutes per week of moderate-intensity exercise and those who spent the same amount of time engaged in vigorous exercise experienced an 88% and 83% increase in insulin sensitivity, respectively; these improvements were not accounted for by weight loss. A meta-analysis of 14 trials (11 of which were randomized; 504 participants) of physical activity interventions lasting 8 weeks or more found that exercise training reduced glycosylated hemoglobin (HbA_{1c}) levels among middle-aged persons with diabetes (Boule et al., 2001). Aerobic exercise interventions—which, on average, consisted of three 53-minute sessions per week of walking or cycling over an 18-week period—were associated with a mean 0.67% reduction in HbA_{1c} level; resistance training (two to three sets ranging from 10 to 20 repetitions at 50% of respondents' repetition maximum) yielded a comparable reduction of 0.64%. These benefits appeared to be independent of change in weight or body composition. In a 10-year observational follow-up of participants with diabetes in the large U.K. Prospective Diabetes Study, each 1% reduction in HbA_{1c} level was associated with a 14% reduction in myocardial infarction, a 37% reduction in microvascular complications, and a 21% reduction in diabetes-related mortality (Stratton et al., 2000).

In prospective studies, walking predicts markedly reduced CVD incidence and CVD mortality among persons with type 2 diabetes. Among Nurses' Health Study participants with diabetes who reported no vigorous exercise, the 14-year relative risks for incident cardiovascular events across increasing quartiles of walking energy expenditure were 1.0 (referent), 0.85, 0.63, and 0.56, after adjustment for BMI and other covariates (Hu et al., 2001). Similar reductions were seen among men with diabetes in the Health Professionals Follow-up Study (Tanasescu et al., 2003). Among 2,449 adults with diabetes in the National Health Interview Survey, walking 2 or more hours per week, compared with not walking, was associated with a 41% reduction in CVD mortality during 8 years of follow-up (Gregg et al., 2003b). In an 18.4-year follow-up of 3,316 Finnish men and women aged 25 to 74 years with diabetes, the adjusted relative risks associated with low, moderate, and high leisure-time physical activity were 1.00 (referent), 0.83, and 0.67 for CVD mortality (Hu et al., 2004c).

A randomized trial from Denmark included 30 minutes of brisk walking three to five times per week as part of a multifactorial approach to the management of type 2 diabetes (Gaede et al., 2003). In this study, 160 patients with diabetes were assigned to receive conventional treatment from their general practitioners or intensive treatment, including a stepwise implementation of behavior modification and pharmacologic therapy, overseen by a physician, nurse, and dietician at the academic center conducting the trial. During 8 years of follow-up, the intensive-treatment group experienced a significant 53% reduction in cardiovascular events compared to the conventional-treatment group. The ongoing Look AHEAD (Action For Health in Diabetes) Study, which has enrolled more than 5,000 participants, should provide additional randomized data on the long-term (11.5 years) effects of sustained weight loss through exercise and decreased energy intake on the risk of CVD in obese persons with type 2 diabetes (Ryan et al., 2003).

Diabetes Incidence

Prospective observational studies have consistently shown a marked reduction in the incidence of type 2 diabetes among physically active or fit individuals as compared with their inactive or unfit peers (*see also* Chapter 11). In the Nurses' Health Study, moderate-intensity activity and more vigorous activity resulted in comparable reductions in diabetes incidence, given equivalent total exercise energy expenditures (Hu et al., 1999). In a cohort of 4,369 middle-aged Finnish women and men followed for 9.4 years, individuals who walked or cycled to work for at least 30 minutes per day experienced a 36% reduction in diabetes incidence compared with their counterparts who did not engage in these activities (Hu et al., 2003). A 6-year follow-up of 1,728 Pima Indians in Arizona, a community with one of the world's highest incidences of type 2 diabetes and a high prevalence of obesity, found that recreational physical activity meeting the 30-minute, moderate-intensity public health guideline was associated with a 26% reduction in diabetes incidence in women and a 12% reduction in men (Kriska et al., 2003). In the Kuopio Ischemic Heart Disease Risk Factor Study, which followed 897 middle-aged men for 4.2 years, men in the lowest quartile of cardiorespiratory fitness were more than four times as likely to develop diabetes as men in the highest two quartiles of fitness (Lynch et al., 1996). In a 14-year follow-up of 4,747 20- to 40-year-old male employees of the Tokyo Gas Company, the relative risks of incident diabetes across increasing quartiles of fitness were 1.0 (referent), 0.78, 0.63, and 0.56 (Sawada et al., 2003). All of these estimates reflect adjustment for the effects of BMI and other covariates.

Intervention studies in high-risk populations also suggest that physical activity lowers the risk of diabetes. In the Da Qing Impaired Glucose Tolerance and Diabetes Study, 577 middle-aged Chinese women and men with impaired glucose tolerance were randomized, by clinic, to one of three treatment groups—diet only, exercise only, or diet plus exercise—or to a control group (Pan et al., 1997). The three interventions were associated with statistically significant reductions of 31%, 46%, and 42% in diabetes risk, respectively, over a 6-year period. Lean and overweight individuals experienced similar reductions in diabetes incidence. In the Finnish Diabetes Prevention Study, 522 middle-aged, overweight women and men with impaired glucose tolerance were randomly assigned to an intensive lifestyle intervention designed to promote healthy eating and exercise patterns or to a control group (Tuomilehto et al., 2001). Members of the diet and exercise intervention group lost significantly more weight than did the control group (3.5 vs. 0.8 kg) and, over 3 years, reduced their risk of developing diabetes by 58%. The U.S. Diabetes Prevention Program, a 3-year follow-up of 3,234 women and men aged 25 to 85 years with impaired glucose tolerance and BMI of 24 kg/m^2 or more, also reported a 58% reduction in diabetes risk among the intervention group, whose members, on average, engaged in moderate-intensity exercise for 30 minutes per day and lost 5% to 7% of their body weight during the trial (Knowler et al., 2002). This study oversampled older individuals, as well as individuals of ethnic groups that suffer disproportionately from diabetes (black Americans, Hispanic Americans, Asian Americans, Pacific Islanders, and American Indians), and found that the intervention was effective in reducing diabetes risk in all age and ethnic groups and in both genders.

Recent data suggest that the protective effect of physical activity on insulin action and diabetes risk may result partly from its favorable influence on adipokines, which are biologically active proteins such as leptin, adiponectin, resistin, and tumor necrosis factor-α that are synthesized by adipose tissue (Franks et al., 2003; Monzillo et al., 2003). More research is needed to elucidate this potential pathway.

Dyslipidemia

In contrast to the findings for insulin sensitivity and hypertension, strong dose–response associations between exercise intensity and blood lipids—specifically, triglyceride and HDL cholesterol levels—have been reported in observational studies (Leon and Sanchez, 2001). An 8-month randomized trial that assigned middle-age sedentary men and women with dyslipidemia to various exercise programs or to a control group found that although exercise did not lower plasma levels of low-density lipoprotein (LDL) cholesterol, it did favorably alter various LDL subfractions in addition to the expected improvements in HDL cholesterol and triglycerides (Kraus et al., 2002). These effects were far more pronounced among the "high-amount/high-intensity" exercise group, who expended the energy equivalent of jogging 20 miles per week, than among the "low-amount/high-intensity" and "low-amount/moderate-intensity" groups, who expended the equivalent of jogging or walking 12 miles per week, respectively. A comparison of the latter two exercise groups showed that they experienced similar improvements in lipoprotein profile to each other. On the basis of these results, the investigators suggest that lipoprotein profiles are more strongly related to amount, rather than intensity, of physical activity. Beneficial effects of aerobic exercise (walking at 70% heart rate reserve for three 50-minute sessions per week) and resistance training on plasma lipoprotein levels were also found in a 10-week randomized trial of women aged 70 to 87 years, providing further evidence that physical activity can improve cardiovascular risk factors, even in the elderly (Fahlman et al., 2002).

Inflammation

Regular physical activity may favorably modulate inflammatory responses and immune system function, critical processes in the pathogenesis of CVD. Dose–response relationships between physical activity or fitness and inflammatory markers, including C-reactive protein (CRP), interleukin-6, and white blood cell count, have been observed in large, population-based samples unselected for CVD. In the National Health and Nutrition Examination Survey III, for example, the adjusted relative risks for elevated CRP (defined as ≥85th percentile of the sex-specific distribution) were 0.98, 0.85, and 0.53 for respondents who engaged in light, moderate, and vigorous leisure-time activity, respectively, during the previous month compared with those engaging in no leisure-time activity during that time (Ford, 2002). In an analysis limited to respondents without CHD, diabetes, or other chronic conditions, frequency of physical activity was also associated in a dose-dependent manner with CRP level (Abramson and Vaccarino, 2002). Compared with those engaging in leisure-time physical activity three or fewer times per month, persons who engaged in such activity 4 to 21 and 22 or more times per month were 23% and 37% less likely, respectively, to have an elevated CRP level. In the Aerobics Center Longitudinal Study, the relative risks of having an elevated CRP were 1.00, 0.43, 0.33, 0.23, and 0.17 for men in the lowest (least fit) to the highest (most fit) quintile, respectively (Church et al., 2002). Data from the British Regional Heart Study, a 20-year follow-up of 3,810 men aged 40 to 59 years, suggest that exercise must be current to confer an anti-inflammatory effect; men who were active in mid-life but became inactive in later life had CRP levels comparable to those of continuously inactive men, whereas men who took up even light activity in later life had CRP levels approaching those of continuously inactive men (Wannamethee et al., 2002). Results from small non-randomized intervention studies also suggest that regular exercise can reduce inflammation (Mattusch et al., 2000, Smith et al., 1999).

Metabolic Syndrome

The metabolic syndrome is a clustering of metabolic abnormalities defined by the National Cholesterol Education Program as the presence of at least three of the following: abdominal obesity, hypertension, hypertriglyceridemia, low HDL cholesterol, and fasting hyperglycemia. (Elevated CRP levels are also common among persons with the metabolic syndrome.) A powerful risk factor for CVD, the syndrome is present in an estimated 27% of adults (Ford et al., 2004) and 10% of adolescents (de Ferranti et al., 2004) in the United States. Although much evidence implicates low activity or fitness levels as risk factors for the individual components of the metabolic syndrome, only recently have longitudinal data become available that link these exposures to the development of the metabolic syndrome itself.

In the Kuopio Ischemic Heart Disease Risk Factor Study, sedentary men had a twofold increase in the risk of developing the metabolic syndrome over a 4-year period compared with men who engaged in at least 3 hours per week of moderate or vigorous leisure-time physical activity (Laaksonen et al., 2002). In the Coronary Artery Risk Development in Young Adults Study, a 15-year follow-up of 2,478 women and men aged 18 to 30 years, participants in the bottom quintile of fitness were twice as likely to develop the metabolic syndrome than participants in the top two quintiles of fitness (Carnethon et al., 2003). Among 9,007 men in the 20-year Aerobics Center Longitudinal Study, the risk of metabolic syndrome was 26% lower for those in the middle tertile of fitness and 53% lower for those in the top tertile, compared with those in the bottom tertile (LaMonte et al., 2005). Among the 1,491 women in this study, the corresponding figures were 20% and 63%. Each of these studies adjusted for baseline BMI and other covariates. These observational findings are supported by randomized data from the U.S. Diabetes Prevention Program, which found that the incidence of the metabolic syndrome was reduced by 41% in the lifestyle intervention group compared with the control group (Orchard et al., 2005).

Hemostasis

Physical activity may also favorably influence hemostatic factors. In a cross-sectional study of 1,507 women and men aged 25 to 64 years in the Northern Sweden Monitoring of Trends and Determinants in Cardiovascular Disease Study (MONICA), tissue plasminogen activator (tPA) activity increased linearly with greater leisure-time physical activity, whereas plasminogen activator inhibitor-1 activity decreased (Eliasson et al., 1996). In a cross-sectional analysis of data from the British Regional Heart Study, habitual leisure-time physical activity showed significant and inverse dose–response relationships with fibrinogen, plasma and blood viscosity, platelet count, coagulation factors VIII and IX, von Willebrand factor, fibrin D-dimer, and tPA antigen, which persisted after adjustment for potential confounders (Wannamethee et al., 2002). Randomized intervention studies have consistently found that regular moderate-intensity exercise improves fibrinolytic capacity in formerly sedentary individuals. However, limited and inconsistent data from trials testing the effect of regular physical activity performed at varying intensities on blood coagulation and platelet reactivity do not allow firm conclusions regarding these two pathways (Lee and Lip, 2003).

Endothelial Function

Data from large epidemiologic studies on the relationship between regular physical activity and endothelial function in apparently healthy individuals are sparse, although modest inverse associations between habitual exercise and circulating levels of cellular adhesion molecules have been reported in both men (Rohde et al., 1999) and women (Demerath et al., 2001). Small intervention studies in men at usual risk of CVD have not consistently demonstrated beneficial effects of exercise on endothelial parameters. However, trials in male patients with hypertension, hypercholesterolemia, diabetes, coronary artery disease, or heart failure have indicated that aerobic exercise training increases nitrous oxide and prostacyclin availability and improves endothelial-dependent vasodilatation (Moyna and Thompson, 2004). Because the vascular endothelium is also involved in other aspects of cardiovascular health, such as mediating the balance between fibrinolytic and prothrombotic processes, controlling inflammatory responses, and regulating blood pressure, it is likely an important pathway by which exercise exerts multiple cardioprotective effects.

Future Directions

Data from observational studies and clinical trials suggest that as little as 30 minutes per day of moderate-intensity physical activity can reduce the incidence of clinical cardiovascular events in populations with low levels of baseline activity. Regular physical activity also appears to slow the initiation or progression of asymptomatic atherosclerosis. The mechanisms responsible for these protective effects likely include the regulation of body weight; the reduction of adiposity, blood pressure, insulin resistance, atherogenic dyslipidemia, and inflammation; and the enhancement of insulin sensitivity, glucose tolerance, and fibrinolytic and endothelial function. Despite recent advances in basic and clinical research, however, our understanding of the physiologic connections between physical activity and CVD is imperfect. Physical inactivity has been associated with so many vascular risk factors that scientists have not fully disentangled the more important and the less important pathways by which exercise affects disease risk. Nevertheless, whether or not a complete picture of the relevant physiology is ultimately realized, the identification of strategies for facilitating sustained exercise at a level sufficient to result in measurable improvements to public health should be a top priority. In largely sedentary societies such as the United States, an urgent task facing health-care providers and policymakers is determining how best to promote appropriate levels of habitual physical activity to their patients and the general public, respectively.

Personal Perspective

Based on a review of available scientific findings, as well as a balancing of efficacy and feasibility concerns, we strongly believe that the clinical and public health message regarding exercise for the prevention of CVD should remain "30 minutes per day of moderate-intensity activity is desirable; and more is better, to a reasonable extent." Although scientific debate continues on the exact amount of physical activity required for optimal cardiovascular health, such a debate serves little purpose if the general public cannot be persuaded to adopt a physically active lifestyle. We do not want to run the risk of allowing the perfect to be the enemy of the good. According to a well-established epidemiologic principle (Rose, 1992), the overall disease burden in a given population generally undergoes a more dramatic reduction when a large segment of the population adopts modest improvements in health behaviors than when a modest segment of the population adopts large improvements.

References

Abramson JL, Vaccarino V. 2002. Relationship between physical activity and inflammation among apparently healthy middle-aged and older US adults. *Arch Intern Med* 162: 1286–92.

American College of Sports Medicine. 1978. American College of Sports Medicine position statement on the recommended quantity and quality of exercise for developing and maintaining fitness in healthy adults. *Med Sci Sports* 10: vii-x.

Bijnen FC, Caspersen CJ, Feskens EJ, Saris WH, Mosterd WL, Kromhout D. 1998. Physical activity and 10-year mortality from cardiovascular diseases and all causes: The Zutphen Elderly Study. *Arch Intern Med* 158: 1499–505.

Blair SN, LaMonte MJ, Nichaman MZ. 2004. The evolution of physical activity recommendations: how much is enough? *Am J Clin Nutr* 79: 913S-20S.

Boule NG, Haddad E, Kenny GP, Wells GA, Sigal RJ. 2001. Effects of exercise on glycemic control and body mass in type 2 diabetes mellitus: a meta-analysis of controlled clinical trials. *JAMA* 286: 1218–27.

Carnethon MR, Gidding SS, Nehgme R, Sidney S, Jacobs DR, Jr., Liu K. 2003. Cardiorespiratory fitness in young adulthood and the development of cardiovascular disease risk factors. *JAMA* 290: 3092–100.

Centers for Disease Control and Prevention. 2001. Physical activity trends—United States, 1990–1998. *MMWR* 50: 166–9.

Centers for Disease Control and Prevention. 2004. Trends in intake of energy and macronutrients—United States, 1971–2000. *MMWR* 53: 80–2.

Church TS, Barlow CE, Earnest CP, Kampert JB, Priest EL, Blair SN. 2002. Associations between cardiorespiratory fitness and C-reactive protein in men. *Arterioscler Thromb Vasc Biol* 22: 1869–76.

de Ferranti SD, Gauvreau K, Ludwig DS, Neufeld EJ, Newburger JW, Rifai N. 2004. Prevalence of the metabolic syndrome in American adolescents: findings from the Third National Health and Nutrition Examination Survey. *Circulation* 110: 2494–7.

Demerath E, Towne B, Blangero J, Siervogel RM. 2001. The relationship of soluble ICAM-1, VCAM-1, P-selectin and E-selectin to cardiovascular disease risk factors in healthy men and women. *Ann Hum Biol* 28: 664–78.

Eliasson M, Asplund K, Evrin PE. 1996. Regular leisure time physical activity predicts high activity of tissue plasminogen activator: The Northern Sweden MONICA Study. *Int J Epidemiol* 25: 1182–8.

Engström G, Ogren M, Hedblad B, Wollmer P, Janzon L. 2001. Asymptomatic leg atherosclerosis is reduced by regular physical activity. Longitudinal results from the cohort "Men Born in 1914." *Eur J Vasc Endovasc Surg* 21: 502–7.

Eyre H, Kahn R, Robertson RM, et al. 2004. Preventing cancer, cardiovascular disease, and diabetes: a common agenda for the American Cancer Society, the American Diabetes Association, and the American Heart Association. *Circulation* 109: 3244–55.

Fahlman MM, Boardley D, Lambert CP, Flynn MG. 2002. Effects of endurance training and resistance training on plasma lipoprotein profiles in elderly women. *J Gerontol A Biol Sci Med Sci* 57: B54–60.

Ford ES. 2002. Does exercise reduce inflammation? Physical activity and C-reactive protein among U.S. adults. *Epidemiology* 13: 561–8.

Ford ES, Giles WH, Mokdad AH. 2004. Increasing prevalence of the metabolic syndrome among U.S. adults. *Diabetes Care* 27: 2444–9.

Franks PW, Farooqi IS, Luan J, et al. 2003. Does physical activity energy expenditure explain the between-individual variation in plasma leptin concentrations after adjusting for differences in body composition? *J Clin Endocrinol Metab* 88: 3258–63.

Gaede P, Vedel P, Larsen N, Jensen GV, Parving HH, Pedersen O. 2003. Multifactorial intervention and cardiovascular disease in patients with type 2 diabetes. *N Engl J Med* 348: 383–93.

Gregg EW, Cauley JA, Stone K, et al. 2003a. Relationship of changes in physical activity and mortality among older women. *JAMA* 289: 2379–86.

Gregg EW, Gerzoff RB, Caspersen CJ, Williamson DF, Narayan KM. 2003b. Relationship of walking to mortality among US adults with diabetes. *Arch Intern Med* 163: 1440–7.

Haapanen N, Miilunpalo S, Vuori I, Oja P, Pasanen M. 1997. Association of leisure time physical activity with the risk of coronary heart disease, hypertension and diabetes in middle-aged men and women. *Int J Epidemiol* 26: 739–47.

Hakim AA, Curb JD, Petrovitch H, et al. 1999. Effects of walking on coronary heart disease in elderly men: the Honolulu Heart Program. *Circulation* 100: 9–13.

Hedley AA, Ogden CL, Johnson CL, Carroll MD, Curtin LR, Flegal KM. 2004. Prevalence of overweight and obesity among US children, adolescents, and adults, 1999–2002. *JAMA* 291: 2847–50.

Houmard JA, Tanner CJ, Slentz CA, Duscha BD, McCartney JS, Kraus WE. 2004. Effect of the volume and intensity of exercise training on insulin sensitivity. *J Appl Physiol* 96: 101–6.

Hu FB, Sigal RJ, Rich-Edwards JW, et al. 1999. Walking compared with vigorous physical activity and risk of type 2 diabetes in women: a prospective study. *JAMA* 282: 1433–9.

Hu FB, Stampfer MJ, Colditz GA, et al. 2000. Physical activity and risk of stroke in women. *JAMA* 283: 2961–7.

Hu FB, Stampfer MJ, Solomon C, et al. 2001. Physical activity and risk for cardiovascular events in diabetic women. *Ann Intern Med* 134: 96–105.

Hu FB, Willett WC, Li T, Stampfer MJ, Colditz GA, Manson JE. 2004a. Adiposity as compared with physical activity in predicting mortality among women. *N Engl J Med* 351: 2694–703.

Hu G, Barengo NC, Tuomilehto J, Lakka TA, Nissinen A, Jousilahti P. 2004b. Relationship of physical activity and body mass index to the risk of hypertension: a prospective study in Finland. *Hypertension* 43: 25–30.

Hu G, Eriksson J, Barengo NC, et al. 2004c. Occupational, commuting, and leisure-time physical activity in relation to total and cardiovascular mortality among Finnish subjects with type 2 diabetes. *Circulation* 110: 666–73.

Hu G, Qiao Q, Silventoinen K, et al. 2003. Occupational, commuting, and leisure-time physical activity in relation to risk for type 2 diabetes in middle-aged Finnish men and women. *Diabetologia* 46: 322–9.

Institute of Medicine. 2002. *Dietary reference intakes for energy, carbohydrates, fiber, fat, protein, and amino acids*. Washington DC: The National Academies Press.

Irwin ML, Yasui Y, Ulrich CM, et al. 2003. Effect of exercise on total and intra-abdominal body fat in postmenopasual women: a randomized trial. *JAMA* 289: 323–30.

Kelley GA, Kelley KS. 2000. Progressive resistance exercise and resting blood pressure: a meta-analysis of randomized controlled trials. *Hypertension* 35: 838–43.

Kelley GA, Kelley KS, Tran ZV. 2001a. Aerobic exercise and resting blood pressure: a meta-analytic review of randomized, controlled trials. *Prev Cardiol* 4: 73–80.

Kelley GA, Kelley KS, Tran ZV. 2001b. Walking and resting blood pressure in adults: a meta-analysis. *Prev Med* 33: 120–7.

Klem ML, Wing RR, McGuire MT, Seagle HM, Hill JO. 1997. A descriptive study of individuals successful at long-term maintenance of substantial weight loss. *Am J Clin Nutr* 66: 239–46.

Knowler WC, Barrett-Connor E, Fowler SE, et al. 2002. Reduction in the incidence of type 2 diabetes with lifestyle intervention or metformin. *N Engl J Med* 346: 393–403.

Kraus WE, Houmard JA, Duscha BD, et al. 2002. Effects of the amount and intensity of exercise on plasma lipoproteins. *N Engl J Med* 347: 1483–92.

Kriska AM, Saremi A, Hanson RL, et al. 2003. Physical activity, obesity, and the incidence of type 2 diabetes in a high-risk population. *Am J Epidemiol* 158: 669–75.

Kurl S, Laukkanen JA, Rauramaa R, Lakka TA, Sivenius J, Salonen JT. 2003. Cardiorespiratory fitness and the risk for stroke in men. *Arch Intern Med* 163: 1682–8.

Laaksonen DE, Lakka HM, Salonen JT, Niskanen LK, Rauramaa R, Lakka TA. 2002. Low levels of leisure-time physical activity and cardiorespiratory fitness predict development of the metabolic syndrome. *Diabetes Care* 25: 1612–8.

LaCroix AZ, Leveille SG, Hecht JA, Grothaus LC, Wagner EH. 1996. Does walking decrease the risk of cardiovascular disease hospitalizations and death in older adults? *J Am Geriatr Soc* 44: 113–20.

Lakka TA, Laukkanen JA, Rauramaa R, et al. 2001. Cardiorespiratory fitness and the progression of carotid atherosclerosis in middle-aged men. *Ann Intern Med* 134: 12–20.

LaMonte MJ, Barlow CE, Jurca R, Kampert JB, Church TS, Blair SN. 2005. Cardiorespiratory fitness is inversely associated with the incidence of metabolic syndrome: a prospective study of men and women. *Circulation* 112: 505–12.

Lee CD, Blair SN. 2002. Cardiorespiratory fitness and stroke mortality in men. *Med Sci Sports Exerc* 34: 592–5.

Lee CD, Folsom AR, Blair SN. 2003. Physical activity and stroke risk: a meta-analysis. *Stroke* 34: 2475–81.

Lee IM. 2004. No pain, no gain? Thoughts on the Caerphilly study. *Br J Sports Med* 38: 4–5.

Lee IM, Hennekens CH, Berger K, Buring JE, Manson JE. 1999. Exercise and risk of stroke in male physicians. *Stroke* 30: 1–6.

Lee IM, Rexrode KM, Cook NR, Manson JE, Buring JE. 2001. Physical activity and coronary heart disease in women: is "no pain, no gain" passe? *JAMA* 285: 1447–54.

Lee IM, Sesso HD, Paffenbarger RS, Jr. 2000. Physical activity and coronary heart disease risk in men: does the duration of exercise episodes predict risk? *Circulation* 102: 981–6.

Lee KW, Lip GY. 2003. Effects of lifestyle on hemostasis, fibrinolysis, and platelet reactivity: a systematic review. *Arch Intern Med* 163: 2368–92.

Leon AS, Sanchez OA. 2001. Response of blood lipids to exercise training alone or combined with dietary intervention. *Med Sci Sports Exerc* 33: S502–15.

Lynch J, Helmrich SP, Lakka TA, et al. 1996. Moderately intense physical activities and high levels of cardiorespiratory fitness reduce the risk of non-insulin-dependent diabetes mellitus in middle-aged men. *Arch Intern Med* 156: 1307–14.

Manson JE, Greenland P, LaCroix AZ, et al. 2002. Walking compared with vigorous exercise for the prevention of cardiovascular events in women. *N Engl J Med* 347: 716–25.

Manson JE, Hu FB, Rich-Edwards JW, et al. 1999. A prospective study of walking as compared with vigorous exercise in the prevention of coronary heart disease in women. *N Engl J Med* 341: 650–8.

Mattusch F, Dufaux B, Heine O, Mertens I, Rost R. 2000. Reduction of the plasma concentration of C-reactive protein following nine months of endurance training. *Int J Sports Med* 21: 21–4.

Mayer-Davis EJ, D'Agostino R, Jr., Karter AJ, et al. 1998. Intensity and amount of physical activity in relation to insulin sensitivity: the Insulin Resistance Atherosclerosis Study. *JAMA* 279: 669–74.

Monzillo LU, Hamdy O, Horton ES, et al. 2003. Effect of lifestyle modification on adipokine levels in obese subjects with insulin resistance. *Obes Res* 11: 1048–54.

Mora S, Redberg RF, Cui Y, et al. 2003. Ability of exercise testing to predict cardiovascular and all-cause death in asymptomatic women: a 20-year follow-up of the Lipid Research Clinics Prevalence Study. *JAMA* 290: 1600–7.

Moyna NM, Thompson PD. 2004. The effect of physical activity on endothelial function in man. *Acta Physiol Scand* 180: 113–23.

Murphy M, Nevill A, Neville C, Biddle S, Hardman A. 2002. Accumulating brisk walking for fitness, cardiovascular risk, and psychological health. *Med Sci Sports Exerc* 34: 1468–74.

Nordstrom CK, Dwyer KM, Merz CN, Shircore A, Dwyer JH. 2003. Leisure time physical activity and early atherosclerosis: the Los Angeles Atherosclerosis Study. *Am J Med* 115: 19–25.

Orchard TJ, Temprosa M, Goldberg R, et al. 2005. The effect of metformin and intensive lifestyle intervention on the metabolic syndrome: the Diabetes Prevention Program randomized trial. *Ann Intern Med* 142: 611–9.

Pan XR, Li GW, Hu YH, et al. 1997. Effects of diet and exercise in preventing NIDDM in people with impaired glucose tolerance. The DaQing IGT and Diabetes Study. *Diabetes Care* 20: 537–44.

Pate RR, Pratt M, Blair SN, et al. 1995. Physical activity and public health. A recommendation from the Centers for Disease Control and Prevention and the American College of Sports Medicine. *JAMA* 273: 402–7.

Pereira MA, Folsom AR, McGovern PG, et al. 1999. Physical activity and incident hypertension in black and white adults: the Atherosclerosis Risk in Communities Study. *Prev Med* 28: 304–12.

Pescatello LS, Franklin BA, Fagard R, Farquhar WB, Kelley GA, Ray CA. 2004. American College of Sports Medicine Position Stand. Exercise and hypertension. *Med Sci Sports Exerc* 36: 533–53.

Petrella RJ, Lattanzio CN, Demeray A, Varallo V, Blore R. 2005. Can adoption of regular exercise later in life prevent metabolic risk for cardiovascular disease? *Diabetes Care* 28: 694–701.

Rauramaa R, Halonen P, Väisänen SB, et al. 2004. Effects of aerobic physical exercise on inflammation and atherosclerosis in men: the DNASCO Study: a six-year randomized, controlled trial. *Ann Intern Med* 140: 1007–14.

Rohde LE, Hennekens CH, Ridker PM. 1999. Cross-sectional study of soluble intercellular adhesion molecule-1 and cardiovascular risk factors in apparently healthy men. *Arterioscler Thromb Vasc Biol* 19: 1595–9.

Rosamond W, Flegal K, Friday G, et al. 2007. Heart disease and stroke statistics—2007 update. A report from the American Heart Association Statistics Committee and Stroke Statistics Committee. *Circulation* 115: e69-e171.

Rose G. 1992. *The Strategy of Preventive Medicine*. New York: Oxford University Press.

Ryan DH, Espeland MA, Foster GD, et al. 2003. Look AHEAD (Action for Health in Diabetes): design and methods for a clinical trial of weight loss for the prevention of cardiovascular disease in type 2 diabetes. *Control Clin Trials* 24: 610–28.

Sawada SS, Lee IM, Muto T, Matuszaki K, Blair SN. 2003. Cardiorespiratory fitness and the incidence of type 2 diabetes: prospective study of Japanese men. *Diabetes Care* 26: 2918–22.

Sesso HD, Paffenbarger RS, Ha T, Lee IM. 1999. Physical activity and cardiovascular disease risk in middle-aged and older women. *Am J Epidemiol* 150: 408–16.

Skerrett PJ, Manson JE. 2002. Reduction in risk of coronary heart disease and diabetes. In N Ruderman, JT Devlin, SH Schneider, A Kriska (Eds.), *Handbook of Exercise in Diabetes*, Alexandria, VA: American Diabetes Association.

Slentz CA, Duscha BD, Johnson JL, et al. 2004. Effects of the amount of exercise on body weight, body composition, and measures of central obesity: STRRIDE—a randomized controlled study. *Arch Intern Med* 164: 31–9.

Smith JK, Dykes R, Douglas JE, Krishnaswamy G, Berk S. 1999. Long-term exercise and atherogenic activity of blood mononuclear cells in persons at risk of developing ischemic heart disease. *JAMA* 281: 1722–27.

Stensland-Bugge E, Bonaa KH, Joakimsen O, Njølstad I. 2000. Sex differences in the relationship of risk factors to subclinical carotid atherosclerosis measured 15 years later: the Tromsø Study. *Stroke* 31: 574–81.

Stratton IM, Adler AI, Neil HA, et al. 2000. Association of glycaemia with macrovascular and microvascular complications of type 2 diabetes (UKPDS 35): prospective observational study. *Br Med J* 321: 405–12.

Tanasescu M, Leitzmann MF, Rimm EB, Hu FB. 2003. Physical activity in relation to cardiovascular disease and total mortality among men with type 2 diabetes. *Circulation* 107: 2435–9.

Tanasescu M, Leitzmann MF, Rimm EB, Willett WC, Stampfer MJ, Hu FB. 2002. Exercise type and intensity in relation to coronary heart disease in men. *JAMA* 288: 1994–2000.

Tuomilehto J, Lindström J, Eriksson JG, et al. 2001. Prevention of type 2 diabetes mellitus by changes in lifestyle among subjects with impaired glucose tolerance. *N Engl J Med* 344: 1343–50.

U.S. Department of Health and Human Services. 1996. *Physical activity and health: a report of the Surgeon General*. Atlanta, GA: U.S. Department of Health and Human Services, Centers for Disease Control and Prevention, National Center for Chronic Disease Prevention and Health Promotion.

US Department of Health and Human Services, US Department of Agriculture. 2005. *Dietary Guidelines for Americans, 2005, 6th edition*. Washington DC: US Government Printing Office.

Wannamethee SG, Lowe GD, Whincup PH, Rumley A, Walker M, Lennon L. 2002. Physical activity and hemostatic and inflammatory variables in elderly men. *Circulation* 105: 1785–90.

Wannamethee SG, Shaper AG, Walker M. 1998. Changes in physical activity, mortality, and incidence of coronary heart disease in older men. *Lancet* 351: 1603–8.

Whelton SP, Chin A, Xin X, He J. 2002. Effect of aerobic exercise on blood pressure: a meta-analysis of randomized, controlled trials. *Ann Intern Med* 136: 493–503.

Wildman RP, Schott LL, Brockwell S, Kuller LH, Sutton-Tyrrell K. 2004. A dietary and exercise intervention slows menopause-associated progression of subclinical atherosclerosis as measured by intima-media thickness of the carotid arteries. *J Am Coll Cardiol* 44: 579–85.

Willett WC, Manson JE, Stampfer MJ, et al. 1995. Weight, weight change, and coronary heart disease in women. Risk within the 'normal' weight range. *JAMA* 273: 461–5.

World Health Organization. 2004. *Global strategy on diet, physical activity and health*. Presented at Fifty-seventh World Health Assembly, WHA57.17, Agenda item 12.6, Geneva.

10

Physical Activity and Cancer

The Evidence, The Issues, and the Challenges

Barbara Sternfeld and I-Min Lee

Cancer, a spectrum of diseases that are all characterized by loss of regulation over cell growth and differentiation and acquisition of the ability to metastasize to distant parts of the body, is the second leading cause of death in the United States, accounting for approximately 565,000 deaths, or about 25% of all deaths, each year (American Cancer Society, 2006). Over 700,000 new cases of cancer are diagnosed annually in men, and about 660,000 new cases are diagnosed annually in women. Among men, prostate cancer occurs most commonly, with an age-adjusted annual incidence rate of 180 per 100,000, representing about one-third of all new cases; among women, breast cancer occurs most frequently (32% of all new cases), and has an incidence rate of 134 per 100,000 (Ries LAG et al., 2005). In both men and women, lung cancer and colorectal cancer are the second and third most commonly occurring cancers, respectively. In addition to the individual and social burden of the disease, the direct medical costs of cancer are estimated at 60.9 billion dollars, and indirect morbidity costs are estimated at 15.5 billion dollars (Chang et al., 2004).

Although genetic susceptibility plays a role in cancer etiology, environmental factors are considered far more important and may explain as much as 80% to 90% of the variability in disease occurrence (Lichtenstein et al., 2000). Among the environmental influences, lifestyle factors—specifically, tobacco use, poor nutrition, obesity, and physical inactivity—account for about one-third of all cancers (American Cancer Society, 2006). Although the role of physical activity in cancer prevention has been examined in detail in epidemiological studies only since the mid-1980s, an impressive body of literature has accumulated that is supportive of this hypothesis, particularly for colon cancer and breast cancer.

This chapter reviews data on the associations between physical activity and the development of various site-specific cancers. Because these data come only from observational epidemiologic studies, with no randomized clinical trials available, the observed associations will be considered in terms of generally accepted criteria for inference of causality. Those criteria include: *(1)* strength of the association; *(2)* consistency of the association across different studies in different populations; *(3)* existence of appropriate temporal relations; and *(4)* existence of a dose–response relationship. This chapter also discusses issues of chance, confounding, and bias as alternate explanations for the observed associations and briefly reviews evidence suggesting biological plausibility, all of which are additional important criteria for evaluating causality. Finally, the chapter ends with a consideration of the public health significance of our current knowledge for reducing the risk of cancer through regular physical activity. Because a number of recent, comprehensive reviews of the physical activity and cancer literature are available (Friedenreich and Thune, 2001; Lee and Oguma, 2006; Lee et al., 2001b; McTiernan et al., 1998; Slattery, 2004; Thune and Furberg, 2001), this chapter does not reference every existing study but, rather, refers the reader to the appropriate sources for obtaining the specific references and greater detail about the individual studies. Where appropriate, examples are drawn from recent studies that have not been included in existing review papers.

Physical Activity and Site-Specific Cancers: What is the Evidence?

Colon and Rectal Cancer

One of the earliest investigations of physical activity and the risk of colon cancer, published in 1984, was a population-based case–control study of 2,950 men living in Los Angeles County who were diagnosed with colon cancer between 1972 and 1981 as well as 31,724 controls (Garabrant et al., 1984). This study estimated occupational physical activity, using census codes to rate individual jobs as highly active, moderately active, or sedentary. The age-adjusted odds ratio (OR) associated with sedentary jobs was 1.6 (95% confidence interval [CI], 1.3–1.8) relative to highly active jobs. This study also examined the risk of rectal cancer associated with occupational activity in 1,213 cases and found no association (OR = 1.0; 95% CI, 0.8–1.3).

Although this early study has a number of limitations (including a crude assessment of occupational activity at only one point in time, no assessment of recreational activity, little ability to adjust for confounding factors, and a sample that was limited to men), its findings are remarkably consistent with the large body of literature that accumulated in the following two decades. There are now more than 50 studies of physical activity and colon cancer that include both cohort and case–control study designs and that represent a combined total of more than 40,000 incident cases (Lee and Oguma, 2006; Thune and Furberg, 2001).* The studies have included men and women from many different population groups in North America, Europe, Asia, Australia, and New Zealand. Most studies have relied on self-reporting to assess recreational physical activity and either self-reporting or job title to assess occupational activity, but they have differed greatly in the amount of detail collected and the ability to quantify activity in terms of frequency, duration, and intensity. Generally, the cohort studies have assessed activity level at the time of entry into the cohort (which may vary from young to older adulthood), whereas the case–control studies have assessed the level of activity during the year or two prior to diagnosis (or index date for controls); only a few studies have repeated assessments of physical activity at different points in time or have attempted to assess lifetime physical activity (Slattery, 2004).

Despite the differences in study design and methods, the findings from these studies have been remarkably similar. As illustrated in Figure 10.1, the totality of evidence suggests that active individuals have about a 40% lower risk of developing colon cancer relative to inactive individuals. When findings are stratified by gender, the magnitude of the risk reduction appears somewhat less in men (about 30%) than in women (about 40%) but is still substantial. Although not all studies have observed a statistically significant inverse association, most have. A recent meta-analysis concluded that physical inactivity was associated with a relative risk (RR) of 1.68 (95% CI, 1.55–1.82) in men and women ages 15 to 69 years and accounted for 16% of colon cancer globally (Bull et al., 2004).

* For a complete review of the studies published prior to 2002, please see Lee 2002, Lee & Oguma, 2006

Generally, the magnitude of the observed associations between physical activity and colon cancer is not substantially changed with adjustment for potential confounding factors, such as body mass index (BMI), smoking, dietary factors, use of non-steroidal anti-inflammatory drugs, or family history of colon cancer (Lee and Oguma 2006; Slattery, 2004). However, limited evidence suggests that at least some of these factors may interact with physical activity in relation to colon cancer. For example, in a population-based case–control study conducted by Slattery et al., the inverse association between physical activity and colon cancer was greater in those with a high energy intake than those with a low intake (Slattery and Potter, 2002). The association between physical activity and colon cancer risk in this study also varied depending on glycemic index, dietary fiber, and body size. Similarly, in a recent case–control study conducted in China, the risk associated with a low level of commuting-related physical activity was far greater in those with a high BMI than in those with a low BMI (Hou et al., 2004). In contrast, a family history of colon cancer may attenuate the inverse association with physical activity (La Vecchia et al., 1999; Slattery and Potter, 2002).

The existence of a dose–response relationship between physical activity and colon cancer risk has been discussed extensively in several previous reviews (Lee and Oguma 2006; Slattery, 2004, Thune and Furberg, 2001). Consideration of this issue is complicated because "dose" can be defined either in terms of total amount of physical activity or in

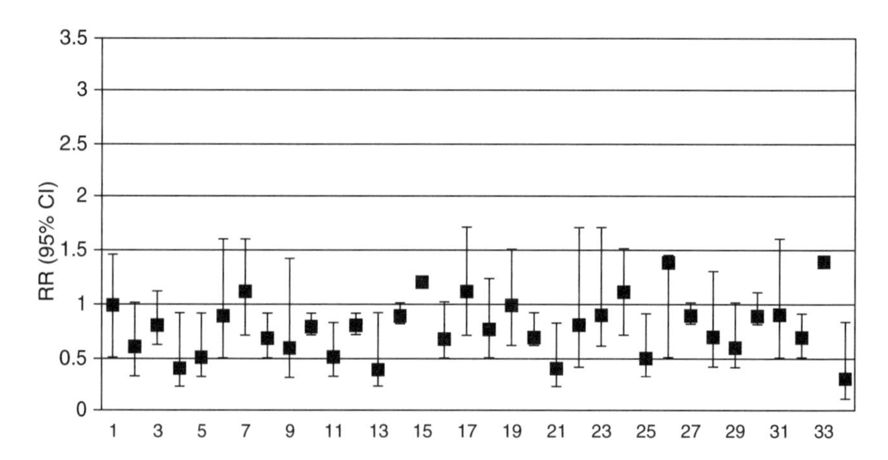

Figure 10.1a Relative risk (RR) and 95% confidence intervals (CIs) from cohort studies of colon cancer and physical activity (most active relative to least active).
Key to Studies: 1. Albanes, 1998; 2. Ballard-Barbash, 1990; 3. Colbert, 2001; 4. Giovannucci, 1995; 5 Lee, 1991; 6. Lee, 1994; 7. Lee, 1997; 6. Severson, 1989; 9. Albanes, 1988; 10. Chow, 1993; 11. Colbert, 2001; 12. Gerhardsson, 1986; 13. Hsing, 1998; 14. Marti, 1989; 15. Paffenbarger, 1987; 16. Severson, 1989; 17. Steenland, 1995; 18. Vena, 1987; 19. Thune, 1996; 20. Will, 1998; 21. Wu, 1987; 22. Albanes, 1989; 23. Ballard-Barbash, 1990; 24. Bostick, 1994; 25. Martinex, 1997; 26. Albanes, 1989; 27. Chow, 1993; 28. Steenland, 1987; 29. Thune, 1996; 30. Will, 1998; 31. Wu, 1987; 32. Chao, 2004; 33. Paffenbarger, 1987; 34. Gerhardsson, 1988.

Notes: A. Citations for all references, with the exception of study 32, may be found in Lee and Oguma, 2006; citation for study 32 may be found in References.
B. Associations refer to recreational activity in men (studies 1–8), occupational activity in men (studies 9–18), total activity in men (studies 19–21), recreational activity in women (studies 22–25), occupational activity in women (studies 26–28), total activity in women (studies 29–31), and recreational activity in men and women combined (studies 32–35).

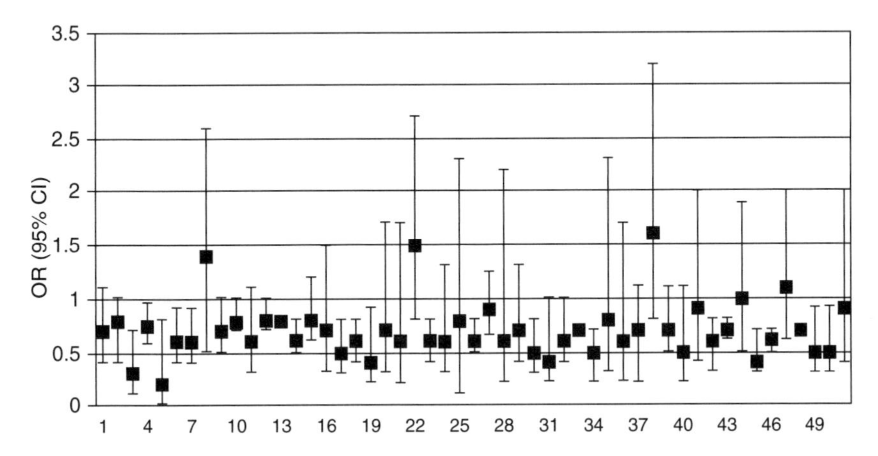

Figure 10.1b Odds ratio (OR) and 95% confidence intervals (CIs) from case–control studies of colon cancer and physical activity (most active relative to least active).
Key to Studies: 1. Hou, 2004; 2. Longnecker, 1995; 3. Slattery, 1988; 4. Slattery, 1997; 5. Tang, 1999; 6. White, 1996; 7. Whittemore, 1990 (U.S.); 8. Whittemore, 1990 (Chinese); 9. Brownson, 1989; 10. Brownson, 1991; 11. Dosemeci, 1993; 12. Fraser, 1993; 13. Fredriksson, 1989; 14. Garabrant, 1984; 15. Hou, 2004; 16. Longnecker, 1985; 17. Marksowitz, 1992; 18. Tavani, 1989; 19. Whittemore, 1990 (U.S.); 20. Whittemore, 1990 (Chinese); 21. Gerhardsson, 1990; 22. Kune, 1990; 23. Le Marchand (1997); 24. Thun, 1992; 25. Hou, 2004; 26. Slattery, 1988; 27. Slattery, 1997; 28. Tang, 1999; 29. White, 1996; 30. Whittemore, 1990 (U.S.); 31. Whittemore, 1990 (Chinese); 32. Hou, 2004; 33. Fredriksoon, 1989; 34. Tavani, 1999; 35. Whittemore, 1990 (U.S.); 36. Whittemore, 1990 (Chinese); 37. Gerhardsson, 1990; 38. Kune, 1990; 39. Le Marchand, 1997; 40. Marcus, 1994; 41. Thun, 1992; 42. Kato, 1990; 43. La Vecchia, 1999 (no family history); 44. La Vecchia, 1999 (family history); 45. Levi, 1999; 46. Slattery, 2002; 47. Arbman, 1993; 48. Benito, 1990; 49. Kato, 1990; 50. Levi, 1999; 51. Peters, 1989.

Notes: A. Citations for all references, with the exception of studies 1, 15, 25, 32, and 46, may be found in Lee and Oguma, 2006 or in Thune and Furberg, 2001; citations for exceptions are in References.
B. Associations refer to recreational activity in men (studies 1–8), occupational activity in men (studies 9–20), total activity in men (studies 21–24), recreational activity in women (studies 25–31), occupational activity in women (studies 32–36), total activity in women (studies 37–41), recreational activity in men and women combined (studies 42–48), and occupational activity in men and women combined (studies 47–51).

terms of any of the component parts (intensity, frequency, and duration) that contribute to total activity. Most studies simply have not had detailed enough assessments of physical activity to allow for evaluation of a dose–response relationship other than in the most general sense of low, medium, and high activity. Nevertheless, although many of those studies did not statistically test for trend (Lee and Oguma, 2006), the results—particularly among men—are consistent with a graded dose–response relationship in which risk declines as activity increases (Thune and Furberg, 2001). A smaller number of studies have assessed physical activity more quantitatively in terms of either hours per week or energy expenditure (metabolic equivalent [MET]-hours per week or kilocalories per week) (Giovannucci et al., 1995; Lee et al., 1991; Martinez et al., 1997; Slattery et al., 1997), but the evidence for a precise dose–response relationship from these studies is not consistent. For example, in the Harvard Alumni Health Study, expenditure of 1,000 kcal/week (equivalent to about

2.5 hours/week of moderate intensity activity) was associated with decreased risk, with little additional risk reduction at higher levels of energy expenditure (Lee et al., 1991). In contrast, the Health Professionals Follow-up Study found a dose–response relationship, with a significantly reduced risk among the most active men who reported approximately 12 hours/week of moderate intensity activity (Giovannucci et al., 1995). In the Nurses' Health Study II (Martinez et al., 1997), a smaller dose of activity (at least 21 MET-hours/week or about 5 hours/week of moderate-intensity activity) was associated with a decreased risk. Still other studies have suggested that intensity, rather than duration, is the more influential factor; a recent report from the Cancer Prevention Study II Nutrition Cohort observed that walking even 7 or more hours per week was not associated with significantly reduced risk (Chao et al., 2004), and in the case–control studies of Slattery et al., vigorous intensity activity resulted in greater reductions in risk than moderate-intensity activity, and the inverse association observed with moderate-intensity physical activity was attributed to the vigorous activity performed by those who also reported moderate activity (Slattery, 2004). As this discussion illustrates, the minimal amount of physical activity required to reduce the risk of colon cancer remains unclear, but at least 30 to 60 minutes/day of moderate- to vigorous-intensity physical activity appears to be a reasonable estimate.

Although the appropriate temporal relationship between exposure and outcome (i.e., exposure precedes outcome) exists in all of the studies of physical activity and colon cancer, the specific relevant time frame of exposure remains largely unknown. In one study of women, activity during early adulthood was not associated with reduced risk (Marcus et al., 1994), suggesting that the susceptible period of exposure may be later in life. A study of Italian men and women examining the risk of colon cancer in relation to activity at different ages (15–19, 30–39, and 50–59 years) observed reduced risk with higher levels of physical activity at all of the ages, perhaps indicating an effect of sustained physical activity throughout adulthood, rather than at any specific point in time (Tavani et al., 1999). The Harvard Alumni Health Study, which failed to find an association between colon cancer and activity assessed either in 1962 through 1966 or in 1977, but found significantly reduced risk in men who were active at both time-points (Lee et al., 1991), also suggested the importance of sustained physical activity. A similar finding was reported in the Cancer Prevention Study II Nutrition Cohort by Chao et al., who observed a significant inverse relationship between colon cancer and physical activity reported in the 1990s in those who also reported moderate or heavy exercise in 1982 but no association in those who were inactive at the earlier time (Chao et al., 2004). Because colon cancer, like most cancers, develops over an extended period of time (during which various factors may either promote or inhibit the progression of the cancer), these findings are consistent with colon cancer biology. An alternate explanation of course is that because these studies depended on self-reported physical activity, the findings might merely reflect better assessment of "true" activity levels when multiple assessments were taken into account.

Many of both the cohort and case–control studies of physical activity and colon cancer have also examined risk of rectal cancer. Similar to the studies of colon cancer, the studies of rectal cancer have been conducted in both men and women and in many countries throughout the world (Thune and Furberg, 2001). Approximately 80% of those studies have not found any significant association (Thune and Furberg, 2001), and the median RR across all studies for the most active people relative to the least active is 1.0 (Lee and Oguma, 2006). One notable exception to this general consensus is a population-based case–control study of 952 incident rectal cancer cases and 1,205 age- and sex-matched controls conducted by Slattery et al., (Slattery et al., 2003). Both occupational and recreational physical activity were associated with a statistically significant 40% to 50% decrease in risk in both men and women, and this relationship was particularly strong for recent vigorous-intensity physical activity as well as for vigorous-intensity activity performed over many years. Although these findings are not consistent with most of the literature, it is possible that many previous studies had insufficient statistical power to detect a relationship that might, in fact, exist. Several other studies with more substantial numbers of rectal cancer cases have also reported reduced risk in association with physical activity (Chao et al., 2004; Gerhardsson et al., 1986), although this observation is not consistent (Brownson et al., 1991; Garabrant et al., 1984).

Breast Cancer

The role of physical activity in preventing the development of breast cancer has been studied extensively, particularly over the past decade. The literature now consists of more than 60 cohort and case–control studies from North America, Europe, Asia, and Australia that collectively include both pre- and postmenopausal women and number well over 100,000 cases (Lee and Oguma, 2006; Thune and Furberg, 2001). Although many of the study samples from North America and Europe have consisted largely of white women, women of other race/ethnicities have also been studied. Two recent population-based case–control studies from California have included sizeable numbers of African Americans, Latinas, and Asians (John et al., 2003; Yang et al., 2003). The studies of physical activity and breast cancer have considered both recreational and occupational physical activity, usually by means of self-reporting, but with widely differing methods of ascertainment ranging from a single, global question (Albanes et al., 1989) to quantitative questionnaires asking for details regarding type, intensity, frequency, and duration of different activities (Bernstein et al., 1994; Friedenreich et al., 2001a). Activity at some point in adulthood has been most frequently assessed, and some studies have examined activity around the time of puberty or young adulthood; still others have attempted to assess lifetime activity or activity at various times of life.

Although the findings for breast cancer are not as consistent as the findings for colon cancer, overall, the data (shown graphically in Fig. 10.2) suggest a reasonably clear, modest reduction of about 20% to 30% in risk of breast cancer for active women compared to sedentary women (Lee and Oguma, 2006; Lee, 2003). The risk reduction appears greater for postmenopausal women than premenopausal women, and a meta-analysis concluded that the RR associated with inactivity was only 1.25 (95% CI, 1.20–1.30) for women ages 15 to 44 years but 1.34 (95% CI, 1.29–1.39) for women ages 45 to 69 years (Bull et al., 2004).

The large majority of the studies of physical activity and breast cancer have collected information on a variety of potential confounding variables, including BMI, dietary factors, reproductive factors (age at menarche, age at menopause, use of oral contraceptives and hormone therapy, and parity), demographic factors, smoking, and family history of breast cancer. Adjustment for these factors has not substantially altered the unadjusted risk estimates.

However, the inverse relationship between physical activity and breast cancer appears to be modified by menopausal status and, perhaps, by other factors. As indicated earlier, the risk reduction is larger among postmenopausal women (Lee and Oguma, 2006; Thune and Furberg, 2001) and, in at least some studies, is not even evident among premenopausal women (Colditz et al., 2003; Friedenreich et al., 2001b; Rockhill et al., 1998). In the Norwegian-Swedish Women's Lifestyle and Health Cohort Study, where 99,504 women ages 30 through 49 years were followed for an average of 9.1 years, no association was observed between breast cancer incidence and physical activity at ages 14, 30, or enrollment (Margolis et al., 2005). This finding raises the possibility that the risk of breast cancer occurring during the perimenopausal years may also be less affected by physical activity.

The interaction between physical activity and menopausal status, like the frequently observed interaction with body fat (obesity is inversely related to premenopausal breast cancer but is a risk factor for postmenopausal disease), provides support for the idea that pre- and postmenopausal breast cancer are etiologically different diseases.

The evidence regarding effect modification of the physical activity–breast cancer relationship by other factors, such as BMI, weight gain during adulthood, parity, and family history of breast cancer, is inconsistent (Lee and Oguma, 2006). For example, the risk reduction with physical activity was essentially limited to the leanest women in the Women's Health Initiative Cohort (McTiernan et al., 2003), as in a large Norwegian cohort (Thune et al., 1997), but in a population-based case–control study, the risk reduction was greatest in the heaviest women at age 18 years (Shoff et al., 2000). Although no overall relationship between physical activity and breast cancer was observed in the Nurses' Health Study II, stratification by oral contraceptive use revealed a non-significant inverse association in current users (Colditz et al., 2003). In contrast, a non-significant interaction ($p = 0.09$) between physical activity and hormone therapy was observed in the American Cancer Society Cancer Prevention Study II Nutrition Cohort that suggested a marginally greater decrease in risk with physical activity among women who were not current hormone users (Patel et al., 2003). This study also stratified analyses by stage of disease and reported a significant reduction in risk with increasing physical activity only for local disease but not *in situ*

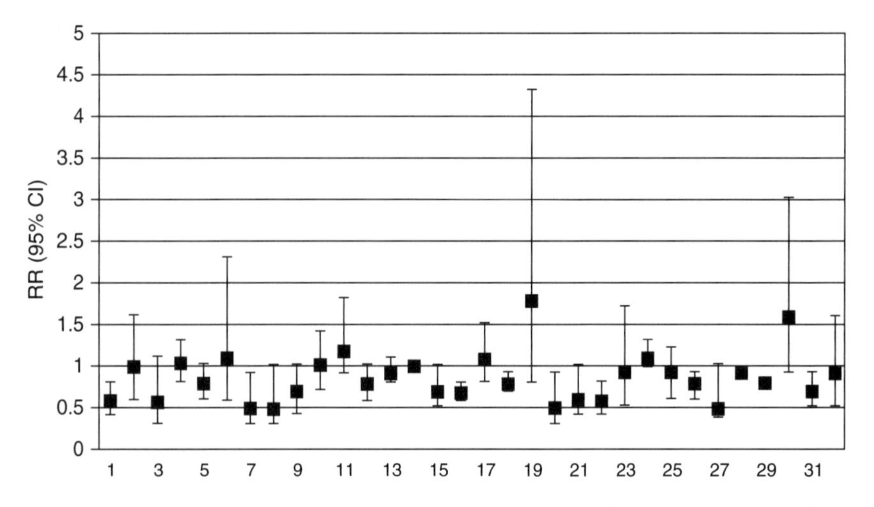

Figure 10.2a Relative risk (RR) and 95% confidence intervals (CIs) from cohort studies of breast cancer and physical activity (most active relative to least active).
Key to studies: 1. Adams-Campbell, 2001; 2. Albanes, 1989; 3. Breslow, 2001; 4. Colditz, 2003; 5. Dirx, 2001; 6. Dorn, 2003 (premenopausal); 7. Dorn, 2003 (postmenopausal; 8. Frisch, 1985; 9. Lee, 2001; 10. Luoto, 2000; 11. Margolis, 2005; 12. McTiernan, 2003; 13. Moore, 2000; 14. Paffenbarger, 1987; 15. Patel, 2003; 16. Pukkala, 1993; 17. Rockhill, 1998; 18. Rockhill, 1999; 19. Sesso, 1998 (premenopausal); 20. Sesso, 1998 (postmenopausal); 21. Thune, 1997; 22. Wyshak, 2000; 23. Albanes, 1989; 24. Calle, 1998; 25. Luoto, 2000; 26. Moradi, 1999; 27. Thune, 1997; 28. Vena, 1987; 29. Zheng, 1993; 30. Dorgan, 1994; 31. Frasier, 1997; 32. Steenland, 1995.

Notes: A. Citations for all references, with the exception of studies 4, 6, 7, 11, 12, and 15, may be found in Lee and Oguma, 2006; citations for exceptions are in References.
B. Associations refer to recreational activity (studies 1–22), occupational activity (studies 23–29), and total activity (studies 30–32).

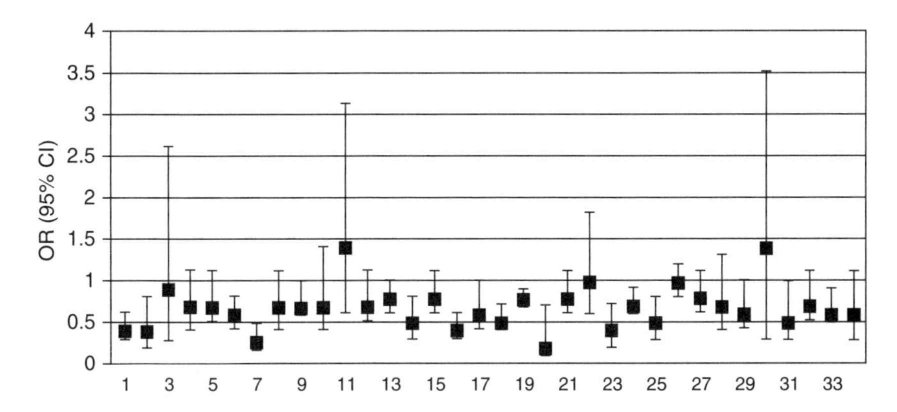

Figure 10.2b Odds ratio (OR) and 95% confidence intervals (CI) from case–control studies of breast cancer and physical activity (most active relative to least active).
Key to studies: 1. Bernstein, 1994; 2. Carpenter, 1999; 3. Chen, 1997; 4. D'Avanzo, 1997; 5. Friedenreich, 1995; 6. Friedenreich, 2001; 7. Gilliland, 2001 (Hispanics); 8. Gilliland, 2001 (non-Hispanics); 9. Hirose, 1995; 10. Hu, 1997 (premenopausal); 11. Hu, 1997 (post-menopausal); 12. John, 2003 (premenopausal); 13. John, 2003; (postmenopausal); 14. Levi, 1999; 15. Marcus, 1999; 16. Matthews, 2001; 17. McTiernan, 1996; 18. Mittendorf, 1995; 19. Moradi, 2000; 20. Shoff, 2000; 21. Steindorf, 2003; 22. Taioli, 1995; 23. Ueji, 1998; 24. Verloop, 2000; 25. Yang, 2003; 26. Coogan, 1996; 27. Coogan, 1997; 28. Coogan, 1999; 29. D'Avanzo, 1997; 30. Dosemeci, 1993; 31. Levi, 1999; 32. Mezzetti, 1998 (pre-menopausal); 33. Mezzetti, 1999 (postmenopausal); 34. Ueji, 1998.

Notes: A. Citations for all references, with the exception of studies 12, 13, 21, and 25, may be found in Lee and Oguma 2006; citations for exceptions are in References.
B. Associations refer to recreational activity (studies 1–25) and occupational activity (studies 26–34).

breast cancer or regional or distant disease. At least two studies have reported no interaction with estrogen- and/or progesterone-receptor status (Enger et al., 2000; Lee et al., 2001a).

As with colon cancer, the question of whether physical activity has a dose–response relationship with breast cancer incidence is complicated by the multidimensionality of the concept of dose. Most of the studies have categorized physical activity into at least three levels, and in more than half of these, there is either a statistically significant trend of decreasing risk with increasing activity, or risk estimates consistent with such a trend (Lee and Oguma, 2006). There is little information related to the intensity of activity required. Some evidence suggests that breast cancer risk is reduced with higher levels of vigorous-intensity, but not moderate-intensity, activity (Adams-Campbell et al., 2001; Bernstein et al., 1994; Mittendorf et al., 1995; Thune et al., 1997). However, in some instances, only vigorous-intensity activities were ascertained (Bernstein et al., 1994; Dorn et al., 2003; McTiernan et al., 2003; Mittendorf et al., 1995), whereas in other instances, categories combined more vigorous activity with greater frequency of activity (Thune et al., 1997), making it difficult to isolate the effect of intensity *per se*. In the Nurses' Health Study II (Colditz et al., 2003), running or jogging 2 or more hours a week was associated with a (non-significant) reduction in breast cancer incidence, whereas walking 4 or more hours a week was not. Similarly, in a case–control study of premenopausal German women, there was no association with MET-hours per week of walking, although this study also failed to observe any association with MET-hours per week of sports activity (Steindorf et al., 2003). In contrast, among Asian American women in Los Angeles, there was a significant inverse dose–response relationship with walking (Yang et al., 2003), and in the multiethnic case–control study from the San Francisco Bay area, walking and bicycling were associated with decreased risk among premenopausal women (John et al., 2003). In the Women's Health Initiative (WHI) Cohort Study (McTiernan et al., 2003), although total activity was associated with decreased risk, strenuous activity was not; this finding may be attributable more to the low level of participation in strenuous activity than to the intensity of activity. Finally, in at least one study, specifically designed to address the issue of intensity (Friedenreich et al., 2001b), there was a strong, inverse dose–response relationship with moderate-intensity activity but only a non-significant trend toward decreasing risk for either light-intensity or vigorous-intensity activity.

The literature is also unclear regarding the total amount of activity associated with reduced breast cancer incidence. Estimates associated with a reduced risk range from as little as 1 hour/week to 7 or more hours/week (Lee and Oguma, 2006), whereas one study of activity at age 18 years suggested that daily vigorous activity was necessary (Mittendorf et al., 1995). In the WHI Cohort Study, breast cancer risk was significantly reduced by 18% with as little as 5.1 MET-hours per week (less than 2 hours of moderate-intensity activity a week) but was reduced even more (22% risk reduction) with 40 or more MET-hours per week (about 10 hours/week of moderate-intensity activity) (McTiernan et al., 2003). A similar amount of activity (>42 MET-hours/week) was associated with a similar reduction in risk (29%) in the Cancer Prevention Study II Nutrition Cohort (Patel et al., 2003). Although the evidence is unclear, a rough estimate of 4 to 7 hours of moderate- to vigorous-intensity activity may be considered the minimal amount needed to influence breast cancer risk (Lee and Oguma, 2006).

A final important question about the relationship between physical activity and breast cancer occurrence is the appropriate time frame of exposure. The period from puberty to first childbirth may be a particularly susceptible time as breast cells continue to develop and differentiate. However, studies that have focused on physical activity around the time of puberty or in young adulthood (Marcus et al., 1999; McTiernan et al., 2003; Mittendorf et al., 1995; Steindorf et al., 2003) have generally observed weaker associations than those focusing on current activity. A number of studies have found strong inverse associations between lifetime activity and breast cancer risk (Dorn et al., 2003; Friedenreich et al., 2001a; John et al., 2003; Matthews et al., 2001; Yang et al., 2003), suggesting that consistent participation in physical activity throughout adulthood may influence breast cancer risk more than activity at any specific point in time.

Prostate Cancer

The evidence regarding physical activity and risk of prostate cancer is much less consistent than for either colon or breast cancer. Among more than 36 studies from North America, Europe, and Asia, slightly more than half have observed an inverse association, with the remaining studies finding either significantly increased risk with increased activity or no association (Fig. 10.3; Friedenreich and Thune, 2001; Lee et al., 2001b; Lee, 2003; Thune and Furberg, 2001). Across all the studies, the median RR is 0.9, indicating little difference in prostate cancer risk between active and inactive men (Lee, 2003). Although the median RR is slightly lower across case–control studies (0.8) than cohort studies (0.9) (Lee and Oguma, 2006), findings of a direct relationship between physical activity and prostate cancer have been reported as frequently with a case–control study design as with a cohort study design. Similarly, findings of inverse, null, and direct associations appear to occur with the same frequency regardless of whether the exposure of interest was occupational or recreational physical activity (Lee et al., 2001b).

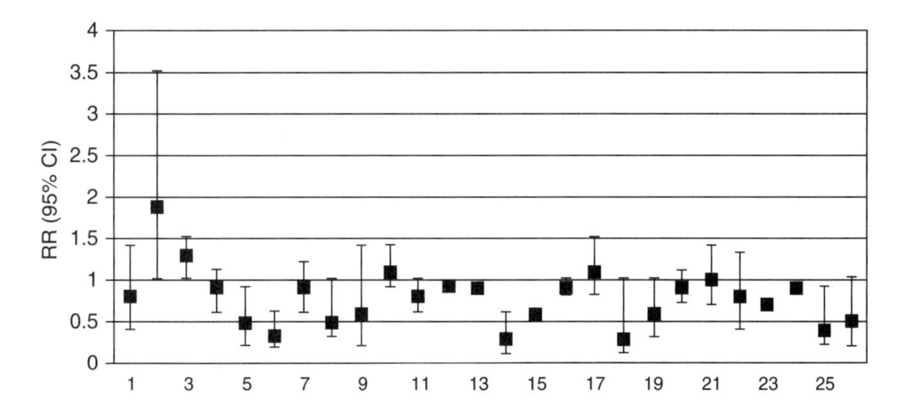

Figure 10.3a Relative risk (RR) and 95% confidence intervals (CIs) from cohort studies of prostate cancer and physical activity (most active relative to least active).
Key to studies: 1. Albanes, 1989; 2. Cerhan, 1987; 3. Gann, 1995; 4. Giovannucci, 1998 (all disease); 5. Giovannucci, 1998 (metastatic disease); 6. Giovannucci, 2005; 7. Lee, 1992 (age: less than 70 years); 8. Lee, 1992 (age: 70 years and older); 9. Lee, 1994; 10. Liu, 2000; 11. Lund Nilsen, 2000; 12. Norman, 2002 (cohort 1); 13. Norman, 2002 (cohort 2); 14. Oliveria, 1996; 15. Paffenbarger, 1987; 16. Patel, 2005; 17. Severson, 1989; 18. Wannamethee, 2001; 19. Albanes, 1989; 20. Hsing, 1994; 21. Severson, 1989; 22. Steenland, 1995; 23. Paffenbarger, 1989; 24. Vena, 1987; 25. Hartman, 1998; 26. Thune, 1994

Notes: A. Citations for all references, with the exception of studies 6 and 16, may be found in Lee and Oguma, 2006; citations for exceptions are in References.
B. Associations refer to recreational activity (studies 1–18), occupational activity (studies 19–24), and total activity (studies 25–26).

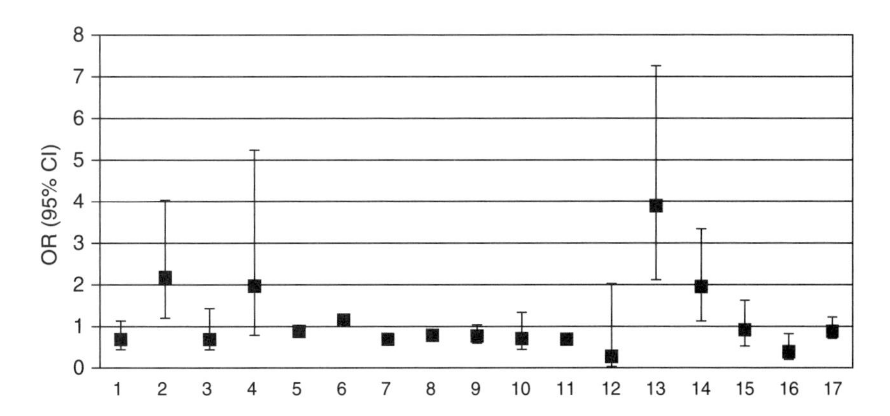

Figure 10.3b Odds ratio (OR) and 95% confidence intervals (CIs) from case–control studies of prostate cancer and physical activity (most active relative to least active).
Key to studies: 1. Andersson, 1995; 2. Sung, 1999; 3. Vileneuve, 1999; 4. West, 1991; 5. Whittemore, 1995 (Caucasians); 6. Whittemore, 1995 (African-Americans); 7. Whittemore, 1995 (Chinese-Americans); 8. Whittemore, 1995 (Japanese-Americans); 9. Yu, 1998 (Caucasians); 10. Yu, 1998 (African-Americans); 11. Brownson, 1991; 12. Doesmeci, 1993; 13. Ilic, 1996; 14. Le Marchand, 1991; 15. Vileneuve, 1999; 16. Bairati, 2000; 17. Friedenreich, 2004.

Notes: A. Citations for all references, with the exception of study 17, may be found in Lee and Oguma, 2006; the citation for study 17 is in References.
B. Associations refer to recreational activity (studies 1–10), occupational activity (studies 11–16), and total activity (studies 17).

Given this lack of consistency in study findings, it is not surprising to find inconsistency regarding the existence of a dose–response relationship. Among the studies that have assessed the incidence of prostate cancer across at least three levels of activity, a few have observed a significant decrease in risk with increasing activity, but others have observed the opposite trend, and still others have observed no trend (Friedenreich and Thune, 2001; Lee et al., 2001b). Even within a single study, observation of a dose–response relationship may vary depending on the assessment of physical activity. For example, a recent population-based case–control study from Canada (Friedenreich et al., 2004) that assessed lifetime physical activity by domain (occupational, household, and recreational activity) found a significant trend of increasing prostate cancer risk with increasing household activity but a marginally significant ($p = 0.06$) trend of decreasing risk with increasing recreational activity. And in the Aerobics Center Longitudinal Study, there was a significant inverse dose–response for fitness levels, with men in the highest level of cardiorespiratory fitness having more than a 70% reduction in prostate cancer (Oliveria et al., 1996). However, for physical activity, there was no dose–response relationship; men expending only 1000 to 2000 kcal/week in recreational physical activity had the same magnitude of risk reduction as those expending 3,000 or more kcal/week.

Some of the inconsistency in study findings may have resulted from detection bias. Since the late 1980s and early 1990s, screening for prostate-specific antigen has been widely introduced, resulting in the detection of many early stage prostate cancers that can be slow-growing and never otherwise detected. If physically active men are more health conscious and, therefore, more likely to seek screening than less active men, then a positive relationship between physical activity and prostate cancer might appear to exist that is, in fact, not true. In the Harvard Alumni Health Study, a high level of physical activity was strongly associated with reduced incidence of prostate cancer in older men for cases diagnosed prior to 1988, but there was no association with cases diagnosed after 1988 (Lee and Oguma, 2006), perhaps reflecting the impact of detection bias. Data from at least two other cohorts have also suggested that differences in screening practices may be responsible for some of the inconsistencies in the literature. In the Health Professionals' Follow-up Study (Giovannucci et al., 1998; Giovannucci et al., 2005) and the American Cancer Society Cancer Prevention Study II Nutrition Cohort (Patel et al., 2005), physical activity was associated with reduced risk of more advanced disease, which is generally diagnosed because of symptoms, but not with risk of early stage disease, which is generally detected through screening. Detracting from this argument, however, was an examination of prostate cancer screening rates by level of physical activity in the 2005 analysis of the Health Professionals' Follow-up Study (Giovannucci et al., 2005), where no clear differences were noted in the screening rates.

Except for age and race/ethnicity, risk factors for prostate cancer are poorly understood. As a result, it is difficult to assess to what extent confounding by unknown factors has contributed to the inconsistent findings regarding physical activity. However, many of the studies with conflicting results have adjusted for variables such as BMI, smoking, alcohol consumption, diet, medical history, and family history of prostate cancer. Effect modification by these factors has generally not been examined, and few subgroup analyses have been conducted (Friedenreich and Thune, 2001). Because prostate cancer is generally more aggressive when it develops at an earlier age, genetic susceptibility may play a more important role than environmental factors, such as physical activity, for early onset disease. However, in the studies that have stratified on age, the results are not consistent (Friedenreich and Thune, 2001; Lee and Oguma, 2006). Also, despite greater risk for prostate cancer in African-American men relative to white men, little is known about how the association with physical activity varies by race/ethnicity (Lee and Oguma, 2006).

Lung Cancer

Only about half as many studies have examined the relationship between physical activity and lung cancer (at least 23) as have examined the other sites discussed earlier (Lee and Oguma, 2006). Several large cohort studies, including a population-based Norwegian cohort of 53,242 men and 28,274 women, ages 20 to 49 years at entry (Thune and Lund, 1997), and the Harvard Alumni Health Study (Lee et al., 1999) have observed a statistically significant 30% to 40% decrease in risk with increasing physical activity. Several case–control studies have also reported inverse relationships of similar magnitude. Although a number of both cohort and case–control studies have not found statistically significant associations with physical activity, overall, the evidence suggests a median RR of 0.8 for a comparison of the most with the least active (Lee and Oguma, 2006).

Because smoking is the single-most important factor in the etiology of lung cancer, confounding could be responsible for an observed inverse association with physical activity. Although many of the studies controlled for cigarette smoking, confounding by factors that affect the degree of exposure, such as depth of inhalation and second-hand smoke, could remain. In a large, population-based case–control study from Canada (Mao et al., 2003), stratification by smoking status revealed a significant interaction, with an inverse dose–response relationship between physical activity and lung cancer risk among smokers that was particularly strong among current smokers but was not apparent among people who had never smoked ("never smokers"). This study also reported a stronger dose–response relationship among the heavier smokers than among smokers with less than 20 pack-years of exposure. In contrast, a recent study that included only current and former smokers found reduced risk in those with 20 to 44 pack-years of smoking (representing the lesser exposure) but no relationship in those who reported 45 to 185 pack-years (Alfano et al., 2004), which may suggest residual confounding. However, in another study of male smokers, no association between physical activity and risk of lung cancer was noted, regardless of the years of smoking or the number of cigarettes a day (Colbert et al., 2002). In an effort to minimize the effect of smoking, the Harvard Alumni Health Study examined physical activity and lung cancer risk only in never and former smokers (as a single group because of insufficient cases among never smokers), and still reported a significant, inverse dose–response relationship (Lee et al., 1999).

Limited and conflicting evidence exists to suggest effect modification by several other factors, such as gender, BMI, and histologic type. Case–control studies of physical activity and lung cancer that have found inverse associations have largely been conducted among women. However, in the Norwegian cohort study, the inverse relationship was significant only among men but not women (Thune and Lund, 1997), whereas in the Canadian case–control study (Mao et al., 2003), decreased risk with increased activity was observed in both women and men but was significant only with moderate-intensity activity in women and only with vigorous-intensity activity in men. This latter study also found that the inverse association was limited to men and women with a BMI less than 30 (Mao et al., 2003). Finally, differences by histologic type are unclear; in the Canadian study, inverse associations were found only for small cell lung cancer in men and squamous cell cancer in women (Mao et al., 2003), whereas lower risk with physical activity was seen only for adenocarcinoma in the Norwegian men (Thune and Lund, 1997).

Endometrial and Ovarian Cancer

About 15 studies, including both cohort and case–control study designs, have published data on the association between physical activity and risk of endometrial cancer (Lee and

Oguma, 2006). Although an independent, inverse relationship was reported in some studies, others did not find this. Two recently published cohort studies exemplify the inconsistencies. In the Netherlands Cohort Study on Diet and Cancer, 62,573 women were followed from 1986 to 1995. After adjustment for BMI and other risk factors for endometrial cancer, 90 minutes a day of non-occupational physical activity was associated with a significant, 46% reduction in risk, and there was a significant inverse dose–response relationship (Schouten et al., 2004). However, no risk reduction was associated with particular modes and intensity of activity, such as sports/exercise, gardening, and recreational biking and walking, although biking and walking to work and shopping were related to reduced risk. In contrast, in the 23,369 women enrolled in the Breast Cancer Detection Demonstration Project Follow-Up Study, higher levels of physical activity were not significantly associated with decreased incidence of endometrial cancer, nor was there any evidence of a dose–response relationship, although a comparison of women at the lowest level of physical activity with all others revealed a marginally significant reduction in risk among those with activity above the lowest level (Colbert et al., 2003). As these findings suggest, it is presently unclear whether or not an inverse relationship between physical activity and endometrial cancer exists; the magnitude of the association if one does exist; and the total amount, intensity, or mode of physical activity that might reduce risk.

The data regarding physical activity and risk of ovarian cancer are even more limited and inconsistent, with only about 10 studies addressing this question. At least two large cohort studies (the Iowa Women's Study and the Nurses' Health Study II) have reported a direct relationship (Anderson et al., 2004; Bertone et al., 2001). Data from the prospective Breast Cancer Detection Demonstration Project are suggestive of an inverse relationship between activity and ovarian cancer risk (Hannan et al., 2004), whereas results from a case–control study in China strongly indicate increased risk in association with increased sedentary behavior (Zhang et al., 2004). Further investigation of this cancer is needed to clarify the relationship.

Pancreatic Cancer

Although data regarding physical activity and incidence of pancreatic cancer are very sparse (fewer than 10 studies; Lee and Oguma, 2006), there is some suggestion of an inverse relationship. For example, in a population-based case–control study from Canada (Hanley et al., 2001), the risk of pancreatic cancer was decreased by almost 45% in men who spent more than 36.6 hours a month in moderate or vigorous physical activity, and, in women risk was marginally reduced as participation in vigorous activity increased. Similarly, in a prospective cohort study of Finnish male smokers, the incidence of pancreatic cancer was lower in men with at least a minimal level of occupational and leisure-time activity, relative to completely sedentary men (Stolzenberg-Solomon et al., 2002). Data from the Nurses' Health Study II and the Health Professionals' Follow-Up Study also suggest an inverse association. With the two cohorts combined, 10.8 MET-hours per week of moderate activity (equivalent to approximately 2–3 hours/week of brisk walking) was associated with a 55% reduction in risk, and there was a significant inverse trend of decreasing risk with increasing activity (Michaud et al., 2001). Analyses stratified by BMI indicated that the risk reduction associated with physical activity was confined to overweight individuals. At this point, any conclusion about whether physical activity is inversely related to risk of pancreatic cancer is premature, given the small number of existing studies.

Testicular Cancer

Only a handful of studies have examined physical activity in relation to testicular cancer (McTiernan et al., 1998; Thune and Furberg, 2001), and the findings, which were reviewed by Thune and Furberg (2001) have been inconsistent. Neither of two cohort studies observed any significant association (Thune and Furberg, 2001), and one case–control study of occupational activity reported an inverse association, whereas the other did not. Of three case–control studies of recreational activity, two found an inverse association with increased activity—particularly during young adulthood—but the third saw an increased risk. An early hospital-based case–control study reported that bicycle and horseback riding were associated with greater likelihood of testicular cancer, possibly resulting from trauma (Coldman et al., 1982).

Other Cancers

The few studies of renal cancer have generally not observed any relationship with physical activity, although the Netherlands Cohort Study reported a non-significant inverse association in men but not women (van Dijk et al., 2004). Generally null associations have been observed for non-Hodgkins lymphoma (Cerhan et al., 2002), and there is essentially no evidence of any association between physical activity and a variety of other site-specific cancers, including stomach, bladder, larynx, and cervix (Lee and Oguma, 2006).

Chance, Confounding, and Bias: Do They Explain the Observed Associations?

Well-designed and -conducted randomized, clinical trials can answer definitively whether a causal relationship exists, such as that between physical activity and lower cancer risk. However, such trials are not always feasible. In particular, it is difficult to imagine conducting a trial with good compliance for physical activity for the length of time required for cancer to develop. In the absence of data from randomized, clinical trials of physical activity and the development of cancer, the interpretation of data from observational epidemiologic studies requires consideration of the roles of chance, confounding, and bias.

To evaluate the role of chance in epidemiologic studies, statistical significance is conventionally set at the level of $p = 0.05$. Therefore, although many of the studies of physical activity and colon cancer indicate statistically significant inverse associations, there is a 5% chance that these are not true inverse associations. However, given the consistency of the association observed between physical activity and lower colon cancer risk, the probability of these findings resulting from chance is very unlikely. Although the literature on breast cancer is less consistent than for colon cancer, the accumulated evidence also suggests that chance is an unlikely explanation, especially because several plausible biologic mechanisms can explain why physical activity should be protective (*see* discussion of Biological Plausibility below).

With regard to confounding, many of the studies—particularly those that examined the major cancer sites—adjusted for a full range of potential confounding variables, including age, body size, dietary factors, alcohol and tobacco use, and health status. The associations between physical activity and colon cancer were generally unaffected by such adjustment, and those for breast cancer, although often attenuated, were still apparent. Nevertheless, statistical adjustment may not completely control for differences between physically active and physically inactive individuals, and those remaining differences may well influence cancer risk. Therefore, the existence of residual confounding as an explanation for the observed decrease in risk cannot be completely ruled out. On the other hand, confounding by unmeasured factors may actually attenuate protective associations that, in fact, exist. An example of this is the failure of many studies of female reproductive cancers to adjust for hormone therapy use (Lee and Oguma, 2006). Because physically active women may be more health conscious than sedentary women, they may have been more likely to use hormone therapy in the past, a factor that could increase risk of both breast and endometrial cancer (if unopposed estrogen was used). Without adjustment for this factor, a true protective effect of physical activity on these cancers could be diluted, or even obscured completely.

The potential confounding effect of body fat deserves particular attention. Because obesity is implicated as a risk factor for many cancers (colon, postmenopausal breast, endometrial, pancreatic cancers), and because physical activity is generally associated with lower levels of body fat, obesity may be an important confounding factor that explains many of the observed associations between physical activity and site-specific cancers. However, with the exception of studies that relied on existing large databases, such as those that examined cancer risk and occupational activity using census information, the vast majority of studies of physical activity and cancer accounted for body fat in one way or another. Most frequently, findings were statistically adjusted for or stratified by body fat. As noted earlier, this adjustment did not generally affect the inverse associations with physical activity. In other instances, investigators explicitly stated that adjustment for body fat did not alter the findings. On the other hand, many investigators have argued that adjustment should not be made for body fat, because body fat may be on the causal pathway between physical activity and reduced cancer risk. The point is made that adjustment for body fat would underestimate the influence of physical activity, because decreased body fat is a beneficial byproduct of being physically active.

Bias is a particularly difficult issue to evaluate with regard to epidemiologic studies of physical activity, largely because of the imprecision of exposure measurement. All of the studies of physical activity and cancer, with the exception of those using database linkages (which are unable to control for many confounding variables) or those based on knowledge of college athletic status, relied on self-reporting for the ascertainment of physical activity or estimated physical activity levels based on job titles. In case–control studies, measurement of exposure based on self-reporting is prone to recall bias, where cases may recall their exposure (physical activity in this case) differently from controls (Armstrong et al., 1994) because of their disease status. However, generally, the findings from case–control studies of physical activity and cancer risk have not differed substantially from the findings from cohort studies, although the magnitude of the association is often greater in the former studies, perhaps indicating some degree of recall bias. Cohort studies are less prone to biased recall of physical activity, because in a prospective cohort study, participants report their physical activity when they are free of cancer at baseline. Thus, their recall cannot be biased by disease.

On the other hand, bias may arise in cohort studies, as well as case–control studies from measurement *error* in the assessment of physical activity. Such error can result from the inability of participants to accurately recall or report their physical activity, incomplete assessment of relevant aspects of physical activity behavior, or failure to assess physical activity during the appropriate period of exposure. If the measurement error occurs equally among those who develop cancer and those who do not—which would seem likely—this would not so much bias the findings as it would attenuate the findings towards the null. Because some degree of measurement error is almost certain, it is likely that the observed associations between physical activity and lower risk of colon and breast cancers are actually of greater magnitude.

Biological Plausibility

Much of the interest in and impetus for the studies of physical activity and cancer described earlier arose because, despite an imperfect understanding of cancer development, several plausible biological mechanisms exist that suggest a protective effect of physical activity. The hypothesized mechanisms include primarily hormonal effects, changes in energy balance and body fat, and enhanced immune function (Lee and Oguma, 2006). Other purported mechanisms, such as increased bowel transit time, also may apply to particular site-specific cancers. Each of these is discussed more fully below in the sections on Hormonal Milieu, Obesity and Body Fat, Immune Function, and Other Potential Mechanisms.

Hormonal Milieu

A single bout of exercise results in acute hormonal responses and regular participation in physical activity—particularly more vigorous exercise—leads to alterations in the resting hormonal milieu. Most relevant in terms of a potential protective effect for hormone-related cancers, such as breast, prostate, endometrial, and ovarian cancers, are the lower resting levels of sex steroid hormones—specifically estrogens and testosterone—associated with physical activity. For example, young girls and women who train vigorously, especially in activities such as ballet dancing and distance running, frequently experience a later age at menarche (Frisch et al., 1980; Merzenich et al., 1993; Moisan et al., 1991), various changes in menstrual function (including a longer luteal phase and longer overall cycle length, more anovulatory cycles, and a greater prevalence of oligomenorrhea and amenorrhea) (Loucks, 1990), and have lower levels of circulating estrogen and progesterone (Ellison and Lager, 1986). Initiation of a strenuous training program by previously untrained women appears to result in similar, although reversible, disruptions of menstrual function (Bullen et al., 1985).

Even more moderate levels of activity may impact menstrual cycles. In high school girls, 600 kcal/week of physical activity, or about 2 hours/week of an activity such as aerobics class or tennis, was associated with greater prevalence of anovulatory cycles (Bernstein et al., 1987). Similarly, among two community-based cohorts of premenopausal women, whose overall level of physical activity was relatively low, those who reported greater amounts of physical activity had longer menstrual cycles than the more sedentary women (Sternfeld et al., 2002).

The implication of such changes in hormone levels and menstrual cyclicity is a lower lifetime exposure to cyclic estrogen and progesterone. Given the known proliferative effects of estrogen and progesterone on breast tissue, this lower level of lifetime exposure among active women could translate to reduced risk of breast cancer (Henderson et al., 1991). Similarly, less exposure to estrogen may reduce the risk of endometrial cancer, and fewer ovulatory cycles may result in less stimulation of ovarian cells and a lower risk of ovarian cancer (McTiernan et al., 1998).

In men, the androgens—particularly testosterone—play a parallel role to estrogen by stimulating growth of the prostate gland, and higher levels of plasma testosterone have been associated with increased prostate cancer risk (Gann et al., 1996; McTiernan et al., 1998), and higher levels of sex hormone-binding globulin (SHBG), which indicate lower levels of bio-available testosterone, have been associated with decreased risk. Some evidence suggests that despite an acute increase in androgen levels following exercise, resting androgen levels are lower in trained men compared to sedentary men, independently of differences in body fat (Lee and Oguma, 2006). However, the evidence is not consistent, and a decline in androgen levels may only be apparent with a high level of vigorous physical training (Lee and Oguma, 2006).

Obesity and Body Fat

Obesity is a risk factor for several cancers, and physical activity is generally inversely associated with BMI, other measures of body fat, and increases in body weight over time (Irwin et al., 2003; Sternfeld et al., 2004; Williamson et al., 1993). Although this might suggest that the inverse associations between physical activity and various site-specific cancers are confounded by obesity, as discussed previously, adjustment for body fat generally shows physical activity to be independently associated with reduced cancer risk. In addition, the effect modification by body fat of the physical activity/cancer relation, seen in a number of studies, raises the possibility that physical activity might reduce the risk of cancer through a direct effect on metabolic factors that often accompany obesity. For example, hyperinsulinemia, which is often a consequence of obesity, leads to an increase in insulin-like growth factors (IGFs), which are stimulatory throughout the body and have been associated with increased risk of premenopausal breast cancer and prostate cancer (Renehan et al., 2004). Physical activity, however, helps normalize insulin levels (even in the absence of significant weight loss; Despres et al., 1991) and increases production of the binding protein for IGF-1 (IGFBP-3), thereby resulting in decreased IGF activity. This, in turn, results in increased hepatic production of SHBG and lower levels of bio-available estrogen and testosterone (McTiernan et al., 1998), which, as discussed earlier, can reduce the risk of the hormone-related cancers as well as colon cancer. Finally, body fat may actually lie directly on the causal pathway between physical activity and reduced incidence of some cancers. Reduction in fat stores, where adrenal androgens are converted to estrogens, which provides the greatest source of estrogens for postmenopausal women, is an example of how physical activity can reduce the occurrence of some cancers by acting directly on body fat.

Immune Function

One of the primary functions of the innate immune system is to recognize and kill foreign cells, such as tumor cells (Slattery, 2004). Because immune function declines with age, and many cancers develop more frequently in older individuals, as well as others with compromised immune function, the immune system is considered a first-line defense against the development and spread of malignancies (Imai et al., 2000). Several key components of the innate immune system that appear responsive to physical activity are the natural killer (NK) cells, cytotoxic T lymphocytes, and monocytes and macrophages (Westerlind, 2003). (For a more detailed summary of the effects of physical activity on these immune system parameters, *see* Westerlind, 2003.) Briefly, the number of NK cells and cytotoxic T lymphocytes increase greatly following a bout of high-intensity exercise, but then rapidly fall below pre-exercise levels. Moderate-intensity exercise also leads to an increase in the NK cells without the subsequent decline, and exercise training, both in previously sedentary people and in athletes, tends to enhance NK cell activity. Finally, although acute exercise increases the number of monocytes and macrophages in peripheral blood, the functional significance of this increase is uncertain. In general, many questions remain regarding the immune system response to physical activity, and the importance of this response for explaining the observed relationships between physical activity and reduced cancer incidence is uncertain.

Other Potential Mechanisms

The earliest explanation for the observed association between physical activity and decreased colon cancer rates was faster bowel transit time that resulted in less exposure of the colon to colonic contents, bile acids and other potential carcinogenic factors. However, the evidence suggesting that physical activity actually causes a decrease in transit time is limited and inconsistent (Coenen et al., 1992; Rao et al., 2004). Increased secretion of the prostaglandins that inhibit tumor growth and increase gut motility has also been offered as an explanation for the decreased risk of colon cancer associated with physical activity (Slattery, 2004). Improved defenses against free radical damage as a result of chronic exercise and increased synthesis of vitamin D, which plays an important role in cell cycle regulation and apoptosis (Friedenreich and Thune, 2001; Lee et al., 2001b; McTiernan et al., 1998; Slattery, 2004) are yet other postulated mechanisms. Finally, improved ventilation and lung perfusion from physical activity that could reduce the concentration and length of exposure to carcinogens in the airways has been offered as a mechanism by which physical activity might reduce the risk of lung cancer (Mao et al., 2003).

Physical Activity and Survival in Patients With Cancer

This chapter has focused on physical activity in the primary prevention of cancer. However, several of the mechanisms postulated to be responsible for the benefit of physical activity in cancer prevention, such as decreased hormonal levels and lower body fat, are also prognostic factors for better survival among patients already diagnosed with cancer (Brown et al., 2003). Thus, it is plausible that physical activity promotes better survival among those who have been treated for cancer. At the moment, however, there are few direct data on this issue. Although numerous studies have suggested better quality of life and reduced weight gain with breast cancer treatment among physically active patients with cancer (Brown et al., 2003; Schmitz et al., 2005), very few studies have directly documented better survival. In one study of women with stage I to III breast cancer, those who participated in moderate or vigorous activity for more than 1 hour/week had a reduced risk of both recurrence and breast cancer mortality (Holmes et al., 2005). Among those who carried out the equivalent of at least 3 hours/week of a moderate- or vigorous-intensity activity, the risk of breast cancer mortality was 40% to 50% less than among those who were inactive. Two other studies of men and women with stage I to III colorectal cancer indicated reduced risks of cancer recurrence (approximately 30%–60% reduction) and overall mortality (approximately 30%–60% reduction) with 18 MET-hours/week or more (approximately 4–5 hours/week of moderate-intensity activity) (Meyerhardt et al., 2006b; Meyerhardt et al., 2006a). Clearly, this is a question that demands more research.

Future Research

Further research in several areas would enhance our understanding of physical activity and cancer prevention. First, although several plausible biologic mechanisms have been proposed, we remain uncertain about the precise underlying mechanisms by which physical activity can reduce risk of various cancers. Randomized, clinical trials of physical activity among healthy persons that target intermediate endpoints, serving as markers of cancer risk (e.g., colon polyps, mammographic density), would be helpful in this respect because it is not feasible to conduct trials with cancer itself as the endpoint of interest. Second, sparse epidemiologic data exist on the relationship between physical activity and risks of the less common cancers. Additionally, the associations for some of the more common cancers, specifically prostate and endometrial cancers, remain unclear and require elucidation. Third, although a clear inverse relationship exists between physical activity and both colon and breast cancer, details regarding the relationship—such as the minimum dose of activity required, the dose–response relationship, the appropriate time frame(s) for exposure, and the effect of changing activity levels over time—are less clear. Fourth, as discussed earlier, very little is known about physical activity and survival among patients who already have cancer. Finally, there is a clear need for better measurement of physical activity in epidemiologic studies. This topic is discussed in detail in Chapter 3.

Personal Perspective

A large and compelling body of evidence exists to indicate that physically active men and women can expect some 30% to 40% reduction in risk of colon cancer, and active women can expect some 20% to 30% reduction in risk of breast cancer. These reductions in risk are likely to be causally related to physical activity. However, from a public health perspective, the amount and intensity of activity needed is still unknown. Despite this lack of clarity regarding dose, the available data suggest that between 30 and 60 minutes/day of moderate-intensity physical activity will provide some degree of risk reduction. This level of physical activity is sufficient for many important health benefits, including a reduction in the risk of cardiovascular disease and diabetes. Clinicians and public health professionals need to recognize not only the benefits of this very minimal amount of physical activity but also that this minimal amount is achievable for most people, given appropriate individual- and environmental-level support and encouragement for this behavior. Our pursuit of the "magic bullet" for cancer prevention has led to several recent disappointments in chemoprevention, most notably for β-carotene (Cook et al., 2000), vitamin E (Lee et al., 2005), and low-dose aspirin (Cook et al., 2005). Perhaps the magic bullet—or at least one of them—really has been known and available to us for many years, dating as far back as the days of Hippocrates: —namely, physical activity.

References

Adams-Campbell LL, Rosenberg L, Rao RS, Palmer JR. 2001. Strenuous physical activity and breast cancer risk in African-American women. *J Natl Med Assoc* 93(7–8): 267–75.

Albanes D, Blair A, Taylor PR. 1989. Physical activity and risk of cancer in the NHANES I population. *Am J Public Health* 79: 744–50.

Alfano CM, Klesges RC, Murray DM, et al. 2004. Physical activity in relation to all-site and lung cancer incidence and mortality in current and former smokers. *Cancer Epidemiol Biomarkers Prev* 13(12): 2233–41.

American Cancer Society. 2006. *Cancer Facts and Figures—2006*. Atlanta, GA: American Cancer Society.

Anderson JP, Ross JA, Folsom AR. 2004. Anthropometric variables, physical activity, and incidence of ovarian cancer: The Iowa Women's Health Study. *Cancer* 100(7): 1515–21.

Armstrong BK, White E, Saracci R. 1994. *Principles of Exposure Measurement in Epidemiology*. Oxford: Oxford University Press.

Bernstein L, Henderson BE, Hanisch R, Sullivan-Halley J, Ross RK. 1994. Physical exercise and reduced risk of breast cancer in young women. *J Natl Cancer Inst* 86: 18: 1403–8.

Bernstein L, Ross RK, Lobo RA, Hanisch R, Krailo MD, Henderson BE. 1987. The effects of moderate physical activity on menstrual cycle patterns in adolescence: implications for breast cancer prevention. *Br J Cancer* 55: 681–5.

Bertone ER, Willett WC, Rosner BA, et al. 2001. Prospective study of recreational physical activity and ovarian cancer. *J Natl Cancer Inst* 93(12): 942–8.

Brown JK, Byers T, Doyle C, et al. 2003. Nutrition and physical activity during and after cancer treatment: an American Cancer Society guide for informed choices. *CA Cancer J Clin* 53(5): 268–91.

Brownson RC, Chang JC, Davis JR, Smith CA. 1991. Physical activity on the job and cancer in Missouri. *Am J Public Health* 81: 639–42.

Bull FC, Armstrong TP, Dixon SH NA, Pratt M. 2004. Comparative Quantification of Health Risks: Global and Regional Burden of Disease due to Selected Major Risk Factors. *Physical Activity* 2: 729.

Bullen BA, Skrinar GS, Beitins IZ, von Mering G, Turnbull BA, McArthur JW. 1985. Induction of menstrual disorders by strenuous exercise in untrained women. *N Engl J Med* 312: 1349–53.

Cerhan JR, Janney CA, Vachon CM, et al. 2002. Anthropometric characteristics, physical activity, and risk of non-Hodgkin's lymphoma subtypes and B-cell chronic lymphocytic leukemia: a prospective study. *Am J Epidemiol* 156(6): 527–35.

Chang S, Long SR, Kutikova L, et al. 2004. Estimating the cost of cancer: results on the basis of claims data analyses for cancer patients diagnosed with seven types of cancer during 1999 to 2000. *J Clin Oncol* 22(17): 3524–30.

Chao A, Connell CJ, Jacobs EJ, et al. 2004. Amount, type, and timing of recreational physical activity in relation to colon and rectal cancer in older adults: the Cancer Prevention Study II Nutrition Cohort. *Cancer Epidemiol Biomarkers Prev* 13(12): 2187–95.

Coenen C, Wegener M, Wedmann B, Schmidt G, Hoffmann S. 1992. Does physical exercise influence bowel transit time in healthy young men? *Am J Gastroenterol* 87(3): 292–5.

Colbert LH, Hartman TJ, Tangrea JA, et al. 2002. Physical activity and lung cancer risk in male smokers. *Int J Cancer* 98(5): 770–3.

Colbert LH, Lacey JV, Jr., Schairer C, Albert P, Schatzkin A, Albanes D. 2003. Physical activity and risk of endometrial cancer in a prospective cohort study (United States). *Cancer Causes Control* 14(6): 559–67.

Colditz GA, Feskanich D, Chen WY, Hunter DJ, Willett WC. 2003. Physical activity and risk of breast cancer in premenopausal women. *Br J Cancer* 89(5): 847–51.

Coldman AJ, Elwood JM, Gallagher RP. 1982. Sports activities and risk of testicular cancer. *Br J Cancer* 46(5): 749–56.

Cook NR, Le IM, Manson JE, Buring JE, Hennekens CH. 2000. Effects of beta-carotene supplementation on cancer incidence by baseline characteristics in the Physicians' Health Study (United States). *Cancer Causes Control* 11(7): 617–26.

Cook NR, Lee IM, Gaziano JM, et al. 2005. Low-dose aspirin in the primary prevention of cancer: the Women's Health Study: a randomized controlled trial. *JAMA* 294(1): 47–55.

Despres JP, Pouliot MC, Moorjani S, et al. 1991. Loss of abdominal fat and metabolic response to exercise training in obese women. *Am J Physiol* 261(2 Pt 1): E159-67.

Dorn J, Vena J, Brasure J, Freudenheim J, Graham S. 2003. Lifetime physical activity and breast cancer risk in pre- and postmenopausal women. *Med Sci Sports Exerc* 35(2): 278–85.

Ellison PT, Lager C. 1986. Moderate recreational running is associated with lowered salivary progesterone profiles in women. *Am J Obstet Gynecol* 154: 1000–3.

Enger SM, Ross RK, Paganini-Hill A, Carpenter CL, Bernstein L. 2000. Body size, physical activity, and breast cancer hormone receptor status: results from two case-control studies. *Cancer Epidemiol Biomarkers Prev* 9(7): 681–7.

Friedenreich C, Thune I. 2001. A review of physical activity and prostrate cancer risk. *Cancer Causes Control* 12: 461–75.

Friedenreich CM, Courneya KS, Bryant HE. 2001a. Influence of physical activity in different age and life periods on the risk of breast cancer. *Epidemiology* 12(6): 604–12.

Friedenreich CM, Courneya KS, Bryant HE. 2001b. Relation between intensity of physical activity and breast cancer risk reduction. *Med Sci Sports Exerc* 33(9): 1538–45.

Friedenreich CM, McGregor SE, Courneya KS, Angyalfi SJ, Elliott FG. 2004. Case-control study of lifetime total physical activity and prostate cancer risk. *Am J Epidemiol* 159(8): 740–9.

Frisch RE, Wyshak G, Vincent L. 1980. Delayed menarche and amenorrhea in ballet dancers. *N Engl J Med* 303: 17–9.

Gann PH, Hennekens CH, Ma J, Longcope C, Stampfer MJ. 1996. Prospective study of sex hormone levels and risk of prostate cancer. *J Natl Cancer Inst* 88(16): 1118–26.

Garabrant DH, Peters JM, Mack TM, Bernstein L. 1984. Job activity and colon cancer risk. *Am J Epidemiol* 119: 6: 1005–14.

Gerhardsson M, Norell SE, Kiviranta H, Pederson NL, Ahlbom A. 1986. Sedentary jobs and colon cancer. *Am J Epidemiol* 123: 5: 775–80.

Giovannucci E, Ascherio A, Rimm EB, Colditz GA, Stampfer MJ, Willett WC. 1995. Physical activity, obesity, and risk for colon cancer and adenoma in men. *Ann Intern Med* 122(5): 327–34.

Giovannucci E, Leitmann M, Spiegelman D, et al. 1998. A prospective study of physical activity and prostate cancer in male health professionals. *Cancer Res* 58: 5117–22.

Giovannucci EL, Liu Y, Leitzmann MF, Stampfer MJ, Willett WC. 2005. A Prospective Study of Physical Activity and Incident and Fatal Prostate Cancer. *Arch Intern Med* 165(9): 1005–10.

Hanley AJ, Johnson KC, Villeneuve PJ, Mao Y. 2001. Physical activity, anthropometric factors and risk of pancreatic cancer: results from the Canadian enhanced cancer surveillance system. *Int J Cancer* 94(1): 140–7.

Hannan LM, Leitzmann MF, Lacey JV, Jr., et al. 2004. Physical activity and risk of ovarian cancer: a prospective cohort study in the United States. *Cancer Epidemiol Biomarkers Prev* 13(5): 765–70.

Henderson BE, Ross RK, Pike MC. 1991. Toward the primary prevention of cancer. *Science* 254: 1131–8.

Holmes MD, Chen WY, Feskanich D, Kroenke CH, Colditz GA. 2005. Physical activity and survival after breast cancer diagnosis. *JAMA* 293(20): 2479–86.

Hou L, Ji BT, Blair A, Dai Q, Gao YT, Chow WH. 2004. Commuting physical activity and risk of colon cancer in Shanghai, China. *Am J Epidemiol* 160(9): 860–7.

Imai K, Matsuyama S, Miyake S, Suga K, Nakachi K. 2000. Natural cytotoxic activity of peripheral-blood lymphocytes and cancer incidence: an 11-year follow-up study of a general population. *Lancet* 356(9244): 1795–9.

Irwin ML, Yasui Y, Ulrich CM, et al. 2003. Effect of exercise on total and intra-abdominal body fat in postmenopausal women: a randomized controlled trial. *JAMA* 289(3): 323–30.

John EM, Horn-Ross PL, Koo J. 2003. Lifetime physical activity and breast cancer risk in a multiethnic population: the San Francisco Bay area breast cancer study. *Cancer Epidemiol Biomarkers Prev* 12(11 Pt 1): 1143–52.

La Vecchia C, Gallus S, Talamini R, Decarli A, Negri E, Franceschi S. 1999. Interaction between selected environmental factors and familial propensity for colon cancer. *Eur J Cancer Prev* 8(2): 147–50.

Lee I-M, Oguma Y. 2006. Physical Activity. In D Schottenfeld and JF Fraumeni Jr, (Eds.), *Cancer Epidemiology and Prevention*, New York, NY: Oxford University Press. pp. 449–467.

Lee I-M, Paffenbarger RS, Jr., Hsieh C. 1991. Physical activity and risk of developing colorectal cancer among college alumni. *J Natl Cancer Inst* 83: 1324–9.

Lee I-M, Sesso HD, Paffenbarger RS. 1999. Physical activity and risk of lung cancer. *Int J Epidemiol* 28: 620–5.

Lee IM. 2003. Physical activity and cancer prevention—data from epidemiologic studies. *Med Sci Sports Exerc* 35(11): 1823–7.

Lee IM, Cook NR, Gaziano JM, et al. 2005. Vitamin E in the primary prevention of cardiovascular disease and cancer: the Women's Health Study: a randomized controlled trial. *JAMA* 294(1): 56–65.

Lee IM, Cook NR, Rexrode KM, Buring JE. 2001a. Lifetime physical activity and risk of breast cancer. *Br J Cancer* 85(7): 962–5.

Lee IM, Sesso HD, Chen JJ, Paffenbarger RS, Jr. 2001b. Does physical activity play a role in the prevention of prostate cancer? *Epidemiol. Rev* 23(1): 132–7.

Lichtenstein P, Holm NV, Verkasalo PK, et al. 2000. Environmental and heritable factors in the causation of cancer—analyses of cohorts of twins from Sweden, Denmark, and Finland. *N Engl J Med* 343(2): 78–85.

Loucks AB. 1990. Effects of exercise training on the menstrual cycle: existence and mechanisms. *Med Sci Sports Exerc* 22: 275–80.

Mao Y, Pan S, Wen SW, Johnson KC. 2003. Physical activity and the risk of lung cancer in Canada. *Am J Epidemiol* 158(6): 564–75.

Marcus PM, Newcomb PA, Storer BE. 1994. Early adulthood physical activity and colon cancer risk among Wisconsin women. *Cancer Epidemiol Biomarkers Prev* 3(8): 641–4.

Marcus PM, Newman B, Moorman PG, et al. 1999. Physical activity at age 12 and adult breast cancer risk (United States). *Cancer Causes Control* 10(4): 293–302.

Margolis KL, Mucci L, Braaten T, et al. 2005. Physical activity in different periods of life and the risk of breast cancer: the Norwegian-Swedish Women's Lifestyle and Health cohort study. *Cancer Epidemiol Biomarkers Prev* 14(1): 27–32.

Martinez ME, Giovannucci E, Spiegelman D, Hunter DJ, Willett WC, Colditz GA. 1997. Leisure-time physical activity, body size, and colon cancer in women. *J Natl Cancer Inst* 89: 948–55.

Matthews CE, Shu XO, Jin F, et al. 2001. Lifetime physical activity and breast cancer risk in the Shanghai Breast Cancer Study. *Br J Cancer* 84(7): 994–1001.

McTiernan A, Kooperberg C, White E, et al. 2003. Recreational physical activity and the risk of breast cancer in postmenopausal women: the Women's Health Initiative Cohort Study. *JAMA* 290(10): 1331–6.

McTiernan A, Ulrich C, Slate S, Potter J. 1998. Physical activity and cancer etiology: associations and mechanisms. *Cancer Causes Control* 9: 487–509.

Merzenich H, Boeing H, Wahrendorf J. 1993. Dietary fat and sports activity as determinants for age at menarche. *Am J Epidemiol* 138: 217–24.

Meyerhardt JA, Giovannucci EL, Holmes MD, et al. 2006a. Physical activity and survival after colorectal cancer diagnosis. *J Clin Oncol* 24(22): 3527–34.

Meyerhardt JA, Heseltine D, Niedzwiecki D, et al. 2006b. Impact of physical activity on cancer recurrence and survival in patients with stage III colon cancer: findings from CALGB 89803. *J Clin Oncol* 24(22): 3535–41.

Michaud DS, Giovannucci E, Willett WC, Colditz GA, Stampfer MJ, Fuchs CS. 2001. Physical activity, obesity, height, and the risk of pancreatic cancer. *JAMA* 286(8): 921–9.

Mittendorf R, Longnecker MP, Newcomb PA, et al. 1995. Strenuous physical activity in young adulthood and risk of breast cancer (United States). *Cancer Causes Control* 6: 347–53.

Moisan J, Meyer F, Gingras S. 1991. Leisure physical activity and age at menarche. *Med Sci Sports Exerc* 25: 1170–5.

Oliveria SA, Kohl HWI, Trichopoulos D, Blair SN. 1996. The association between cardiorespiratory fitness and prostate cancer. *Med Sci Sports Exerc* 28: 97–104.

Patel AV, Callel EE, Bernstein L, Wu AH, Thun MJ. 2003. Recreational physical activity and risk of postmenopausal breast cancer in a large cohort of US women. *Cancer Causes Control* 14(6): 519–29.

Patel AV, Rodriguez C, Jacobs EJ, Solomon L, Thun MJ, Calle EE. 2005. Recreational physical activity and risk of prostate cancer in a large cohort of U.S. men. *Cancer Epidemiol Biomarkers Prev* 14(1): 275–9.

Rao KA, Yazaki E, Evans DF, Carbon R. 2004. Objective evaluation of small bowel and colonic transit time using pH telemetry in athletes with gastrointestinal symptoms. *Br J Sports Med* 38(4): 482–7.

Renehan AG, Zwahlen M, Minder C, O'Dwyer ST, Shalet SM, Egger M. 2004. Insulin-like growth factor (IGF)-I, IGF binding protein-3, and cancer risk: systematic review and meta-regression analysis. *Lancet* 363(9418): 1346–53.

Ries LAG, Eisner MP KCHBMBCL, Mariotto A, Feuer EJ, Edwards BD (Eds). 2005. *SEER Cancer Statistics Review, 1975—2002.*

Rockhill B, Willett WC, Hunter DJ, et al. 1998. Physical activity and breast cancer risk in a cohort of young women. *J Natl Cancer Inst* 90: 1155–60.

Schmitz KH, Holtzman J, Courneya KS, Masse LC, Duval S, Kane R. 2005. Controlled physical activity trials in cancer survivors: a systematic review and meta-analysis. *Cancer Epidemiol Biomarkers Prev* 14(7): 1588–95.

Schouten LJ, Goldbohm RA, van den Brandt PA. 2004. Anthropometry, physical activity, and endometrial cancer risk: results from the Netherlands Cohort Study. *J Natl Cancer Inst* 96(21): 1635–8.

Shoff SM, Newcomb PA, Trentham-Dietz A, et al. 2000. Early-life physical activity and postmenopausal breast cancer: effect of body size and weight change. *Cancer Epidemiol Biomarkers Prev* 9(6): 591–5.

Slattery ML. 2004. Physical activity and colorectal cancer. *Sports Med* 34(4): 239–52.

Slattery ML, Edwards S, Curtin K, et al. 2003. Physical activity and colorectal cancer. *Am J Epidemiol* 158(3): 214–24.

Slattery ML, Edwards SL, Ma KN, Friedman GD, Potter JD. 1997. Physical activity and colon cancer: a public health perspective. *Ann Epidemiol* 7(2): 137–45.

Slattery ML, Potter JD. 2002. Physical activity and colon cancer: confounding or interaction? *Med Sci Sports Exerc* 34(6): 913–9.

Steindorf K, Schmidt M, Kropp S, Chang-Claude J. 2003. Case-control study of physical activity and breast cancer risk among premenopausal women in Germany. *Am J Epidemiol* 157(2): 121–30.

Sternfeld B, Jacobs MK, Quesenberry CP, Jr., Gold EB, Sowers M. 2002. Physical activity and menstrual cycle characteristics in two prospective cohorts. *Am J Epidemiol* 156(5): 402–9.

Sternfeld B, Wang H, Quesenberry CP, Jr., et al. 2004. Physical activity and changes in weight and waist circumference in midlife women: findings from the Study of Women's Health Across the Nation. *Am J Epidemiol* 160(9): 912–22.

Stolzenberg-Solomon RZ, Pietinen P, Taylor PR, Virtamo J, Albanes D. 2002. A prospective study of medical conditions, anthropometry, physical activity, and pancreatic cancer in male smokers (Finland). *Cancer Causes Control* 13(5): 417–26.

Tavani A, Braga C, La Vecchia C, et al. 1999. Physical activity and risk of cancers of the colon and rectum: an Italian case-control study. *Br J Cancer* 79(11–12): 1912–6.

Thune I, Brenn T, Lund E, Gaard M. 1997. Physical activity and the risk of breast cancer. *N Engl J Med* 336: 1269–75.

Thune I, Furberg AS. 2001. Physical activity and cancer risk: dose-response and cancer, all sites and site-specific. *Med Sci Sports Exerc* 33(6 Suppl): S530-50.

Thune I, Lund E. 1997. The influence of physical activity on lung-cancer risk. a prospective study of 81,516 men and women. *Int J Cancer* 70: 57–62.

van Dijk BA, Schouten LJ, Kiemeney LA, Goldbohm RA, van den Brandt PA. 2004. Relation of height, body mass, energy intake, and physical activity to risk of renal cell carcinoma: results from the Netherlands Cohort Study. *Am J Epidemiol* 160(12): 1159–67.

Westerlind KC. 2003. Physical activity and cancer prevention—mechanisms. *Med Sci Sports Exerc* 35(11): 1834–40.

Williamson DF, Madans J, Anda RF, Kleinman JC, Kahn HS, Byers T. 1993. Recreational physical activity and 10-year weight change in a US national cohort. *Int J Obes Relat Metab Disord.* 17: 279–86.

Yang D, Bernstein L, Wu AH. 2003. Physical activity and breast cancer risk among Asian-American women in Los Angeles: a case-control study. *Cancer* 97(10): 2565–75.

Zhang M, Xie X, Lee AH, Binns CW. 2004. Sedentary behaviours and epithelial ovarian cancer risk. *Cancer Causes Control* 15(1): 83–9.

11

Physical Activity, Fitness, and the Prevention of Type 2 Diabetes

Gang Hu, Timo A. Lakka,
and Jaakko Tuomilehto

Diabetes is one of the most costly and burdensome chronic diseases and one of the fastest growing public health problems in the world. It has been estimated that the number of adults age 20 years or older who suffer from diabetes will double from the current 171 million in 2000 to 366 million in 2030 (Wild et al., 2004). Recent data have shown that the lifetime risk of type 2 diabetes is over 30% in the United States and over 40% to 50% in Europe and Asia (Centers for Disease Control and Prevention, 2003; DECODE Study Group, 2003; Qiao et al., 2003). In addition, whereas type 2 diabetes was previously considered to be a disease of middle and late adulthood, it is also now increasingly prevalent in children and adolescents (Arslanian, 2002).

The development of type 2 diabetes involves an interaction between genetics and lifestyle factors (Neel, 1962). A sedentary lifestyle and obesity are two important lifestyle risk factors for type 2 diabetes (Wing et al., 2001). Results from prospective cohort studies (Bjornholt et al., 2001; Burchfiel et al., 1995; Carnethon et al., 2003; Dotevall et al., 2004; Eriksson and Lindgarde, 1996; Folsom et al., 2000; Haapanen et al., 1997; Helmrich et al., 1991; Hsia et al., 2005; Hu et al., 2001; Hu et al., 2003a; Hu et al., 1999; Hu et al., 2004b; Hu et al., 2003b; James et al., 1998; Kriska et al., 2003; Lynch et al., 1996; Manson et al., 1992; Manson et al., 1991; Meisinger et al., 2005; Meisinger et al., 2002; Nakanishi et al., 2004; Okada et al., 2000; Perry et al., 1995; Sawada et al., 2003; Schranz et al., 1991; Wannamethee et al., 2000; Wei et al., 1999; Weinstein et al., 2004) and clinical trials (Davey Smith et al., 2005; Eriksson and Lindgarde, 1991; Knowler et al., 2002; Pan et al., 1997; Tuomilehto et al., 2001) have shown that moderate or high levels of physical activity or physical fitness and changes in lifestyle (including dietary modification, increase in physical activity, and weight loss) can prevent type 2 diabetes. Plausible biological mechanisms support the findings from these epidemiologic studies. Physical activity may slow the initiation and progression of type 2 diabetes via favorable effects on body adiposity, insulin sensitivity, glycemic control, blood pressure, lipid profile, hemostatic factors, endothelial function, inflammatory defense systems, and developing metabolic syndrome. In this chapter, we examine the current evidence regarding the role of physical activity and physical fitness in the primary prevention of type 2 diabetes.

Physical Activity and Type 2 Diabetes: Data From Prospective Cohort Studies

Table 11.1 summarizes the results of 25 prospective cohort studies of physical activity and the risk of developing type 2 diabetes.

Early Studies

The first study investigating the association between physical activity and the risk of type 2 diabetes was carried out in 5,990 male alumni from the University of Pennsylvania (Helmrich et al., 1991). This study indicated that higher levels of leisure-time physical activity were associated with lower risk of developing type 2 diabetes. For each 500-kcal/week increment in leisure-time physical activity, the age-adjusted risk of developing diabetes declined by 6%. The association remained after adjustment for obesity, hypertension, and parental history of diabetes. Subsequently, a 2-year follow-up study in Malta showed that low overall physical activity during work, leisure time, and commuting was associated with a 3.7-fold increase in age-standardized risk of type 2 diabetes and impaired glucose tolerance compared to high physical activity among participants with normal or impaired glucose tolerance at baseline (Schranz et al., 1991).

Soon after the publication of these early studies, two other large studies reported similar findings. The Nurses' Health Study investigated the association of physical activity and type 2 diabetes among 87,253 U.S. women, ages 34 to 59 years, who were free of diabetes, cardiovascular disease, and cancer at baseline (Manson et al., 1991). During 8 years of follow-up (1980–1988), 1,303 cases of self-reported type 2 diabetes developed. Women who engaged in vigorous exercise at least once per week had a 33% reduced age-adjusted risk of type 2 diabetes compared to women who did not exercise weekly. Multivariable adjustment for age, family history of diabetes, body mass index (BMI), and other variables did not alter the observed risk reduction. The Physicians' Health Study of 21,271 U.S. men ages 40 to 84 years indicated that those who exercised vigorously at least once a week had a multivariable-adjusted relative risk (RR) of type 2 diabetes of 0.71 during a 5-year follow-up from 1982 to 1988 (Manson et al., 1992). In updated analyses of the Nurses' Health Study, which extended the period of follow-up from 1986 to 1994, and in the Health Professionals' Follow-up Study of 37,918 men ages 40 to 75 years who were followed from 1986 to 1996, investigators found a progressive reduction in the multivariable-adjusted RR of type 2 diabetes across increasing quintiles of leisure-time physical activity, with risks that were 26% to 38% lower in the highest vs. lowest quintile (Hu et al., 2001; Hu et al., 1999).

Subsequent Studies in Men Only

Several other studies of men in different countries subsequently confirmed the association between higher levels of physical activity and lower risk of developing type 2 diabetes. In the Honolulu Heart Program, the multivariable-adjusted risk of type 2 diabetes was inversely related to total physical activity during a follow-up of 2 to 6 years among 6,815 Japanese-American men ages 45 to 68 years (Burchfiel et al., 1995). The results from the British Regional Heart Study indicated that men who engaged in moderate levels of physical activity had a substantially reduced risk of type 2 diabetes (60% risk reduction) compared to physically inactive men, after adjustment for age, BMI, systolic blood pressure, high-density lipoprotein (HDL) cholesterol, smoking, alcohol intake, and prevalent coronary heart disease (CHD) (Perry et al., 1995).

Table 11.1 Prospective Cohort Studies of Physical Activity and the Risk of Type 2 Diabetes

Study (reference)	*Subjects*	*Age range (years)*	*No. of incident cases; duration of study*	*Physical activity comparison groups*	*Relative risk (95% confidence interval)*	*Adjustment factors*
College Alumni Health Study (Helmrich et al., 1991)	5990 men	39–68	202 cases; 14 years	500-kcal/week increments in leisure-time physical activity	0.94 (0.90–0.98)	Age, parental history of diabetes, BMI, and history of hypertension
Nurses' Health Study (Manson et al., 1991)	87,253 women	34–59	1303 cases; 8 years	Vigorous exercise in leisure time at least once weekly vs. less than once weekly	0.67 (0.60–0.75) 0.84 (0.75–0.94)	Age Age, family history of diabetes, BMI, hypertension, high serum cholesterol, smoking, and alcohol consumption
Population sample in Malta (Schranz et al., 1991)	196 men and women	>20	37 cases; 2 years	Low overall physical activity (including work, leisure time and commuting) vs. high activity, among subjects with normal glucose or IGT at baseline	3.7 times higher risk of IGT and diabetes	Age
Physicians' Health Study (Manson et al., 1992)	21,271 men	40–84	285 cases; 5 years	Vigorous exercise in leisure time at least once weekly vs. less than once weekly	0.64 (0.51–0.82) 0.71 (0.54–0.94)	Age Age, BMI, hypertension, high serum cholesterol, smoking, and alcohol consumption
Honolulu Heart Program (Burchfiel et al., 1995)	6815 men	45–68	391 cases; 6 years	Highest quintile of physical activity index vs. lower four quintiles	0.55 (0.41–0.75) 0.49 (0.34–0.72)	Age Age, parental history of diabetes, BMI, systolic blood pressure, triglycerides, glucose, and hematocrit

Continued

Table 11.1 Prospective Cohort Studies of Physical Activity and the Risk of Type 2 Diabetes *(Continued)*

Study (reference)	*Subjects*	*Age range (years)*	*No. of incident cases; duration of study*	*Physical activity comparison groups*	*Relative risk (95% confidence interval)*	*Adjustment factors*
British Regional Heart Study (Perry et al., 1995)	7735 men	40–59	194 cases; 12.8 years	Moderate activity (including leisure time and commuting) vs. inactivity	0.4 (0.2–0.8)	Age, BMI, systolic blood pressure, HDL cholesterol, smoking, alcohol consumption, and prevalent CHD
Malmö Preventive Trial (Eriksson and Lindgarde, 1996)	4637 men	48–54	116 cases; 6 years	Physical activity score (including walking or cycling to work and leisure activity) among men who subsequently developed diabetes vs. men who did not	16% lower mean value of physical activity score	Unadjusted
Kuopio Ischemic Heart Disease Risk Factor Study (Lynch et al., 1996)	897 men	42–60	46 cases; 4 years	Leisure-time physical activity of intensity ≥5.5 METs for at least 40 min/week vs. less activity	0.44 (0.22–0.88)	Age, parental history of diabetes, BMI, triglycerides, baseline glucose, and alcohol consumption
Population sample from northeastern Finland (Haapanen et al., 1997)	891 men and 973 women	35–63	118 cases, 10 years	Total weekly leisure-time and commuting physical activity: low (0-1100 kcal/week) vs. high (>1900 kcal/week) in men; low (0-900 kcal/week) vs. high (>1500 kcal/week) in women	Men: 1.54 (0.83–2.84) Women: 2.64 (1.28–5.44)	Age
Pitt County Study (James et al., 1998)	598 men and 318 women	30–55	78 cases, 5 years	Moderate physical activity vs. inactivity (based on vigorous exercise or work, walking, and home maintenance)	0.35 (0.12–0.98)	Age, sex, BMI, waist-to-hip ratio, and education

Nurses' Health Study (Hu et al., 1999)	70,102 women	40–65	1419 cases; 8 years	At least 21.8 MET-hours/week of leisure-time physical activity (highest quintile) vs. ≤2.0 (lowest quintile)	0.74 (0.62–0.89)	Age, parental history of diabetes, BMI, history of hypertension, history of high cholesterol, smoking, menopausal status, and alcohol consumption
				At least 10.8 MET-hours/week of walking (highest quintile) vs. ≤0.5 (lowest quintile)	0.74 (0.59–0.93)	
Iowa Women's Health Study (Folsom et al., 2000)	34,257 women	55–69	1997 cases; 12 years	Any leisure-time physical activity vs. no physical activity	0.86 (0.78–0.95)	Age, parental history of diabetes, BMI, waist-to-hip ratio, smoking, education, alcohol consumption, energy intake, whole intake, and Keys score
				Physical activity index	Low: 1.00 (referent) Moderate: 0.91 (0.82–1.02) High: 0.79 (0.70–0.90)	
Osaka Health Survey (Okada et al., 2000)	6013 men	35–60	444 cases; 10 years	Leisure-time physical activity at least once/week vs. less often	0.75 (0.61–0.93)	Age, parental history of diabetes, BMI, blood pressure, smoking, and alcohol consumption
				Vigorous activity once at weekend vs. sedentary	0.55 (0.35–0.88)	
British Regional Heart Study (Wannamethee et al., 2000)	5159 men	40–59	196 cases; 16.8 years	Moderate or vigorous activity during leisure time and commuting vs. no physical activity	Moderate: 0.53 (0.31–0.92) Moderately vigorous to vigorous: 0.51 (0.30–0.89)	Age, BMI, smoking, alcohol consumption, social class, pre-existing CHD, and insulin
Health Professionals' Follow-up Study (Hu et al., 2001)	37,918 men	40–75	1058 cases; 10 years	At least 40.9 MET-hours/week of leisure-time physical activity (highest quintile) vs. <6.0 (lowest quintile)	0.62 (0.50–0.76)	Age, parental history of diabetes, BMI, smoking, alcohol consumption
				Each 10 MET-hours/week increase in walking	0.89 (0.82–0.96)	
				Each 2 hours/day increase in time spent watching TV	1.20 (1.08–1.32)	

Continued

Table 11.1 Prospective Cohort Studies of Physical Activity and the Risk of Type 2 Diabetes *(Continued)*

Study (reference)	*Subjects*	*Age range (years)*	*No. of incident cases; duration of study*	*Physical activity comparison groups*	*Relative risk (95% confidence interval)*	*Adjustment factors*
MONICA/KORA Augsburg Cohort Study (Meisinger et al., 2002)	3052 men and 3114 women	35–74	213 cases, 7.6 years	Inactive during leisure time vs. active	Men: 1.81 (1.04–3.16) Women: 1.20 (0.83–1.74)	Age, BMI
Nurses' Health Study (Hu et al., 2003a)	68,497 women	45–70	1515 cases; 6 years	Each 2 hours/day increase in time spent watching TV	1.14 (1.05–1.23)	Age, family history of diabetes, BMI, smoking, dietary covariate, and alcohol consumption
FIN-MONICA Study (Hu et al., 2003b)	6898 men and 7392 women	35–64	373 cases, 12 years	Work, leisure-time and commuting physical activity	See Table 11.2	See table 2
Pima Indians Community Study (Kriska et al., 2003)	676 men and 1052 women	15–59	346 cases; 6 years	High leisure-time physical activity (≥16 MET-hours/week) vs. low (<16)	Men: 0.66 (0.45–0.99) Women: 0.70 (0.53–0.92)	Age
Göteborg BEDA Study (Dotevall et al., 2004)	1351 women	39–65	73 cases; 18 years	Sedentary vs. any leisure-time physical activity	2.08 (1.29–3.34)	Age
FIN-MONICA Study (Hu et al., 2004b)	2017 men and 2352 women	45–64	120 cases; 12 years	High vs. low index of combined work, leisure-time and commuting physical activity	0.43 (0.25–0.74)	Age, sex, BMI, systolic blood pressure, smoking, and education

Japanese Male Office Workers Survey (2004) (Nakanishi et al., 2004)	2924 men	35–59	168 cases, 7	Daily energy expenditure; quartile 4 vs. quartile 1	0.41 (0.24–-0.71)	Age, family history of diabetes, BMI, blood pressure, smoking, HDL cholesterol, triglycerides, and alcohol consumption
Women's Health Study (Weinstein et al., 2004)	37 878 women	45 or more	1361 cases, 6.9 years	Active vs. inactive (≥1000 vs. <1000 kcal/week in leisure-time activity)	0.85 (0.75–0.97)	Age, family history of diabetes, hypertension, smoking, high cholesterol, alcohol consumption, and dietary factors
				At least 4 hours/week of walking (highest quintile) vs. none (lowest quintile)	0.64 (0.53–0.78)	
MONICA/KORA Augsburg Cohort Study (Meisinger et al., 2005)	4069 men and 4034 women	25–74	227 cases, 7.4 years	High vs. no activity	Men: 0.83 (0.50–1.36) Women: 0.24 (0.06–0.98)	Age, parental history of diabetes, BMI, hypertension, dyslipidemia, education, smoking, and alcohol consumption
Women's Health Initiative Observational Study (Hsia et al., 2005)	87,907 women		5.1 years	Quartile 5 vs. quartile 1 of total physical activity	0.78 (0.67–0.91)	Age, BMI, education, alcohol consumption, hypertension, smoking, hypercholesterolemia, and dietary fiber
				Quartile 5 vs. quartile 1 of walking	0.82 (0.70–0.95)	

In Sweden, the Malmö Preventive Trial reported that men who developed type 2 diabetes during a 6-year follow-up had a 16% lower mean value in physical activity score at baseline compared to men who did not develop diabetes (Eriksson and Lindgarde, 1996). In Finland, data from the Kuopio Ischemic Heart Disease Risk Factor Study of 897 middle-age Finnish men showed that vigorous-intensity (≥5.5 metabolic equivalents [METs]) exercise for at least 40 minutes/week was associated with decreased rates of type 2 diabetes after adjusting for age, baseline glucose levels, BMI, and other known risk factors (Lynch et al., 1996).

Additional data on Japanese men, living in Japan, were provided by the Osaka Health Survey, which included 6,013 Japanese men ages 35 to 60 years who were free of diabetes, impaired fasting glycemia, or hypertension at baseline (Okada et al., 2000). Men who participated in regular exercise at least once a week or vigorous activity once a week on weekends had a decreased risk of type 2 diabetes after adjustment for BMI and other potential confounding factors. Another recent study of 2,924 Japanese male office workers, ages 35 to 59 years, who were free of diabetes, impaired fasting glucose, hypertension, or cardiovascular disease at baseline found that physical activity in daily life (expressed in terms of daily energy expenditure) also was inversely associated with the risk of developing impaired fasting glucose or type 2 diabetes after adjustment for BMI and other potential confounding factors (Nakanishi et al., 2004).

Subsequent Studies That Included Women

The inverse relationship between physical activity and type 2 diabetes also has been observed in prospective studies that included women, as well as in studies of women alone, from several different countries. A Finnish prospective study that examined 891 men and 973 women ages 35 to 63 years reported that only women with a higher total amount of physical activity or weekly vigorous exercise had a reduced risk of developing type 2 diabetes during 10 years of follow-up (Haapanen et al., 1997). An age-adjusted RR of 2.6 for type 2 diabetes was found for the lowest third of physical activity compared to the highest third. This association remained statistically significant even after further adjustment for BMI and other potential confounding factors. Among men, risk also was increased, but this was not statistically significant.

We recently investigated 6,898 Finnish men and 7,392 women, ages 35 to 64 years, without a history of stroke, CHD, or diabetes at baseline (Hu et al., 2003b). During a mean follow-up of 12 years, there were 373 incident cases of drug-treated or clinically diagnosed type 2 diabetes. A moderate level of physical activity at work was associated with a 30% reduction in the risk of type 2 diabetes compared to a low level; active work was associated with a 26% reduction (Table 11.2). For leisure-time physical activity, risk reductions were 19% and 16% for moderate and active categories, respectively, compared to the low category. Daily walking or cycling to and from work for more than 30 minutes was also significantly and inversely associated with risk. These associations were independent of age, systolic blood pressure, smoking, education, the two other kinds of physical activity, and BMI.

In a separate analysis, we evaluated the independent and joint associations of physical activity, BMI, and plasma glucose levels with the risk of type 2 diabetes among 2,017 Finnish men and 2,352 women (Hu et al., 2004b). We classified participants into three levels of physical activity: *(1)* low levels of occupational, leisure-time, and commuting physical activity; *(2)* moderate-to-high levels of only one kind of activity; and *(3)* moderate-to-high levels of at least two kinds of activity. Simultaneous engagement in at least two kinds of physical activity (occupational, leisure-time, or commuting) at a moderate or high level was associated with lower risk of type 2 diabetes than engagement in only one kind

Table 11.2 Relative Risks of Type 2 Diabetes According to Different Levels of Occupational, Commuting, and Leisure-Time Physical Activity Among Finns

			Relative risk (95% confidence interval)*		
Physical activity	*No. of cases*	*Person-years*	*Model 1*	*Model 2*	*Model 3*
Occupational physical activity:					
Light	199	67,250	1.00	1.00	1.00
Moderate	63	48,184	0.57 (0.43–0.76)	0.66 (0.49–0.90)	0.70 (0.52–0.96)
Active	111	55,695	0.76 (0.60–0.97)	0.73 (0.56–0.94)	0.74 (0.57–0.95)
p-value for trend			<0.001	0.008	0.020
Walking or cycling to/from work:					
0 minutes/day	242	81,556	1.00	1.00	1.00
1–29 minutes/day	93	54,576	0.75 (0.59–0.96)	0.88 (0.68–1.15)	0.96 (0.74–1.25)
≥ 30 minutes/day	38	34,998	0.42 (0.30–0.59)	0.54 (0.38–0.77)	0.64 (0.45–0.92)
p-value for trend			<0.001	0.003	0.048
Leisure-time physical activity:					
Low	173	56,387	1.00	1.00	1.00
Moderate	166	88,350	0.63 (0.50–0.78)	0.67 (0.53–0.84)	0.81 (0.64–1.02)
Active	34	26,392	0.52 (0.36–0.75)	0.61 (0.41–0.90)	0.84 (0.57–1.25)
p-value for trend			<0.001	0.001	0.186

*Model 1 was adjusted for age, sex, and study year; Model 2 was adjusted for the factors in Model 1, plus systolic blood pressure, smoking status, education, and the two other kinds of physical activity; Model 3 was adjusted for the factors in Model 2, plus body mass index.

(Adapted from Hu et al., 2003b, with permission.)

of activity at a moderate or high level. Level 2 physical activity, compared to level 1, was associated with a 15% reduction in risk of type 2 diabetes; level 3 was associated with a 57% decrease.

When we stratified participants by BMI and glucose homeostasis, inverse associations with physical activity were observed among individuals with BMI less than 30 kg/m^2 and 30 kg/m^2 or greater as well as among those with normal and impaired glucose homeostasis (Figs. 11.1A and 11.1B). We then examined the joint relationships among physical activity, BMI, plasma glucose, and type 2 diabetes (Fig. 11.2). Obese participants with low physical activity and impaired glucose regulation had a substantial, 30-fold increase in risk compared to non-obese persons with high physical activity and normal glucose homeostasis.

Studies of women in other countries have supported the findings among Finnish women. In the Iowa Women's Health Study of 34,257 postmenopausal women ages 55 to 69 years without diabetes, those who participated in any leisure-time physical activity had a 14% lower risk of developing type 2 diabetes compared to sedentary women, after adjustment for age, BMI, and other confounding factors (Folsom et al., 2000). The MONICA/KORA Augsburg Cohort Study examined sex-specific associations between leisure-time physical activity and incident type 2 diabetes among 4,069 German men and 4,034 women ages 25 to 74 years who were followed for 7.4 years (Meisinger et al., 2005; Meisinger et al., 2002).

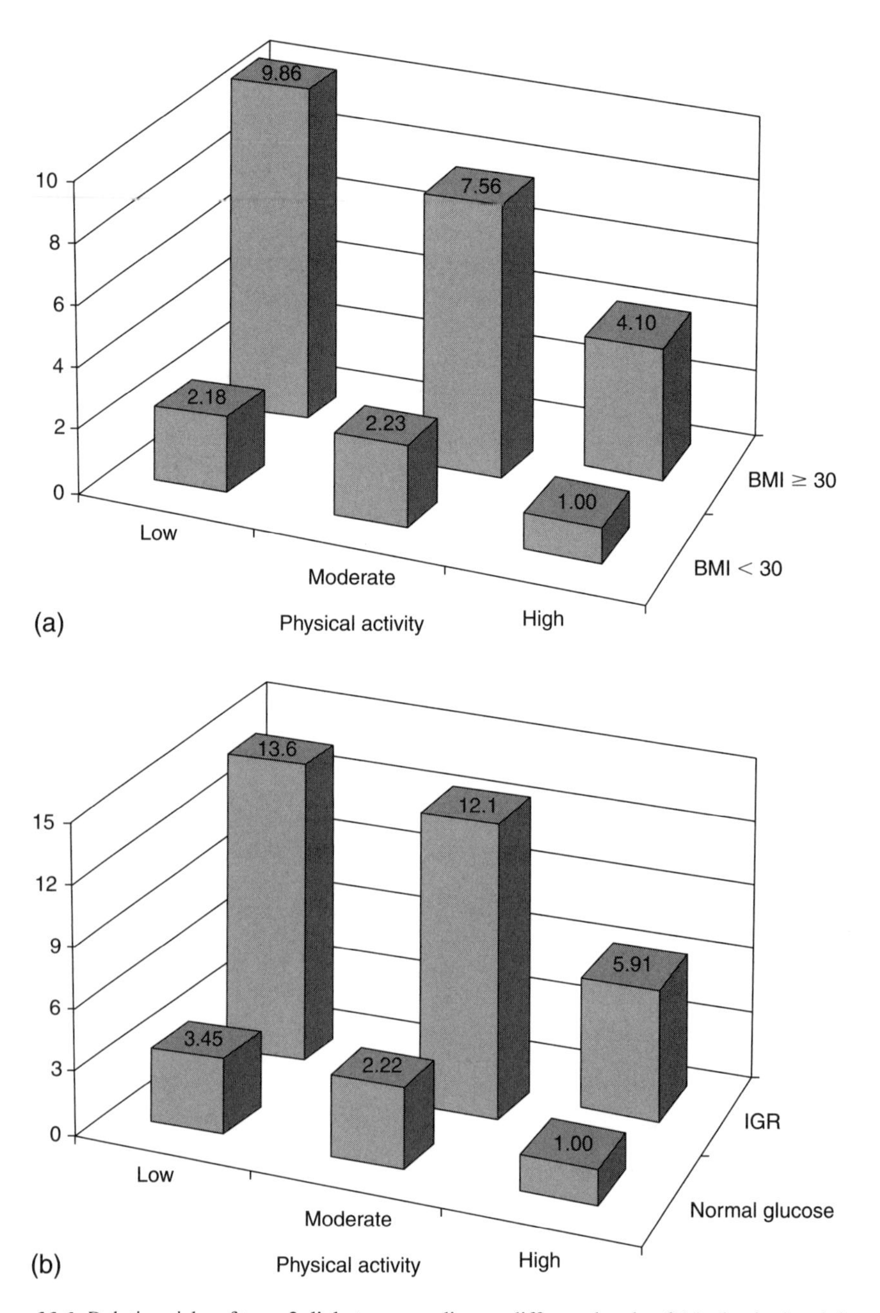

Figure 11.1 Relative risks of type 2 diabetes according to different levels of (a) physical activity and body mass index (BMI; <30 kg/m^2 and ≥ 30 kg/m^2) and (b) physical activity and glucose status (normal glucose, impaired glucose regulation [IGR]). Adjusted for age, sex, study year, systolic blood pressure, smoking status, education, and BMI. "Low" physical activity = low levels of occupational, leisure-time, and commuting physical activity; "moderate" = moderate-to-high levels of only one kind of activity; "high" = moderate-to-high levels of at least two kinds of activity. (Adapted from Hu et al., 2004b, with permission.)

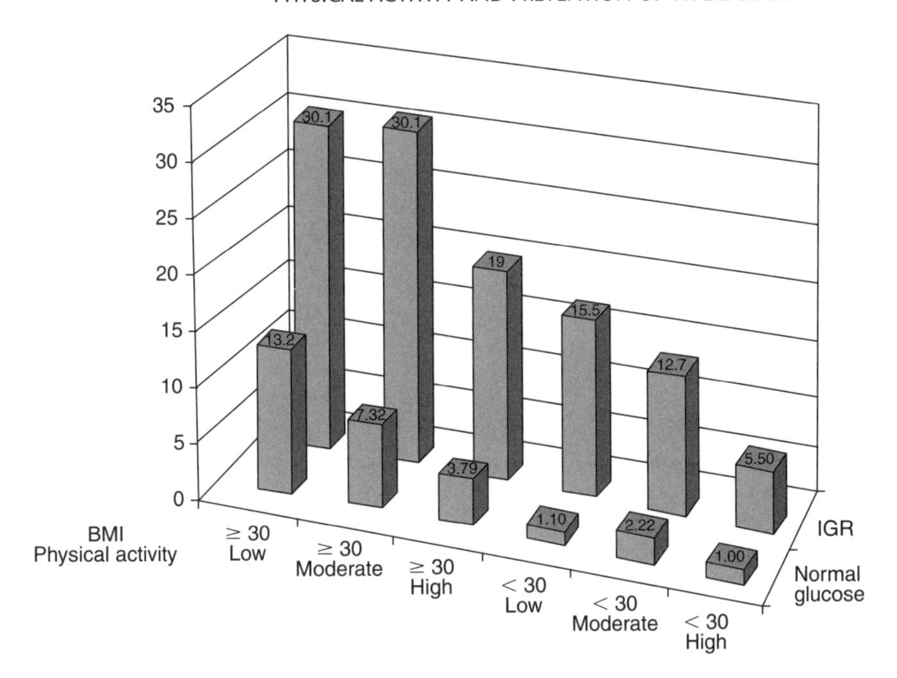

Figure 11.2 Relative risks of type 2 diabetes according to joint levels of physical activity, body mass index, and glucose homeostasis. Adjusted for age, sex, study year, systolic blood pressure, smoking status, and education. IGR, impaired glucose regulation. For definition of physical activity levels, refer to Figure 11.1. (Adapted from Hu et al., 2004b, with permission.)

A significant inverse association between leisure-time physical activity and incident type 2 diabetes was found in both men and women, but more consistently in women, after adjustment for age, BMI, and other confounding factors. Among 2,017 Swedish women in the Gothenburg BEDA Study, investigators observed a significant inverse association between leisure-time physical activity and the risk of type 2 diabetes (Dotevall et al., 2004). Another U.S. study, the Women's Health Study, examined the joint association of leisure-time physical activity and BMI with development of type 2 diabetes among 37,878 women free of cardiovascular disease, cancer, and diabetes who were followed for 6.9 years (Weinstein et al., 2004). BMI and physical inactivity were independent predictors of incident diabetes when examined separately. However, when examined together, BMI was a far more important predictor: the inverse relationship between physical activity and risk of type 2 diabetes was attenuated once BMI was taken into account.

Studies That Included Minority Populations

The inverse relationship between physical activity and lower risk of type 2 diabetes has also been documented in studies that have included minority populations. In the Pitt County Study, African-American men and women who engaged in moderate physical activity had a 65% lower risk of developing type 2 diabetes than their physically inactive counterparts, after adjusting for age, BMI, and other risk factors (James et al., 1998). The Pima Indians Community Study reported in age-adjusted analysis that leisure-time physical activity was associated with lower risk of type 2 diabetes; however, the relationship was weakened after additional adjustment for BMI (Kriska et al., 2003). The Women's Health Initiative

Observational Study evaluated whether physical activity independently predicted the risk of type 2 diabetes among African-American, Hispanic, Asian, and Caucasian women who were postmenopausal (Hsia et al., 2005). After adjusting for age, BMI, and other risk factors, a significant inverse association between total physical activity and risk was apparent in Caucasian women but not among women belonging to the other race/ethnic minority groups (Hsia et al., 2005). The lack of association among non-Caucasian women may have been attributable to the smaller sample sizes of these other groups.

Discussion

These prospective cohort studies, conducted among different populations and assessing different domains of activity, indicate that regular physical activity during occupation, commuting, leisure-time, or daily life reduces the risk of type 2 diabetes by 15% to 60%, with most studies showing a 30% to 50% risk reduction. The benefit of physical activity is apparent in both men and women and in younger and older individuals. Although the data are limited, the inverse relationship also has been observed in minorities as well as in Caucasians.

Several potential limitations need to be discussed in interpreting the results from the prospective cohort studies. First, many of the studies used questionnaires to assess physical activity, which likely resulted in an imprecise measure of habitual activity. However, any misclassification would have been random, leading to an underestimation of the risk reduction associated with physical activity. Additionally, studies that have assessed cardiorespiratory fitness (*see* "Physical Fitness and Type 2 Diabetes" below; a more objective measure) have reported similar inverse associations with risk of type 2 diabetes. Although fitness is, to some extent, genetically determined (*see* Chapter 5), an individual's recent physical activity pattern accounts for up to 70% to 80% of the variance in detailed recordings of physical activity (Paffenbarger et al., 1993).

A second issue to consider is the criteria used for diagnosing diabetes. The use of self-reported diabetes based on medical or treatment history was more common in these studies than the use of glucose tolerance or fasting glucose tests for diagnosis. However, results from studies using self-reported diagnosis and those from studies screening for type 2 diabetes were generally similar.

Third, although most of these observational studies did control for age, BMI, and several other important confounding factors, residual confounding resulting from unmeasured factors may still be present. However, residual confounding is unlikely to be a major concern, in view of the consistency of findings among these prospective studies. Additionally, randomized clinical trials of behavior modification (*see* "Change in Lifestyle, Including Physical Activity, and Type 2 Diabetes" below), where confounding is much less of a concern, have provided results that support the findings of the prospective cohort studies in Table 11.1.

An observation worth noting is that even after adjusting for BMI, many of the studies in Table 11.1 continued to note significant, but attenuated, inverse associations between physical activity and type 2 diabetes. This suggests that physical activity has beneficial effects on the development of the disease, apart from its effects on changing body weight and adiposity (*see* additional discussion in Biological Mechanisms).

How much physical activity is required for a reduction in risk of type 2 diabetes? Although the data are sparse, it appears that even 30 minutes per day of moderate-intensity physical activity (such as brisk walking) is sufficient to reduce the risk. This amount is supported by data from clinical trials of lifestyle intervention and risk of developing type 2 diabetes among high-risk individuals (*see* "Change in Lifestyle, Including Physical Activity, and Type 2 Diabetes" below). In the Nurses' Health Study (Hu et al., 1999), the Health Professionals' Follow-up Study (Hu et al., 2001), the Japanese Male Office Workers Survey (Nakanishi et al., 2004), the Women's Health Study (Weinstein et al., 2004), and the Women's Health Initiative Observational Study (Hsia et al., 2005), the magnitude of the inverse association between walking and risk of type 2 diabetes was similar to that between vigorous-intensity leisure activity and risk. Additionally, decreasing the amount of time spent watching television is helpful for reducing risk. Each 2-hour increment in TV watching per day was shown to be associated with a 14% to 20% increase in the risk of type 2 diabetes among men and women in two large studies (Hu et al., 2001; Hu et al., 2003a).

Although 30 minutes of moderate activity daily appears sufficient to reduce the risk of diabetes, this amount may not be adequate for weight control (*see* Chapter 15 for additional discussion). A major, independent risk factor for type 2 diabetes is obesity, which is an important health problem today (*see* Chapter 12). Regular physical activity can reduce body weight and fat mass without dietary caloric restriction in overweight individuals. An increase in total energy expenditure appears to be the most important determinant of successful exercise-induced weight loss. The best long-term results may be achieved when physical activity produces an energy expenditure of at least 2500 kcal/week (approximately 60 minutes/day of moderate-intensity activity). However, the optimal approach in weight reduction programs appears to be a combination of regular physical activity and caloric restriction. A minimum of 60 minutes/day, but more likely 80 to 90 minutes/day, of moderate-intensity physical activity may be needed to avoid or limit weight regain in formerly overweight or obese individuals. Regular moderate-intensity physical activity, a healthy diet, and avoiding unhealthy weight gain are effective and safe ways to prevent and treat type 2 diabetes; additionally, these behaviors also can prevent cardiovascular diseases and reduce premature mortality (Blair et al., 2001; Dubbert et al., 2002; Erlichman et al., 2002; Hu et al., 2004a; Hu et al., 2004c; Hu et al., 2005; Katzmarzyk et al., 2003; Pate et al., 1995; Wannamethee and Shaper, 2001; Willett et al., 1999). Particular attention should be paid to individuals who are physically inactive, have unhealthy diets, or are prone to weight gain. To combat the epidemic of overweight at a population level, it is important to develop strategies to increase habitual physical activity and to prevent overweight and obesity in collaboration with communities, families, schools, work sites, health-care professionals, media, and policymakers (Lakka and Bouchard, 2005).

Physical Fitness and Type 2 Diabetes: Data From Prospective Cohort Studies

There is a much smaller body of evidence on the role of physical fitness in preventing type 2 diabetes. Only six prospective cohort studies have assessed the association of physical fitness with the risk of type 2 diabetes (Bjornholt et al., 2001; Carnethon et al., 2003; Eriksson and Lindgarde, 1996; Lynch et al., 1996; Sawada et al., 2003; Wei et al., 1999; Table 11.3). Five of the studies used glucose tolerance or fasting glucose tests to screen for diabetes among participants at baseline (Bjornholt et al., 2001; Carnethon et al., 2003; Eriksson and Lindgarde, 1996; Lynch et al., 1996; Wei et al., 1999) and during follow-up (Carnethon et al., 2003; Eriksson and Lindgarde, 1996; Lynch et al., 1996; Sawada et al., 2003; Wei et al., 1999).

Data from a Swedish study, the Malmö Preventive Trial, found that poor physical fitness, measured by vital capacity and maximal oxygen uptake, was inversely associated with the risk of type 2 diabetes in men (Eriksson and Lindgarde, 1996). In the Kuopio Ischemic Heart Disease Risk Factor Study, Finland, high compared to low levels of cardiorespiratory fitness (maximal oxygen uptake of ≥31.0 vs. <25.8 mL/kg/minutes) among men

Table 11.3 Prospective Cohort Studies of Physical Fitness and the Risk of Type 2 Diabetes

Study (reference)	*Subjects*	*Age range (years)*	*No. of incident cases; duration of study*	*Physical fitness comparison groups*	*Relative risk (95% confidence interval)*	*Adjustment factors*
Malmö Preventive Trials (Eriksson and Lindgarde, 1996)	2673 men	48–54	60 cases; 6 years	Each unit increase in physical fitness	0.51 (0.37–0.69)	Fasting blood glucose, BMI, 40-minute insulin increment, and 2-hour insulin
Kuopio Ischemic Heart Disease Risk Factor Study (Lynch et al., 1996)	751 men	42–60	39 cases; 4 years	Cardiorespiratory fitness; ≥31.0 vs. <25.8 mL of oxygen per kilogram per minute	0.26 (0.08–0.82)	Age, parental history of diabetes, BMI, triglycerides, baseline glucose, and alcohol consumption
Aerobics Center Longitudinal Study (Wei et al., 1999)	8633 men	30–79	149 cases; 6 years	Lowest 20% of cardiorespiratory fitness vs. highest 40%	2.6 (1.6–4.2)	Age, parental history of diabetes, BMI, high blood pressure, high levels of HDL cholesterol, total cholesterol, and triglycerides, smoking, and alcohol consumption
Oslo Healthy Men Study (Bjornholt et al., 2001)	1947 men	40–59	143 cases; 22.5 years	Each unit increase in fitness	0.46 (0.31–0.67)	Age, parental history of diabetes, sex, BMI, blood pressure, cholesterol, triglycerides, glucose disappearance rate, and fasting glucose
CARDIA Study (Carnethon et al., 2003)	4464 men and women	18–30	156 cases; 15 years	Each minute decrease in test duration	1.12 (1.03–1.22)	Age, parental history of diabetes, sex, BMI, and smoking
Tokyo Gas Company Study (Sawada et al., 2003)	4747 men	20–40	280 cases; 14 years	Quartile 3 vs. quartile 1 of cardiorespiratory fitness	0.63 (0.45–0.89)	Age, parental history of diabetes, BMI, systolic blood pressure, smoking, and alcohol consumption
				Quartile 4 vs. quartile 1 of cardiorespiratory fitness	0.56 (0.37–0.84)	

BMI: body mass index.

ages 42 to 60 years also was associated with a 74% lower risk, after adjusting for age, baseline glucose levels, and other risk factors (Lynch et al., 1996). In a Norwegian study, the Oslo Healthy Men Study, investigators reported that each unit increase in physical fitness was associated with a 54% decrease in the risk of type 2 diabetes after adjustment for confounding factors (Bjornholt et al., 2001). The Aerobics Center Longitudinal Study, conducted among 8,633 U.S. men ages 30 to 79 years, indicated that men with low cardiorespiratory fitness (the least fit 20%) had a 3.7-fold increase in risk of developing type 2 diabetes during follow-up compared to men with high fitness (the most fit 40%) (Wei et al., 1999). In Japan, the Tokyo Gas Company Study investigated 4,747 Japanese men ages 20 to 40 years at baseline and reported that low cardiorespiratory fitness (measured by a cycle ergometer test and maximal oxygen uptake) was associated with an increased risk of incident type 2 diabetes (Sawada et al., 2003).

The only study to include women, the Coronary Artery Risk Development in Young Adults Study, enrolled 4,487 U.S. men and women ages 18 to 30 years and assessed whether low fitness (estimated by short duration on a maximal treadmill test) predicted the development of type 2 diabetes or the metabolic syndrome and whether improving fitness over time (as assessed by increase in treadmill test duration between examinations) was associated with risk reduction (Carnethon et al., 2003). After adjustment for age, race, sex, smoking, family history of diabetes, and BMI, participants with low fitness (bottom 20%) were about twice as likely to develop type 2 diabetes or the metabolic syndrome than those with high fitness (top 40%). Moreover, increasing fitness level during the 7-year study was associated with a 60% reduction in risk of type 2 diabetes and 50% reduction in risk of the metabolic syndrome.

These studies of physical fitness—primarily in men—have shown similar findings to the studies of physical activity but with generally larger magnitudes of association. This may have resulted from fitness measurements being less prone to measurement error and misclassification. In addition, factors other than physical activity may influence both physical fitness and health through related biological factors (Blair et al., 2001).

Physical Activity or Physical Fitness and the Metabolic Syndrome: Data From Prospective Cohort Studies

Several studies have assessed the association of physical activity or physical fitness with the risk of developing the metabolic syndrome. The Kuopio Ischemic Heart Disease Risk Factor Study reported that men engaging in more than 3 hours/week of moderate or vigorous leisure-time physical activity were half as likely as sedentary men to have the metabolic syndrome after adjustment for major confounders (age, BMI, smoking, alcohol, and socioeconomic status) and potentially mediating factors (insulin, glucose, lipids, and blood pressure), especially in high-risk men (Laaksonen et al., 2002). The study also showed that poor cardiorespiratory fitness is associated with all components of the metabolic syndrome and suggested that poor fitness also be considered a feature of the metabolic syndrome (Lakka et al., 2003). In another study, investigators examined to what extent the longitudinal development of fatness, cardiopulmonary fitness, and lifestyle variables from age 13 to 36 years determined the occurrence of the metabolic syndrome at age 36 years (Ferreira et al., 2005). Participants with the metabolic syndrome at age 36 years, compared to those without the syndrome, had a more marked decrease in cardiopulmonary fitness levels, a more marked increase in light- to moderate-intensity physical activity, but a more marked decrease in hard physical activity. In a recent analysis from the Aerobics Center Longitudinal Study, including 9,007 U.S. men and 1,491 women ages 20 to 80 years without the metabolic syndrome at baseline, investigators found that cardiorespiratory fitness was inversely associated with incident metabolic syndrome in both men and women (LaMonte et al., 2005).

Change in Lifestyle, Including Physical Activity, and Type 2 Diabetes: Data From Clinical Trials

In recent years, five clinical trials have assessed whether regular physical activity, with or without dietary intervention, can reduce progression to type 2 diabetes among adults with impaired glucose tolerance (Eriksson and Lindgarde, 1991; Knowler et al., 2002; Pan et al., 1997; Tuomilehto et al., 2001) or with high cardiovascular risk (Davey Smith et al., 2005). Two early reports from Sweden and China (Eriksson and Lindgarde, 1991; Pan et al., 1997) indicated that a change in lifestyle (physical activity, with our without diet change) could prevent type 2 diabetes. However, these data were limited because the Swedish study was a non-randomized trial, and the Chinese study randomized clinics, rather than the individual subject, to intervention and control groups. Subsequently, two well-designed, randomized, controlled trials in Finland and the United States (Knowler et al., 2002; Tuomilehto et al., 2001) confirmed the earlier Swedish and Chinese findings. The details of these trials follow.

The Swedish study, the Malmö Study, targeted increased physical activity and weight loss as major intervention strategies to prevent and delay type 2 diabetes in a non-randomized clinical trial conducted among participants with impaired glucose tolerance (Eriksson and Lindgarde, 1991). Subjects participating in the exercise program had less than half the risk of developing type 2 diabetes during a 5-year follow-up compared to those who did not participate. In the Chinese study, 577 individuals from Da Qing with impaired glucose tolerance were randomized by clinic into one of the four groups: exercise only, diet only, diet plus exercise, and a control group (Pan et al., 1997). The cumulative incidence of type 2 diabetes during 6 years was significantly lower in the exercise group (41%), diet group (44%), and diet plus exercise group (46%) compared to the control group (68%). These differences remained significant even after adjusting for differences in baseline BMI and fasting glucose.

In the Finnish Diabetes Prevention Study (DPS), 522 middle-age (mean age: 55 years) men (33%) and women (67%) who were overweight (mean BMI: 31 kg/m^2) and had impaired glucose tolerance were randomized either to an intensive lifestyle intervention group or a control group (Eriksson et al., 1999; Tuomilehto et al., 2001). The participants in the intervention group had frequent consultation visits with a nutritionist (seven times during the first year). They received individual advice about how to achieve the intervention goals, which were: *(1)* reduction in body weight of 5% or more, *(2)* total fat intake less than 30% of energy consumed, *(3)* saturated fat intake less than 10% of energy consumed, *(4)* fiber intake of at least 15 g per 1000 kcal, and *(5)* moderate exercise for at least 30 minutes/day. After the intensive intervention period, there was a maintenance phase that included a counselling session every 3 months. At each of these counselling sessions, exercise habits were discussed, all kinds of physical activity were strongly recommended, and increased physical activity was considered an essential part of a successful weight -loss program. Endurance exercise, including walking, jogging, swimming, aerobic ball games, and skiing, was recommended to increase aerobic capacity and cardiorespiratory fitness. Participants were also offered an opportunity to attend supervised, progressive, individually tailored circuit-type resistance training sessions. The moderate-intensity and medium- to high-volume programs were designed to improve the functional capacity and strength of the large muscle groups of the upper and lower body. The mean amount of weight lost between baseline and the end of year two was 3.5 kg in the intervention group and 0.8 kg in the control group. The cumulative incidence of type 2 diabetes after 4 years was 11% in the intervention group and 23% in the control group ($p < 0.001$). During the entire trial, the risk of diabetes was reduced by 58% in the intervention group compared to the control group ($p < 0.001$). The reduction in the incidence of diabetes was directly associated with changes in lifestyle; there was a strong inverse correlation between the number of intervention goals achieved (0–5) and the incidence of diabetes. In fact, none of the participants achieving four or five of the five intervention goals developed diabetes. Physical activity was clearly important; among participants who did not meet the weight loss goal, the risk of developing diabetes in those who exercised more than 4 hours/week, compared to those who were sedentary, was reduced (intervention group, RR = 0.2, 95% CI, 0.1–0.6; control group, RR= 0.6, 95% CI, 0.3–1.1).

In additional analyses of data from the Finnish DPS, the role of leisure-time physical activity in preventing type 2 diabetes was evaluated by examining the association of changes in leisure-time physical activity with the incidence of diabetes among participants in both the combined intervention and control groups (Laaksonen et al., 2005). The change in total leisure-time physical activity was strongly associated with risk of incident diabetes (Table 11.4). Adjusting for age, sex, intervention group, smoking, and major risk factors for

Table 11.4 Relative Risks* (95% Confidence Interval) of Developing Type 2 Diabetes, According to Tertiles of Change in Leisure-Time Physical Activity Among Finns in the Diabetes Prevention Study

Tertiles† *(hours/week)*	*Model 1*	*Model 2*	*Model 3*
	Change in total leisure-time physical activity		
–3.2 (–35 through –0.5)	1.00	1.00	1.00
0.5 (–0.5 through 1.7)	0.47 (0.28–0.79)	0.48 (0.28–0.82)	0.52 (0.31–0.89)
3.8 (1.8–19)	0.26 (0.15–0.47)	0.29 (0.16–0.53)	0.34 (0.19 0.62)
p-trend	<0.001	<0.001	<0.001
	Change in moderate-to-vigorous leisure-time physical activity (≥3.5 METs)		
–1.5 (–13.5 through –0.1)	1.00	1.00	1.00
0.5 (–0.1 through 1.3)	0.78 (0.46–1.33)	0.86 (0.49–1.48)	0.95 (0.54–1.65)
2.6 (1.3–14.4)	0.35 (0.18–0.65)	0.40 (0.21–0.76)	0.51 (0.26 0.97)
p-trend	0.001	0.004	0.037
	Change in low-intensity leisure-time physical activity (<3.5 METs)		
–3.2 (–34 through –1.0)	1.00	1.00	1.00
0.8 (–0.9 through 1.1)	0.83 (0.47–1.45)	0.85 (0.47–1.53)	0.63 (0.34–1.17)
3.1 (1.1–15.0)	0.38 (0.20–0.70)	0.41 (0.22–0.77)	0.36 (0.19 0.67)
p- trend	0.001	0.003	0.001

* Model 1 was adjusted for age, sex, group, baseline physical activity. For moderate-to vigorous activity, adjustment was also made for baseline low-intensity activity and change in low-intensity activity. Model 2 was adjusted for variables in Model 1, plus baseline values and changes in dietary intake of energy, total fat, saturated fat, and fiber. Model 3 was adjusted for variables in model 2, plus baseline values and change in BMI.

†The median (range) of the change in leisure-time physical activity is shown.

BMI: body mass index; MET: metabolic equivalent.

(From Laaksonen et al., 2005, with permission.)

diabetes at baseline (including BMI, fasting and 2-hour plasma glucose and insulin levels, family history of diabetes, and total leisure-time physical activity), participants in the upper third of the change in total leisure-time physical activity were 66% less likely to develop diabetes than those in the lower third. Participants who were in the upper third of change in moderate-to-vigorous leisure-time physical activity were 49% less likely to develop diabetes than those who were in the lower third, after adjustment for confounding factors (including low-intensity leisure-time physical activity and its change). The upper third of change in low-intensity leisure-time physical activity predicted a 64% reduction in the risk of incident diabetes compared to the lower third, even with adjustment for moderate-to-vigorous leisure-time physical activity and its change.

A similar randomized clinical trial of lifestyle change and the risk of developing type 2 diabetes among persons at high risk was conducted in the United States. In the Diabetes Prevention Program (DPP), 3,234 non-diabetic persons with elevated fasting and postload plasma glucose concentrations were randomized to a placebo group, a group assigned metformin, or a group assigned to a lifestyle-modification program with the goals of at least a 7% weight loss and at least 150 minutes of physical activity per week (Knowler et al., 2002). The mean age of participants was 51 years, the mean BMI was 34.0 kg/m^2. Women comprised 68% of the participants, and 45% were members of non-Caucasian ethnic groups. The physical activity intervention emphasized brisk walking, but other activities with equivalent intensity, including aerobic dance, bicycle riding, skating, and swimming, were also recommended. Participants were advised to distribute their physical activity throughout the week, with sessions lasting at least 10 minutes. Voluntary, supervised physical activity sessions were offered at least twice per week throughout the study, including group walks, aerobic classes, and one-to-one personal training. After an average follow-up of 2.8 years, the incidence of diabetes was 11.0, 7.8, and 4.8 cases per 100 person-years in the placebo, metformin, and lifestyle groups, respectively. The lifestyle intervention reduced the incidence of type 2 diabetes by 58% (95% CI, 48%–66%) and metformin by 31% (17%–43%), compared to placebo. Noteworthy was the finding that the lifestyle intervention was significantly more effective than metformin in the prevention of type 2 diabetes. The effect of lifestyle intervention on diabetes risk was highly effective in all baseline BMI subgroups (for BMI <30, 30 to <35, and ≥35 kg/m^2, risk reductions were 65%, 61%, and 51%, respectively).

Additional analyses of the U.S. DPP data examined the effect of intensive lifestyle intervention and metformin therapy on the incidence of the metabolic syndrome among adults without the syndrome at baseline (Orchard et al., 2005). After a mean follow-up of 3.0 years, the cumulative incidence per 100 person-years of the metabolic syndrome was 61% in the placebo group, 50% in the metformin group, and 38% in the lifestyle group. Compared to placebo, the incidence of the metabolic syndrome was reduced by 41% in the lifestyle group ($p < 0.01$) and 17% in the metformin group ($p = 0.03$).

Finally, the Multiple Risk Factor Intervention Trial (MRFIT) enrolled 12,866 middle-age U.S. men, ages 35 to 57 years, who were at high risk for CHD and delivered either special intervention or usual care over 6 to 7 years (Davey Smith et al., 2005). This trial, initiated in 1973, was originally designed to examine CHD as the outcome of interest. The special intervention group was counseled to change diet (reduce saturated fat, cholesterol, and calorie intake), stop smoking, and increase physical activity. Recently, the data from MRFIT were analyzed to investigate the role of such a comprehensive intervention program in preventing type 2 diabetes in men without impaired glucose tolerance. Among 11,827 men without diabetes or impaired glucose tolerance at baseline, a total of 666 men (11.5%) in the intervention group and 616 men (10.8%) in the usual care group met the criteria for diabetes during 6 years of follow-up. Among nonsmokers, the intervention program resulted in a statistically significant 18% reduction in the incidence of diabetes compared to the usual care group. In smokers, however, the risk increased significantly by 26% in the intervention group.

The data from the clinical trials described earlier provide evidence that lifestyle intervention, including counselling for physical activity, nutrition, and body weight, can reduce the risk of type 2 diabetes by 40% to 60% among adults with impaired glucose tolerance and by about 20% among non-smoking men in the general population who are at high risk for CHD.

Biological Mechanisms

Several biological mechanisms have been proposed to explain the reduction in risk of type 2 diabetes with physical activity. A large body of literature demonstrates that regular physical activity can improve insulin sensitivity and other components of the metabolic syndrome (Mayer-Davis et al., 1998; Wannamethee et al., 2000) as well as decrease the risk of developing the metabolic syndrome (Laaksonen et al., 2002). Data from the Insulin Resistance Atherosclerosis Study showed that both vigorous and non-vigorous activities were associated with higher insulin sensitivity among 1,467 men and women ages 40 to 69 years (Mayer-Davis et al., 1998). The British Regional Heart Study examined the role of serum insulin concentration and components of the insulin resistance syndrome in the relationship between physical activity and the incidence of type 2 diabetes among 5,159 men ages 40 to 59 years (Wannamethee et al., 2000). This study observed that physical activity was significantly and inversely associated with serum insulin concentrations and many components of the metabolic syndrome and that these associations partly explained the inverse relationship between physical activity and the incidence of type 2 diabetes.

The lifestyle intervention in the DPS (Lindstrom et al., 2003; Tuomilehto et al., 2001) and the DPP (The Diabetes Prevention Program Research Group, 2005) resulted not only in a marked reduction in the risk of developing type 2 diabetes but also in reduction in fasting and 2-hour glucose and hemoglobin A_{1c}. Additionally, favorable changes in several cardiovascular risk factors, including reduction in body weight, decrease in blood pressure, increase in plasma levels of HDL cholesterol, and decrease in plasma levels of triglycerides, were seen with lifestyle intervention. Systemic inflammation (Haffner, 2003; Willerson and Ridker, 2004) and endothelial dysfunction (Harris and Matthews, 2004; Landmesser et al., 2000; 2004) have been identified to play a central role in the development of atherosclerosis. Inflammation (as measured by C-reactive protein, fibrinogen, and plasminogen activator inhibitor [PAI]) has been related to increased insulin resistance but not impaired insulin secretion (Festa et al., 2003; Temelkova-Kurktschiev et al., 2002).

Physical activity also has beneficial effects on adiposity. As noted earlier, many prospective cohort studies that did adjust for BMI continued to observe significant inverse associations between physical activity or fitness and risk of type 2 diabetes (Tables 11.1 and 11.3). However, the associations generally were attenuated, compared to analyses that did not adjust for BMI, suggesting that the benefit of physical activity on risk is partially mediated through changes in adiposity. Recent research has shown that adipose tissue is an important endocrine organ that plays a key role in the integration of endocrine, metabolic, and inflammatory signals for the control of energy homeostasis (Chandran et al., 2003; Saltiel and Kahn, 2001). The adipocyte has been shown to secrete a variety of bio-active proteins into the circulation. These proteins, termed adipocytokines, include leptin, tumor necrosis factor (TNF)-α, PAI-1, adipsin, resistin, and adiponectin (Chandran et al., 2003). Some of these adipocytokines have been implicated in the development of insulin resistance (Pittas et al., 2004).

Furthermore, inflammation markers (cytokines interleukin [IL]-1β, IL-6, and TNF-α) also have been found to increase the risk of type 2 diabetes (Spranger et al., 2003). Recently, Meigs et al. (2004) reported that endothelial dysfunction, as measured by the biomarkers E-selectin, intercellular adhesion molecule 1, and vascular cell adhesion molecule 1, predicts type 2 diabetes in women independent of other known risk factors, including obesity and subclinical inflammation.

Although the exact mechanisms underlying the association between a low cardiorespiratory fitness and increased risk of type 2 diabetes is unknown, several putative mechanisms have been proposed. Individuals with a low cardiorespiratory fitness tend to have insulin resistance (Sato et al., 1984), as well as fewer glucose transporters, compared to those who are more fit (Ivy and Kuo, 1998). Data from the Kuopio Ischemic Heart Disease Risk Factor Study have suggested that poor cardiorespiratory fitness is not only associated with all components of the metabolic syndrome but might also be considered a feature of the syndrome (Lakka et al., 2003). Finally, low cardiorespiratory fitness is an indication of a sedentary lifestyle, which is associated with increased risk of the metabolic syndrome and type 2 diabetes.

Future Research

The currently available epidemiological evidence from prospective cohort studies and clinical trials indicates that 30 minutes/day of moderate-to-vigorous physical activity can reduce the risk of type 2 diabetes. Physical activity reduces the risk of type 2 diabetes by exerting favorable changes in insulin sensitivity and the metabolic syndrome (including reducing body weight, blood pressure, plasma levels of triglycerides, and inflammation) and increasing plasma levels of HDL cholesterol. Several important research questions in this area remain to be addressed. Lifestyle interventions, including physical activity, have been shown to prevent progression to type 2 diabetes in high-risk individuals. However, it is unclear whether similar lifestyle interventions can prevent type 2 diabetes in the general population at large, in younger and older populations, or in various racial and ethnic groups. Additionally, studies are needed to further clarify the biological mechanisms underlying the physical activity and diabetes association, and any effects of gene–physical activity interaction. Finally, a most important priority should be determining the most effective public health strategies for promoting physical activity in the whole population.

Personal Perspective

Diabetes is one of the fastest growing public health problems in the world, causing economic, social, and personal burdens. Increasing physical activity is an important strategy to help reduce this problem. A variety of organizations, including the U.S. Centers for Disease Control and Prevention and the American College of Sports Medicine (Pate et al., 1995), the National Institutes of Health (NIH Consensus Development Panel on Physical Activity and Cardiovascular Health, 1996) and the World Health Organization (World Health Organization, 2004) have recommended that every U.S. adult should have at least 30 minutes of moderate-intensity physical activity (such as brisk walking, cycling, swimming, home repair, and yard work) on most—preferably all—days of the week. Based on our review of the scientific evidence, a level of physical activity consistent with these recommendations—at least 30 minutes/day of moderate-to-vigorous physical activity—is effective in preventing type 2 diabetes. Regular physical activity should be an important component of a healthy lifestyle for everyone. Public health messages, health-care professionals, and the health-care system should aggressively promote physical activity during occupation, commuting, leisure time, and all aspects of daily life.

References

Arslanian S. 2002. Type 2 diabetes in children: clinical aspects and risk factors. *Horm. Res.* 57 (Suppl 1): 19–28.

Bjornholt JV, Erikssen G, Liestol K, Jervell J, Erikssen J, Thaulow E. 2001. Prediction of Type 2 diabetes in healthy middle-aged men with special emphasis on glucose homeostasis. Results from 22.5 years' follow-up. *Diabet. Med.* 18: 261–7.

Blair SN, Cheng Y, Holder JS. 2001. Is physical activity or physical fitness more important in defining health benefits? *Med Sci Sports Exerc* 33: S379–99.

Burchfiel CM, Sharp DS, Curb JD, et al. 1995. Physical activity and incidence of diabetes: the Honolulu Heart Program. *Am J Epidemiol* 141: 360–8.

Carnethon MR, Gidding SS, Nehgme R, Sidney S, Jacobs DR, Jr., Liu K. 2003. Cardiorespiratory fitness in young adulthood and the development of cardiovascular disease risk factors. *JAMA* 290: 3092–100.

Centers for Disease Control and Prevention. 2003. Prevalence of diabetes and impaired fasting glucose in adults—United States, 1999–2000. *MMWR* 52: 833–7.

Chandran M, Phillips SA, Ciaraldi T, Henry RR. 2003. Adiponectin: more than just another fat cell hormone? *Diabetes Care* 26: 2442–50.

Davey Smith G, Bracha Y, Svendsen KH, Neaton JD, Haffner SM, Kuller LH. 2005. Incidence of type 2 diabetes in the randomized multiple risk factor intervention trial. *Ann Intern Med* 142: 313–22.

DECODE Study Group. 2003. Age- and sex-specific prevalences of diabetes and impaired glucose regulation in 13 European cohorts. *Diabetes Care* 26: 61–9.

Dotevall A, Johansson S, Wilhelmsen L, Rosengren A. 2004. Increased levels of triglycerides, BMI and blood pressure and low physical activity increase the risk of diabetes in Swedish women. A prospective 18-year follow-up of the BEDA*study. *Diabet Med* 21: 615–22.

Dubbert PM, Carithers T, Sumner AE, et al. 2002. Obesity, physical inactivity, and risk for cardiovascular disease. *Am J Med Sci* 324: 116–26.

Eriksson J, Lindstrom J, Valle T, et al. 1999. Prevention of Type II diabetes in subjects with impaired glucose tolerance: the Diabetes Prevention Study (DPS) in Finland. Study design and 1-year interim report on the feasibility of the lifestyle intervention programme. *Diabetologia* 42: 793–801.

Eriksson KF, Lindgarde F. 1991. Prevention of type 2 (non-insulin-dependent) diabetes mellitus by diet and physical exercise. The 6-year Malmo feasibility study. *Diabetologia* 34: 891–8.

Eriksson KF, Lindgarde F. 1996. Poor physical fitness, and impaired early insulin response but late hyperinsulinaemia, as predictors of NIDDM in middle-aged Swedish men. *Diabetologia* 39: 573–9.

Erlichman J, Kerbey AL, James WP. 2002. Physical activity and its impact on health outcomes. Paper 1: The impact of physical activity on cardiovascular disease and all-cause mortality: an historical perspective. *Obes Rev* 3: 257–71.

Ferreira I, Twisk JW, van Mechelen W, Kemper HC, Stehouwer CD. 2005. Development of fatness, fitness, and lifestyle from adolescence to the age of 36 years: determinants of the metabolic syndrome in young adults: the Amsterdam growth and health longitudinal study. *Arch Intern Med* 165: 42–8

Festa A, Hanley AJ, Tracy RP, D'Agostino R, Jr., Haffner SM. 2003. Inflammation in the prediabetic state is related to increased insulin resistance rather than decreased insulin secretion. *Circulation* 108: 1822–30.

Folsom AR, Kushi LH, Hong CP. 2000. Physical activity and incident diabetes mellitus in postmenopausal women. *Am. J. Public Health* 90: 134–8.

Haapanen N, Miilunpalo S, Vuori I, Oja P, Pasanen M. 1997. Association of leisure time physical activity with the risk of coronary heart disease, hypertension and diabetes in middle-aged men and women. *Int. J. Epidemiol.* 26: 739–47.

Haffner SM. 2003. Pre-diabetes, insulin resistance, inflammation and CVD risk. *Diabetes Res Clin Pract* 61 Suppl 1: S9-S18.

Harris KF, Matthews KA. 2004. Interactions between autonomic nervous system activity and endothelial function: a model for the development of cardiovascular disease. *Psychosom Med* 66: 153–64.

Helmrich SP, Ragland DR, Leung RW, Paffenbarger RS, Jr. 1991. Physical activity and reduced occurrence of non-insulin-dependent diabetes mellitus. *N Engl J Med* 325: 147–52.

Hsia J, Wu L, Allen C, et al. 2005. Physical activity and diabetes risk in postmenopausal women. *Am J Prev Med* 28: 19–25.

Hu FB, Leitzmann MF, Stampfer MJ, Colditz GA, Willett WC, Rimm EB. 2001. Physical activity and television watching in relation to risk for type 2 diabetes mellitus in men. *Arch Intern Med* 161: 1542–8.

Hu FB, Li TY, Colditz GA, Willett WC, Manson JE. 2003a. Television watching and other sedentary behaviors in relation to risk of obesity and type 2 diabetes mellitus in women. *JAMA* 289: 1785–91.

Hu FB, Sigal RJ, Rich-Edwards JW, et al. 1999. Walking compared with vigorous physical activity and risk of type 2 diabetes in women: a prospective study. *JAMA* 282: 1433–9.

Hu FB, Willett WC, Li T, Stampfer MJ, Colditz GA, Manson JE. 2004a. Adiposity as compared with physical activity in predicting mortality among women. *N Engl J Med* 351: 2694–703.

Hu G, Lindstrom J, Valle TT, et al. 2004b. Physical activity, body mass index, and risk of type 2 diabetes in patients with normal or impaired glucose regulation. *Arch Intern Med* 164: 892–6.

Hu G, Qiao Q, Silventoinen K, et al. 2003b. Occupational, commuting, and leisure-time physical activity in relation to risk for type 2 diabetes in middle-aged Finnish men and women. *Diabetologia* 46: 322–9.

Hu G, Tuomilehto J, Silventoinen K, Barengo N, Jousilahti P. 2004c. Joint effects of physical activity, body mass index, waist circumference and waist-to-hip ratio with the risk of cardiovascular disease among middle-aged Finnish men and women. *Eur Heart J* 25: 2212–9.

Hu G, Tuomilehto J, Silventoinen K, Barengo NC, Peltonen M, Jousilahti P. 2005. The effects of physical activity and body mass index on cardiovascular, cancer and all-cause mortality among 47 212 middle-aged Finnish men and women. *Int J Obes Relat Metab Disord* 29: 894–902.

Ivy JL, Kuo CH. 1998. Regulation of GLUT4 protein and glycogen synthase during muscle glycogen synthesis after exercise. *Acta Physiol. Scand* 162: 295–304.

James SA, Jamjoum L, Raghunathan TE, Strogatz DS, Furth ED, Khazanie PG. 1998. Physical activity and NIDDM in African-Americans. The Pitt County Study. *Diabetes Care* 21: 555–62.

Katzmarzyk PT, Janssen I, Ardern CI. 2003. Physical inactivity, excess adiposity and premature mortality. *Obes Rev* 4: 257–90.

Knowler WC, Barrett-Connor E, Fowler SE, et al. 2002. Reduction in the incidence of type 2 diabetes with lifestyle intervention or metformin. *N Engl J Med* 346: 393–403.

Kriska AM, Saremi A, Hanson RL, et al. 2003. Physical activity, obesity, and the incidence of type 2 diabetes in a high-risk population. *Am J Epidemiol* 158: 669–75.

Laaksonen DE, Lakka HM, Salonen JT, Niskanen LK, Rauramaa R, Lakka TA. 2002. Low levels of leisure-time physical activity and cardiorespiratory fitness predict development of the metabolic syndrome. *Diabetes Care* 25: 1612–8.

Laaksonen DE, Lindstrom J, Lakka TA, et al. 2005. Physical activity in the prevention of type 2 diabetes: the Finnish diabetes prevention study. *Diabetes* 54: 158–65.

Lakka TA, Bouchard C. 2005. *Physical activity, obesity and cardiovascular diseases. Handb Exp Pharmacol* 170: 137–163.

Lakka TA, Laaksonen DE, Lakka HM, et al. 2003. Sedentary lifestyle, poor cardiorespiratory fitness, and the metabolic syndrome. *Med Sci Sports Exerc* 35: 1279–86.

LaMonte MJ, Barlow CE, Jurca R, Kampert JB, Church TS, Blair SN. 2005. Cardiorespiratory fitness is inversely associated with the incidence of metabolic syndrome: a prospective study of men and women. *Circulation* 112: 505–12.

Landmesser U, Hornig B, Drexler H. 2000. Endothelial dysfunction in hypercholesterolemia: mechanisms, pathophysiological importance, and therapeutic interventions. *Semin Thromb Hemost* 26: 529–37.

Landmesser U, Hornig B, Drexler H. 2004. Endothelial function: a critical determinant in atherosclerosis? *Circulation* 109: II27–33.

Lindstrom J, Louheranta A, Mannelin M, et al. 2003. The Finnish Diabetes Prevention Study (DPS): lifestyle intervention and 3-year results on diet and physical activity. *Diabetes Care* 26: 3230–6.

Lynch J, Helmrich SP, Lakka TA, et al. 1996. Moderately intense physical activities and high levels of cardiorespiratory fitness reduce the risk of non-insulin-dependent diabetes mellitus in middle-aged men. *Arch Intern Med* 156: 1307–14.

Manson JE, Nathan DM, Krolewski AS, Stampfer MJ, Willett WC, Hennekens CH. 1992. A prospective study of exercise and incidence of diabetes among US male physicians. *JAMA* 268: 63–7.

Manson JE, Rimm EB, Stampfer MJ, et al. 1991. Physical activity and incidence of non-insulin-dependent diabetes mellitus in women. *Lancet* 338: 774–8.

Mayer-Davis EJ, D'Agostino R, Jr., Karter AJ, et al. 1998. Intensity and amount of physical activity in relation to insulin sensitivity: the Insulin Resistance Atherosclerosis Study. *JAMA* 279: 669–74.

Meigs JB, Hu FB, Rifai N, Manson JE. 2004. Biomarkers of endothelial dysfunction and risk of type 2 diabetes mellitus. *JAMA* 291: 1978–86.

Meisinger C, Lowel H, Thorand B, Doring A. 2005. Leisure time physical activity and the risk of type 2 diabetes in men and women from the general population. The MONICA/KORA Augsburg Cohort Study. *Diabetologia* 48: 27–34.

Meisinger C, Thorand B, Schneider A, Stieber J, Doring A, Lowel H. 2002. Sex differences in risk factors for incident type 2 diabetes mellitus: the MONICA Augsburg cohort study. *Arch Intern Med* 162: 82–9.

Nakanishi N, Takatorige T, Suzuki K. 2004. Daily life activity and risk of developing impaired fasting glucose or type 2 diabetes in middle-aged Japanese men. *Diabetologia* 47: 1768–75.

Neel JV. 1962. Diabetes mellitus: a "thrifty" genotype rendered detrimental by "progress"? *Am J Hum Genet* 14: 353–62.

NIH Consensus Development Panel on Physical Activity and Cardiovascular Health. 1996. Physical activity and cardiovascular health. NIH Consensus Development Panel on Physical Activity and Cardiovascular Health. *JAMA* 276: 241–6.

Okada K, Hayashi T, Tsumura K, Suematsu C, Endo G, Fujii S. 2000. Leisure-time physical activity at weekends and the risk of Type 2 diabetes mellitus in Japanese men: the Osaka Health Survey. *Diabet Med* 17: 53–8.

Orchard TJ, Temprosa M, Goldberg R, et al. 2005. The effect of metformin and intensive lifestyle intervention on the metabolic syndrome: the Diabetes Prevention Program randomized trial. *Ann Intern Med* 142: 611–9.

Paffenbarger RS, Jr., Blair SN, Lee IM, Hyde RT. 1993. Measurement of physical activity to assess health effects in free-living populations. *Med Sci Sports Exerc* 25: 60–70.

Pan X, Li G, Hu Y, et al. 1997. Effects of diet and exercise in preventing NIDDM in people with impaired glucose tolerance. The Da Qing IGT and Diabetes Study. *Diabetes Care* 20: 537–44.

Pate RR, Pratt M, Blair SN, et al. 1995. Physical activity and public health. A recommendation from the Centers for Disease Control and Prevention and the American College of Sports Medicine. *JAMA* 273: 402–7.

Perry IJ, Wannamethee SG, Walker MK, Thomson AG, Whincup PH, Shaper AG. 1995. Prospective study of risk factors for development of non-insulin dependent diabetes in middle aged British men. *BMJ* 310: 560–4.

Pittas AG, Joseph NA, Greenberg AS. 2004. Adipocytokines and insulin resistance. *J Clin Endocrinol Metab* 89: 447–52.

Qiao Q, Hu G, Tuomilehto J, et al. 2003. Age- and sex-specific prevalence of diabetes and impaired glucose regulation in 11 Asian cohorts. *Diabetes Care* 26: 1770–80.

Saltiel AR, Kahn CR. 2001. Insulin signalling and the regulation of glucose and lipid metabolism. *Nature* 414: 799–806.

Sato Y, Iguchi A, Sakamoto N. 1984. Biochemical determination of training effects using insulin clamp technique. *Horm Metab Res* 16: 483–6.

Sawada SS, Lee IM, Muto T, Matuszaki K, Blair SN. 2003. Cardiorespiratory fitness and the incidence of type 2 diabetes: prospective study of Japanese men. *Diabetes Care* 26: 2918–22.

Schranz A, Tuomilehto J, Marti B, Jarrett RJ, Grabauskas V, Vassallo A. 1991. Low physical activity and worsening of glucose tolerance: results from a 2-year follow-up of a population sample in Malta. *Diabetes Res Clin Pract* 11: 127–36.

Spranger J, Kroke A, Mohlig M, et al. 2003. Inflammatory cytokines and the risk to develop type 2 diabetes: results of the prospective population-based European Prospective Investigation into Cancer and Nutrition (EPIC)-Potsdam Study. *Diabetes* 52: 812–7.

Temelkova-Kurktschiev T, Siegert G, Bergmann S, et al. 2002. Subclinical inflammation is strongly related to insulin resistance but not to impaired insulin secretion in a high risk population for diabetes. *Metabolism* 51: 743–9.

The Diabetes Prevention Program Research Group. 2002. The Diabetes Prevention Program (DPP): description of lifestyle intervention. *Diabetes Care* 25: 2165–71.

The Diabetes Prevention Program Research Group. 2005. Impact of Intensive Lifestyle and Metformin Therapy on Cardiovascular Disease Risk Factors in the Diabetes Prevention Program. *Diabetes Care* 28: 888–94.

Tuomilehto J, Lindstrom J, Eriksson JG, et al. 2001. Prevention of type 2 diabetes mellitus by changes in lifestyle among subjects with impaired glucose tolerance. *N Engl J Med* 344: 1343–50.

Wannamethee SG, Shaper AG. 2001. Physical activity in the prevention of cardiovascular disease: an epidemiological perspective. *Sports Med* 31: 101–14.

Wannamethee SG, Shaper AG, Alberti KG. 2000. Physical activity, metabolic factors, and the incidence of coronary heart disease and type 2 diabetes. *Arch Intern Med* 160: 2108–16.

Wei M, Gibbons LW, Mitchell TL, Kampert JB, Lee CD, Blair SN. 1999. The association between cardiorespiratory fitness and impaired fasting glucose and type 2 diabetes mellitus in men. *Ann Intern Med* 130: 89–96.

Weinstein AR, Sesso HD, Lee IM, et al. 2004. Relationship of physical activity vs body mass index with type 2 diabetes in women. *JAMA* 292: 1188–94.

Wild S, Roglic G, Green A, Sicree R, King H. 2004. Global prevalence of diabetes: estimates for the year 2000 and projections for 2030. *Diabetes Care* 27: 1047–53.

Willerson JT, Ridker PM. 2004. Inflammation as a cardiovascular risk factor. *Circulation* 109: II2–10

Willett WC, Dietz WH, Colditz GA. 1999. Guidelines for healthy weight. *N Engl J Med* 341: 427–34.

Wing RR, Goldstein MG, Acton KJ, et al. 2001. Behavioral science research in diabetes: lifestyle changes related to obesity, eating behavior, and physical activity. *Diabetes Care* 24: 117–23.

World Health Organisation. 2004. Global strategy on diet, physical activity, and health. *Rep. WHA27.17, Agenda Item 12.6*, Geneva.

12

Physical Activity and Weight Control

John M. Jakicic, Amy D.Otto,
Kristen Polzien, and
Kelliann Davis

Ogden et al. (Ogden et al., 2006) recently reported that the prevalence of overweight and obesity continues to increase in the United States. Based on estimates from 2003 to 2004 (Figure 12.1), more than 66% of adults are classified as overweight (body mass index [BMI] ≥ 25.0 kg/m^2), 32% as obese (BMI ≥ 30.0 kg/m^2), and 5% as extremely obese (BMI ≥ 40.0 kg/m^2). These figures reflect a continuous trend toward an increasing prevalence of excess body weight over the past three decades. This trend is concerning because of the established link between excess body weight and increased risks of several chronic diseases, such as type 2 diabetes (McTigue et al., 2006; Weinstein et al., 2004) as well as cardiovascular disease and several types of cancer (National Institutes of Health, 1998).

The issue that is central to weight control is energy balance. Theoretically, when energy intake and expenditure equal each other, body weight is maintained. For weight loss to occur, an energy deficit must occur, with expenditure exceeding intake. The interest in physical activity as a lifestyle strategy to combat the increasing prevalence of overweight and obesity stems from the fact that physical activity is a means to increase energy expenditure and that the levels of physical activity in the United States and many other parts of the world are low (Bull et al., 2004). As highlighted by Ravussin and Bogardus (1989), physical activity is the most variable component of total daily energy expenditure. Therefore, it is important to understand the contribution of physical activity toward weight control.

Although overweight and obesity are also important health concerns in children (Ogden et al., 2006), we limit our discussion in this chapter to adults because the focus of this book is primarily on the adult population. There have been numerous studies investigating the importance of physical activity for weight control in adults. These studies have focused on the role of physical activity in initial weight loss among overweight and obese adults, the maintenance of successful weight loss (i.e., the prevention of weight regain after initial weight loss), and the prevention of weight gain. Of particular interest for public health is the necessary dose of physical activity that will result in optimal weight control. Because the dose(s) of physical activity that appear(s) necessary for these three areas of weight control—initial weight loss, long-term maintenance of the initial weight loss, and prevention of weight gain over time—appear to be different, the role of physical activity in each of these areas of weight control is discussed separately.

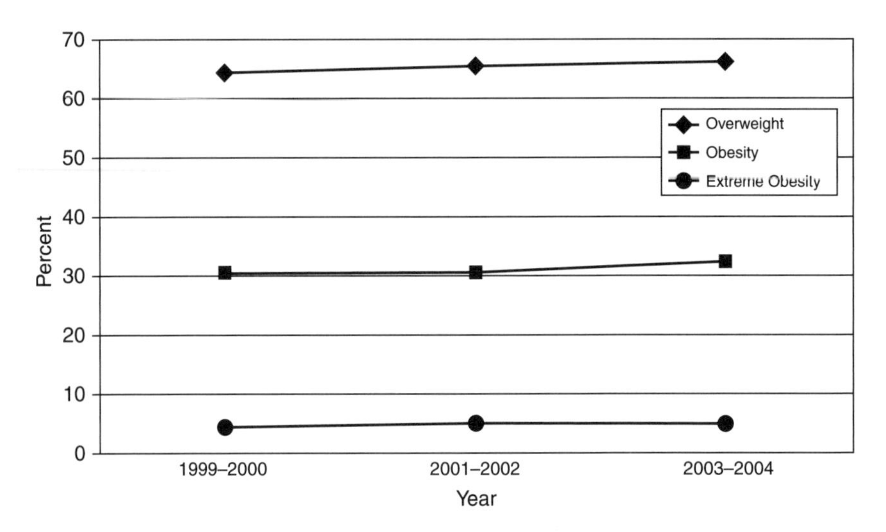

Figure 12.1 Prevalence of overweight, obesity, and extreme obesity in U.S. Adults, 1999–2004. (Based on data from Ogden et al., 2006.)

The Role of Physical Activity in Initial Weight Loss

Physical activity is commonly recommended as part of a comprehensive behavioral weight loss program. However, current evidence from a large number of studies suggests that physical activity has had only a modest impact on the magnitude of weight loss observed in overweight and obese adults over an initial 6-month intervention period, as reflected in the clinical guidelines for weight control published by the U.S. National Institutes of Health (National Institutes of Health, 1998). This report, based primarily on data from randomized clinical trials lasting at least 4 months, concluded that most of the initial weight loss observed in lifestyle intervention studies was achieved through reductions in energy intake, with physical activity having only a modest effect. On average, efforts to achieve weight loss by means of physical activity alone resulted in a 2% to 3% decrease in body weight or BMI. The addition of physical activity to a diet intervention results in only a small amount of additional weight loss, as shown in a recent meta-analysis of 43 randomized, controlled trials including 3,476 overweight or obese adults, which examined the effect of exercise on weight loss (Shaw et al., 2006). In an analysis specifically comparing exercise and diet interventions to diet only interventions (14 trials; 1,049 subjects), an additional 1.1-kg (95% confidence interval [CI], 0.6–1.5) weight loss was found with the combined intervention.

For example, in a study of 154 overweight and obese adults (79% women; mean age: 45.7 years; mean weight; 98.6 kg) at risk for the onset of type 2 diabetes, Wing et al. (1998) randomly assigned subjects to a control group and three lifestyle intervention groups targeting diet alone (goal: 800–1,000 kcal/day with 20% of calories as fat, adjusted to 1,200–1,500 kcal/day over time), exercise alone (goal: 1,500 kcal/week of moderate-intensity activity), and the combination of diet and exercise. At 6 months, weight losses of 1.5 kg, 9.1 kg, 2.1 kg, and 10.3 kg were observed in the control, diet alone, exercise alone, and diet and exercise groups, respectively ($p < 0.001$ among groups). However, these weight losses were not sustained over the long term: By the end of 2 years, changes of –0.3 kg, –2.1 kg, 1.0 kg, and –2.5 kg, respectively, were observed, with no significant differences among groups.

In another study of 131 sedentary, overweight men (ages 30–59 years; mean weight: 94.2 kg), Wood et al. (1988) randomly assigned subjects to a control, diet alone, and exercise alone group. Subjects in the diet group were provided individual diet prescriptions designed to reduce baseline body fat by one-third over a 9-month period, whereas those in the exercise group were provided with individual exercise prescriptions also designed to reduce baseline body fat by one-third over a 9-month period (on average, 18.9 km/week of jogging). Weight loss in the exercise group was 3.0 and 4.0 kg at 7 and 12 months, respectively, which was significantly less than the 7.6 kg and 7.2 kg weight loss observed in the diet group (controls gained 0.2 and 0.6 kg, respectively). In a 12-week study of 96 overweight adults (50% female; mean age: 36.6 years), Hagan et al. (1986) randomly assigned subjects to a control, diet alone (1,200 kcal/day), exercise alone (30 minutes/day of walking/running for 5 days/week), or diet and exercise group. Weight losses of 8.4% and 5.5% for men and women, respectively, were observed in the diet alone intervention; weight losses of 0.3% and 0.6%, respectively, were observed in the exercise alone intervention group; and weight losses of 11.4% and 7.5%, respectively, were observed in the combined diet plus exercise intervention group.

An important consideration is the fact that energy deficits that can be induced through physical activity alone—at least, in amounts tolerable for most individuals—are relatively small, compared to deficits that can be attained through dietary restriction alone. For example, for a 100-kg person, 30 minutes of walking a day at 3 miles/hour, 5 days/week (which is the current recommendation for health; Pate et al., 1995) will result in an approximate energy deficit of 875 kcal/week (assuming diet does not change). In weight loss studies involving dietary modifications, energy deficits of 500 to 700 kcal/day may be asked for (Jakicic et al., 2003), resulting in a far larger magnitude of energy deficit.

When an equivalent energy deficit is induced, whether by means of diet alone or physical activity alone, comparable weight losses appear possible. In a 12-week study of 57 obese, middle-age men, Ross et al. (2000) randomly assigned subjects to four groups: control, diet-induced weight loss, exercise-induced weight loss, and exercise without weight loss. The diet-induced weight loss group was asked to reduce their caloric intake by 700 kcal/day, the exercise-induced weight loss group was required to expend 700 kcal/day in physical activity, and the exercise without weight loss group also had to expend 700 kcal/day in physical activity, as well as maintain their weight, which resulted in an increased intake of approximately 700 kcal/day. All exercise sessions were supervised, with an average compliance of 98%. The exercise was substantial: an average of 63.3 and 60.4 minutes/day of brisk walking/light jogging every day in the exercise-induced weight loss and exercise without weight loss groups, respectively.

After 12 weeks, body weight decreased by comparable amounts, 7.4 to 7.6 kg (8%), in both weight loss groups (Figure 12.2) and did not change in the control and exercise without weight loss groups. Interestingly, total body fat lost was 1.3 kg more in the exercise-induced weight loss group than the diet-induced weight loss group. In the exercise without weight loss group, although weight was maintained, abdominal and visceral fat was significantly decreased. Although this study indicates that comparable weight losses can occur with equivalent energy deficits, whether achieved through diet alone or exercise alone, individuals may be unwilling to agree to substantial amounts of exercise. It is worth noting that of the 101 men randomized into the study, 34 refused participation because of dissatisfaction with their assigned intervention groups.

Therefore, the available data indicate that physical activity alone, at least in amounts palatable for most individuals, has only a modest impact on short-term weight loss in overweight and obese adults and that its effect on weight loss is much smaller than that seen with dietary interventions. A typical exercise intervention might have 1,500 kcal/week of physical activity as its goal; this can be achieved by 30 to 45 minutes/day of moderate-to-vigorous physical activity, 3 to 5 days/week (Klein et al., 2004). Although this modest, feasible amount of physical activity might only result in a 2% to 3% loss of body weight,

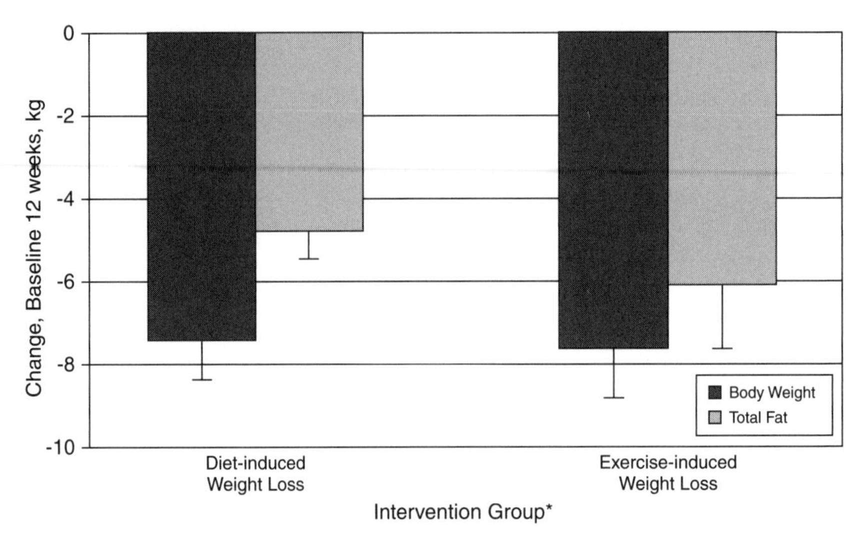

Figure 12.2 Comparable body weight losses achieved by diet or exercise, with comparable energy deficits. (Based on data from Ross et al., 2000.)

physical activity should still be considered an important component of any weight loss program because there is strong evidence that such an increase in physical activity can increase cardiorespiratory fitness, regardless of whether weight loss occurs, and improved cardiovascular fitness enhances the quality of life in overweight patients by improving mood, self-esteem, and physical function in daily activities (National Institutes of Health, 1998). Additionally, although the amount of weight loss may be modest, other health benefits are observed with physical activity. In the meta-analysis referred to earlier (Shaw et al., 2006), compared to the control group, participants in exercise only interventions experienced significant improvements in diastolic blood pressure, serum triglyceride, and fasting serum glucose.

The Role of Physical Activity in the Maintenance of Weight Loss

The maintenance of weight loss, or the prevention of weight regain, is defined as maintaining a weight that is within 2.3 kg (5 lb) of one's current weight after weight loss (St Jeor et al., 1997). Recent estimates have indicated that behavioral interventions that include a combination of energy restriction through diet and increased energy expenditure through physical activity result in a weight loss of approximately 10% of initial body weight within a 6-month period (Wing, 2002). This amount of weight loss is important clinically because it has been demonstrated that a 5% to 10% weight loss is sufficient to improve risk factors for chronic diseases and that a 10% weight loss or greater is associated with improvements in the risk factors being sustained over the long term, reducing the risk of numerous chronic disease conditions (Jakicic et al., 2001; National Institutes of Health, 1998). For example, in the Diabetes Prevention Program (DPP), participants in the lifestyle intervention arm, which had as its goal a 7% weight loss through a combination of healthy diet and increased physical activity, experienced a 58% reduction in the onset of type 2 diabetes over an average of 2.8 years compared to the placebo group (Diabetes Prevention Program Research Group, 2002). In the study by Wing et al. (1998) described earlier, a weight loss of 4.5 kg, whether achieved by diet, exercise, or a combination of both strategies, reduced the onset of type 2 diabetes over 2 years by approximately 30%. Despite the clear importance of weight loss for reducing the risks of various chronic diseases, maintenance of weight loss has been challenging; following an initial weight loss, approximately 33% to 50% of this initial weight loss is regained in the ensuing 12 to 18 months (Wing, 2002).

Although there is a large body of data from randomized clinical trials on the role of physical activity in initial weight loss among overweight and obese adults, most of the data on the role of physical activity in the long-term maintenance of this initial weight loss comes from observational epidemiologic studies, including observational follow-up of participants from randomized, controlled trials (Fogelholm and Kukkonen-Harjula, 2000; Saris et al., 2003). The National Weight Control Registry (NWCR) is a registry of adults who report having lost at least 13.6 kg (30 lb) and maintaining this weight loss for at least 1 year (Klem et al., 1997). In this registry, subjects report on their physical activity and dietary habits over time, thus providing data on the behaviors of individuals who have successfully lost and maintained a large weight loss. Of interest is the pattern of physical activity in this cohort. Using data on self-reported physical activity of 629 women and 155 men in the NWCR, Klem et al. (1997) calculated that subjects expended approximately 2,800 kcal/week in leisure-time physical activity (equivalent to brisk walking for some 5–6 hours/week) to maintain their body weight (Table 12.1). McGuire et al. (1999) further highlighted the importance of physical activity for weight loss maintenance, observing that individuals in the NWCR who regained weight after 1 year in the registry reported greater decreases in energy expenditure compared to individuals in the registry who continued to maintain their large weight loss.

Other studies also have supported the importance of physical activity for maintenance of weight loss. For example, Kayman et al. (1990) interviewed 44 obese women who successfully lost weight but subsequently regained weight ("relapsers"), 30 formerly obese women who maintained weight loss ("maintainers"), and 34 non-obese women who had always remained at the same average weight ("controls"). Ninety percent of maintainers and 82% of controls exercised regularly in contrast to 34% of relapsers. In another study, Leser et al. (2002) followed 27 of 38 women who lost weight with a very-low-calorie diet intervention. At the end of the intervention, subjects lost 20.7 kg (standard deviation [SD]: 9.2), and 3 years after the intervention, they had gained back 13.9 kg (SD: 11.3).

Table 12.1 Physical Activity Patterns* of Men and Women in the National Weight Control Registry+

Energy Expended (kcal/week)	*Men (n = 155)*	*Women (n = 629)*	*Both Sexes (n = 784)*
Walking	201 (192)	185 (196)	188 (195)
Climbing stairs	1237 (2659)	1,054 (1459)	1089 (1750)
Light activities	169 (685)	233 (738)	220 (728)
Moderate activities	635 (1240)	499 (969)	525 (1028)
Vigorous activities	1235 (1845)	688 (1403)	794 (1515)
Total	3476 (3552)	2659 (2533)	2817 (2781)

*Self-reported walking, climbing stairs, and leisure-time activities; mean (standard deviation).

+To enroll in the registry, a minimum weight loss of 13.6 kg (30 lbs), maintained over >1 year, is required.

(Based on data from Klem et al., 1997.)

Self-reported physical activity was inversely correlated ($r = -0.53$; $p = 0.005$) with weight change at the 3-year follow-up. Physical activity also has been shown to predict maintenance of weight loss following an intervention involving pharmacotherapy. In the Sibutramine Trial on Obesity Reduction and Maintenance (van Baak et al., 2003), 605 obese subjects ages 17 to 65 years were enrolled into a 6-month, open-label, run-in phase where all subjects were treated with 10 mg/day of sibutramine and a 600-kcal/day deficient diet. At the end of the 6 months, subjects who lost more than 5% of their initial weight then were randomized to sibutramine (10–20 mg/day) or placebo in a 3:1 ratio for an 18-month maintenance phase. In an observational analysis of the 261 subjects who completed the study, investigators examined the predictors of weight-loss maintenance using regression models. The factors that were significantly predictive of weight-loss maintenance at 24 months were sibutramine treatment, initial change in weight over 6 months, and leisure-time physical activity, with these variables explaining 20% of the variation in weight maintenance between subjects.

These data, as well as data from other studies, led an international expert panel (Saris et al., 2003) to conclude that given the current environment (i.e., typical diet consumed in developed countries and conditions that promote little physical activity), for many individuals "there is compelling evidence that prevention of weight regain in formerly obese individuals requires 60–90 minutes (a day) of moderate intensity activity or lesser amounts of vigorous intensity activity." The 2005 U.S. Dietary Guidelines for Americans (Department of Health and Human Services, 2005) concurred, stating that to sustain weight loss in adulthood, at least 60 to 90 minutes/day of moderate-intensity physical activity is needed without exceeding caloric intake requirements. Additional discussion on the amount of physical activity required for maintenance of weight loss is provided later in "Physical Activity Recommendations for Weight Control."

The Role of Physical Activity in the Prevention of Weight Gain and Obesity

As stated previously, the long-term maintenance of weight loss among overweight and obese persons is challenging (Wing, 2002). Therefore, although it is important to continue to develop effective strategies to address the major public health problem of overweight and obesity, researchers and practitioners increasingly recognize that an emphasis on preventing weight gain over time (i.e., primary prevention) is equally important, so there is not the need to lose the extra and unnecessary weight gained over time in many adults. Compared to data on the role of physical activity in initial weight loss and in prevention of weight regain, data on the role of physical activity in the prevention of weight gain over time are less clear.

There have been many prospective cohort studies examining the relationship of physical activity on weight gain over time in adults (Fogelholm and Kukkonen-Harjula, 2000; Wareham et al., 2005). Many of these studies have assessed physical activity and weight at two or more time-points: baseline and at least one follow-up. The findings on the association of baseline physical activity and weight gain over time are inconsistent. However, the association of physical activity at follow-up, or of change in physical activity between baseline and follow-up, with weight gain at follow-up is more consistent. These data indicate that higher levels of physical activity at follow-up or increases in physical activity between baseline and follow-up are associated with less weight gain. Thus, the interpretation of these data are not clear—the data can either be interpreted as showing that ongoing physical activity is necessary to prevent weight gain or, alternately, that weight gain over time makes individuals less likely to be physically active. Additionally, because the physical activity data from these studies are primarily self-reported, the imprecision associated with the self-reports, in addition to changes in physical activity over time, may also have contributed to the lack of associations observed for baseline physical activity.

For example, in the Health and Retirement Survey (He and Baker, 2004), the average level of self-reported physical activity in 1992 and 1994 was not associated with change in self-reported weight between 1992 and 1996 among 7,391 nationally representative adults ages 51 to 61 years. In this cohort, the mean BMI increased over time in both men and women as well as in all ethnic groups. The Pound of Prevention (POP) Study (Sherwood et al., 2000) was a 3-year randomized trial evaluating the efficacy of mail-based education programs in reducing weight gain with age in a community sample of 826 women and 218 men ages 20 to 45 years. Self-reported physical activity and measured weight were assessed at baseline and annually. As in the national sample from the Health and Retirement Survey, men and women in the POP Study gained weight over time (on average, 1.69 and 1.76 kg, respectively, over 3 years). In observational analyses examining the relationship between physical activity and weight change, the average physical activity level over 3 years was not predictive of weight change in men, although it was in women. However, in both sexes, there was a significant inverse association between change in physical activity and change in weight (i.e., increases in physical activity were associated with less weight gain).

Several prospective cohort studies have assessed sedentary behavior (as opposed to physical activity); their findings have shown positive associations between measures of sedentary behavior and weight change over time (Foster et al., 2006). Sedentary activities reduce the opportunities for physical activity, potentially resulting in an overall reduction in energy expenditure and contributing to weight gain. In the Australian Longitudinal Study on Women's Health, Ball et al. (2002) followed a cohort of 8,726 young women, ages 18 to 23 years, for a period of 4 years to examine predictors of weight maintenance. Weight was reported at baseline and year four, and time spent sitting was reported at year four. Forty-one percent of these young women gained weight (>5% gain from initial body weight) over the 4 years, 44% maintained weight (within 5% of initial weight), and 15% lost weight (>5% loss from initial body weight). With more time spent sitting, the likelihood of weight maintenance decreased. Compared to those sitting less than 33 hours/week, the odds ratios for weight maintenance vs. weight gain were 0.83 (95% CI, 0.73–0.95) and 0.80 (95% CI, 0.70–0.91), respectively, in women who sat for 33 to less than 52 and 52 or more hours/week. In the Nurses' Health Study, Hu et al. (2003) also reported that sedentary behavior was significantly associated with the risk of becoming obese. Among 50,277 women ages 46 to 71 years with BMI less than 30 kg/m^2 in 1992, the average time per week spent watching TV/VCR was reported at baseline. In this analysis, women were followed for 6 years, reporting their follow-up weight on bi-annual questionnaires. For each 2-hour/day increase in time spent watching TV, there was a 23% (95% CI, 17%–30%) increase in the risk of becoming obese. This was contrasted to a 24% (95% CI, 19%–29%) decrease in risk for each 1-hour/day increase in brisk walking.

In addition to studies utilizing self-reported physical activity, which can be imprecise, studies using more objective measures have yielded results that concur with the findings from studies using self-reported data. In the Aerobics Center Longitudinal Study (DiPietro et al., 1998), an analysis of 4,599 men and 724 women (mean age: 43 years) showed significant inverse associations between change in cardiorespiratory fitness, an objective marker of current physical activity, and weight change over an average follow-up of 7.5 years. Cardiorespiratory fitness was measured using maximal exercise testing on the treadmill, and weight also was measured in subjects. For every 1-minute improvement in treadmill time, the odds ratio for a weight gain of 5 kg or greater was 0.86 (95% CI, 0.83–0.89) in men and 0.91 (95% CI, 0.83–1.00) in women. For a weight gain of 10 kg or greater, the corresponding results were 0.79 (95% CI, 0.75–0.84) and 0.79 (95% CI, 0.67–0.93), respectively. In a separate analysis of 2,501 healthy men ages 20 to 55 years with at least four medical examinations where cardiorespiratory fitness and body weight were measured and leisure-time physical activity reported (Di Pietro et al., 2004), investigators estimated the amount of physical activity needed to prevent weight gain over an average of 5 years. Physical activity was estimated as physical activity level (PAL) units, which are multiples of resting metabolic rate averaged over 24 hours. Among men maintaining the same PAL, small curvilinear slopes of weight gain over time were observed. Men who decreased their PAL over time also gained weight. In contrast, a change from low (<1.45 METs per 24 hours) to moderate (1.45–1.60 METs per 24 hours) or high (>1.60 METs per 24 hours) PAL was associated with small weight losses over time. A shift from low to moderate PAL or moderate to high PAL may be achieved by some 45 to 60 minutes/day of moderate-intensity physical activity.

In a study that utilized doubly labeled water (an accurate method for assessment of energy intake and expenditure), indirect calorimetry (to estimate resting metabolic rate), and measured body weight, findings were consistent with those from the Health and Retirement Survey (He and Baker, 2004) described earlier, where self-reported data on physical activity and body weight were collected. Tataranni et al. (2003) studied 64 male and 28 female, non-diabetic Pima Indians with average age 35 years and 35% body fat. After an average of 4 years, follow-up weight measures were available in 74 subjects. Baseline total energy intake was positively and significantly associated with weight change, whereas the association was inverse and also significant for resting metabolic rate. However, as in the Health and Retirement Survey, baseline energy expenditure was unrelated to weight change over the follow-up interval.

Data from randomized, controlled studies of exercise interventions have also provided some information on physical activity and weight change in adults over a short time frame (typically, weeks to months, as contrasted with years of follow-up in the observational studies). If subjects in an exercise intervention arm lose a modest amount of weight over the trial, while controls gain a modest amount of weight, then the net effect of the intervention would be not only the weight loss but also the prevention of weight that would have been gained. For example, in the Studies of Targeted Risk Reduction Interventions through Defined Exercise, Slentz et al. (2004) reported the findings of a randomized controlled trial of 182 sedentary men and women, ages 40 to 65 years, with BMI 25 to 35 kg/m^2, and mild-to-moderate dyslipidemia. Subjects were randomly assigned to a control arm; low-amount, moderate-intensity exercise (equivalent to about 12 miles/week of walking, with subjects allowed to exercise on treadmills, cycle ergometers, and elliptical trainers); low-amount, high-intensity exercise (equivalent to about 12 miles/week of jogging); or high-amount, high-intensity exercise (equivalent to about 20 miles/week of jogging). There was an initial ramp-up period of 2 to 3 months, and the exercise interventions were conducted for 6 months. All exercise sessions were supervised, and 120 subjects completed the study. There was a dose–response relationship between the total amount of exercise carried out and the amount of weight lost, with weight changes of 1.1, –1.3, –1.1, and –3.5 kg in the four arms, respectively. Thus, compared to the control group, which gained a small amount of weight, the net weight changes were –2.4, –2.2, and –4.3 kg in the three exercise-intervention groups, respectively. Diet (as measured by a 3-day food record and a 24-hour dietary recall at baseline and at the end of intervention) was not significantly changed. The investigators concluded that absent of diet changes, weight gain over time can be reversed by a modest amount of exercise equivalent to some 30 minutes/day of walking (i.e., about 12 miles/week) and that greater amounts of weight can be lost with higher doses of exercise.

The data described earlier, although by no means conclusive, suggest that physical activity can play a role in the prevention of weight gain over time in adults. With the majority of the data on long-term (i.e., years) prevention of weight gain available from prospective cohort studies, the lack of certainty comes from many of these studies showing that baseline physical activity levels were inconsistently associated with weight change over time, although follow-up levels were more consistently associated in an inverse fashion (Fogelholm and Kukkonen-Harjula, 2000; Wareham et al., 2005). The available data also are unclear regarding the amount of exercise that might be needed, with many studies collecting information on physical activity that is difficult to translate to practice; for example, in the CARDIA study (Schmitz et al., 2000), physical activity was ascertained as frequency of participation in a list of different activities over the past 12 months, but no data were collected on duration. Based on the limited evidence available, the International Association for the Study of Obesity (Saris et al., 2003) and the 2005 U.S. Dietary Guidelines for Americans (Department of Health and Human Services, 2005) suggest that some 45 to 60 minutes/day of moderate-intensity physical activity appears needed to prevent weight gain.

Methodologic Considerations

Randomized, clinical trials are considered the "gold standard" of research study designs because such studies, when well-designed and -conducted, produce data that are least susceptible to bias and confounding. However, when investigating the role of physical activity in weight control, this study design may not always be the most appropriate choice. Compliance and cost considerations may make it impossible to conduct such studies, particularly if the study duration is long. Thus, although there have been many randomized, clinical trials investigating physical activity and initial weight loss in overweight or obese adults—with such studies typically lasting weeks to months—this study design is less feasible when investigating physical activity and weight maintenance after initial weight loss or prevention of weight gain over the long term, with few such studies existing. An ambitious long-term trial that incorporates physical activity for weight control, the Look AHEAD (Action for Health in Diabetes) study (Wadden et al., 2006) is currently ongoing. This is a multicenter, randomized, controlled trial designed to investigate whether intentional weight loss reduces cardiovascular morbidity and mortality in overweight persons with type 2 diabetes. The study began in 2001 and is planned to conclude in 2012. A total of 5,145 participants were randomly assigned to lifestyle intervention, targeting diet and physical activity (≥175 minutes/week of moderate-intensity activity) with a goal of 7% loss of initial weight or more, or enhanced usual care involving diabetes support and education.

A crucial concern for the validity of results from randomized, controlled trials is compliance, which needs to be good for valid findings to be obtained. Although this may seem a technicality, there is a fine distinction between the assessment of compliance in behavioral intervention trials and in exercise intervention trials. In the former type of trial, the direct target of intervention is behavioral intervention. As an illustration, in the study by Jakicic et al. (2003), all subjects were enrolled in a standard behavioral weight loss intervention based on social cognitive theory, with subjects scheduled to attend behavioral group meetings and receiving scheduled telephone calls. Participants, who all received the same behavioral weight loss intervention, also were randomly assigned to one of four different exercise groups. Thus, the appropriate measure of compliance in this study is the proportion of sessions attended and telephone calls received (these were 71.4% and 75.1%, respectively, over the 12-month trial). The assumption made is that an effective behavioral intervention will translate to increased levels of physical activity. In contrast, exercise intervention trials are designed to directly intervene on the physical activity behavior of subjects, with exercise sessions frequently being directly observed. Compliance in these studies is measured as the proportion of targeted physical activity achieved. For example, the study by Ross et al. (2000) described earlier was an exercise intervention trial with four arms: control, diet-induced weight loss, exercise-induced weight loss, and exercise without weight loss. In both arms involving exercise, all exercise sessions were supervised, with an average compliance of 98% attendance at exercise sessions over the 12-week trial.

Maintaining good compliance for physical activity can be difficult, and less than ideal compliance likely explains the results in studies where physical activity did not produce the expected weight loss. In a study by Byrne et al. (Byrne et al., 2006), subjects achieved an average of two-thirds of the exercise energy expenditure prescribed in a 32-week trial and approximately three-quarters of the target weight loss. Investigators calculated that had subjects achieved the prescribed energy expenditure, the targeted weight loss would have been reached. Where compliance is excellent, the weight loss achieved should equal the calculated caloric deficit. In the study by Ross et al. (2000) described earlier with 98% compliance at exercise sessions, the exercise-induced weight loss group was asked to exercise to expend 700 kcal/day. Over the 12-week trial, this should have resulted in a 58,800 kcal ($700 \times 7 \times 12$) deficit, and a theoretical calculation stated that a 7.6-kg weight loss (3,500 kcal energy deficit = 0.45 kg [1 1b]) should have been attained. The observed weight loss for this arm in the trial was 7.6 kg (Figure 12.2), equal to the calculated amount, attesting to the excellent compliance.

Compliance appears to be better when the physical activity prescribed is of moderate, rather than vigorous, intensity. In a 6-month exercise intervention study by Duncan et al. (2005), subjects were randomly assigned to a control group or one of four walking groups: moderate-intensity and low frequency (3–4 days/week), moderate-intensity and high frequency (5–7 days/week), vigorous-intensity and low frequency, or vigorous-intensity and high frequency. The moderate-intensity prescriptions resulted in better compliance (65.8%) compared to vigorous-intensity prescriptions (57.8%; $p < 0.03$); however, there was little difference in compliance between low and high frequency prescriptions (62.7% and 60.9%, respectively).

Because of the difficulty in maintaining good compliance over a long duration, almost all of the long-term studies on physical activity and weight loss maintenance or prevention of weight gain have been observational epidemiologic studies. General concerns with this study design include confounding, particularly confounding by diet. In addition, the direction of association also can be unclear—in studies of physical activity and prevention of weight gain over time (*see* above in "The Role of Physical Activity in the Prevention of Weight Gain and Obesity" for detailed discussion), baseline physical activity is inconsistently related to weight change at follow-up, whereas physical activity at follow-up is consistently and negatively related to weight change. Thus, it is unclear whether continued physical activity is necessary to prevent weight gain or whether weight gain over time causes individuals to be less active.

In observational studies, as well as behavioral intervention trials, physical activity primarily has been self-reported by subjects (e.g., using questionnaires or activity diaries). This may lead to a bias in observational studies if leaner and heavier individuals report their physical activity differentially. For example, if lean persons accurately report their activity, but heavy persons overreport theirs, the association of physical activity with weight loss will be underestimated. In behavioral intervention trials, although participants are randomized to different arms of the trial, bias may still occur if those successful in losing weight (in any arm) report their activity differently from those who do not lose weight.

Body weight and BMI have commonly been the measures of interest in studies of physical activity and weight control. Although they correlate well with total adiposity in the population, in a particular individual this might not be true (as in the example of an athlete who may have high weight and BMI because of muscle, not fat). The use of weight and BMI, however, is still valid for studies of groups of persons; moreover, these measures are easily understood by the public and easy to measure clinically. In many randomized trials of physical activity and weight loss, besides measuring weight, investigators have also assessed fat distribution because visceral adiposity is strongly related to metabolic risk factors (Fox et al., 2007) and increased risk of coronary heart disease (Li et al., 2006). In some trials where physical activity resulted in only minimal or no weight loss, measures of central adiposity nonetheless were found to improve, supporting the value of physical activity. For example, in the Physical Activity for Total Health Study (Irwin et al., 2003), women in the exercise intervention arm (45 minutes/day of moderate-intensity activity, 5 days/week) lost 1.3 kg and 1.2% total body fat after 12 months compared to baseline. However, the amount of intra-abdominal fat lost was of larger magnitude (5.8%). In the Dose–Response to Exercise in postmenopausal Women Study (Church et al., 2007), women randomly assigned to exercise at 4, 8, or 12 kcal/kg/week (on average, 72, 136, and 192 minutes/week, respectively, of supervised moderate-intensity physical activity was performed) did not lose weight or total body fat after 6 months compared to the control group, yet significant decreases in waist circumference occurred in all exercise groups.

Independent Effect of Physical Fitness or Activity on Health Outcomes

The findings reported earlier indicate that physical activity has a small impact on short-term weight loss but appears to play a more pivotal role in the long-term maintenance of weight loss. However, as discussed earlier, with minimal or even no short-term weight loss, other health benefits, such as decreased visceral adiposity, can occur. Additionally, for clinical endpoints such as cardiovascular disease and premature mortality, physical activity and cardiorespiratory fitness have consistently been shown to reduce the risks of these outcomes, with their effects being independent of body weight. Many of the studies supporting the relationship between higher levels of cardiorespiratory fitness and lower mortality rates, independent of body weight or other measures of adiposity, have come from data collected as part of the Aerobic Center Longitudinal Study (ACLS; Blair et al., 1989). For example, both Barlow et al. (1995) and Farrell et al. (2002) reported that after adjusting for measured BMI, cardiorespiratory fitness was inversely related to all-cause mortality in women. Compared to the least fit 20% of women, the relative risk (RR) of dying during follow-up was 0.49 (95% CI, 0.35–0.69) among those moderately fit (next 40%) and 0.57 (0.40–0.83) among the most fit (top 40%) (Farrell et al., 2002). Similar findings have been noted for men in this study (Lee et al., 1999), with fit men having lower rates of all-cause and cardiovascular mortality, regardless of whether men were lean (<25th percentile body fat based on either hydrostatic weighing or skinfold thickness), normal weight (25th to <75th percentile), or obese (≥75th percentile). Among men with diabetes in the ACLS (Church et al., 2005), higher levels of fitness also were strongly related to lower rates of all-cause mortality among normal weight, overweight, and class I obese men using measured weight and height. These associations are likely to be mediated in part by improvements in metabolic risk factors with higher levels of fitness: In a group of ACLS men undergoing computed tomography or magnetic imaging scans of the abdomen, better fitness was associated with better lipid and blood pressure profiles at any given level of subcutaneous or visceral fat (Lee et al., 2005).

An inherent strength of the ACLS database is the objective measurement of many variables, including cardiorespiratory fitness, body weight, and other measures of adiposity. However, drawing generalizable conclusions based on these data may be limited. For example, there were few participants in the study with extreme levels of obesity; overweight and obese individuals in the study primarily had BMIs in the range of 25 to 29.9 kg/m^2 or 30 to 34.9 kg/m^2 (class I obesity). Therefore, extending the findings to individuals with class II (35–39.9 kg/m^2) or III obesity (≥40 kg/m^2) has yet to be established. Additionally, this study comprises sizeable numbers of individuals who were obese yet possessed high cardiorespiratory fitness; such persons likely do not represent the general population.

Despite these potential limitations, the ACLS findings have been supported by data from other studies with a more representative population, such as the Women's Health Initiative Observational Study (Manson et al., 2002), which also show that higher levels of physical activity, independent of BMI, are associated with lower cardiovascular disease rates. Additionally, several large prospective cohort studies with select populations, such as the Harvard Alumni Health Study (Lee and Paffenbarger, 2000) and the Health Professionals' Follow-up Study (Li et al., 2006) in men, as well as the Nurses' Health Study (Manson et al., 1999) and the Women's Health Study (Lee et al., 2001) in women, all have reported inverse associations between physical activity and risks of cardiovascular disease and all-cause mortality that are independent of BMI.

One specific area in which the different studies do not agree is the following: Data from the ACLS suggest that being unfit is more strongly related to increased risks of all-cause and cardiovascular disease mortality than is being overweight or obese. In an analysis by Lee et al. (1999), compared to lean (<25th percentile body fat) and fit men, lean and unfit men had a multivariate RR for all-cause mortality of 2.07 (1.16–3.69). However, for obese (≥75th percentile) but fit men, this was 0.92 (0.65–1.31), indicating no adverse effect from obesity if men were fit. The corresponding findings for cardiovascular mortality were 3.16 (1.12–8.92) and 1.35 (0.66–2.76), respectively, also indicating no significant adverse effect from obesity, if men were fit. In contrast, data from the Harvard Alumni Health Study (Lee and Paffenbarger, 2000), the Health Professionals' Follow-up Study (Li et al., 2006), the Nurses' Health Study (Hu et al., 2004), Women's Health Initiative Observational Study (Manson et al., 2002), and the Women's Health Study (Lee et al., 2001) all indicate that obesity is an independent risk factor of approximately equal magnitude to physical inactivity and that high levels of physical activity do not totally ameliorate the increased risks associated with obesity as suggested by the ACLS. For example, in the Harvard Alumni Health Study (Fig. 12.3), the RRs of all-cause mortality among inactive, overweight men, inactive but normal weight men, active overweight men, and active men of normal weight

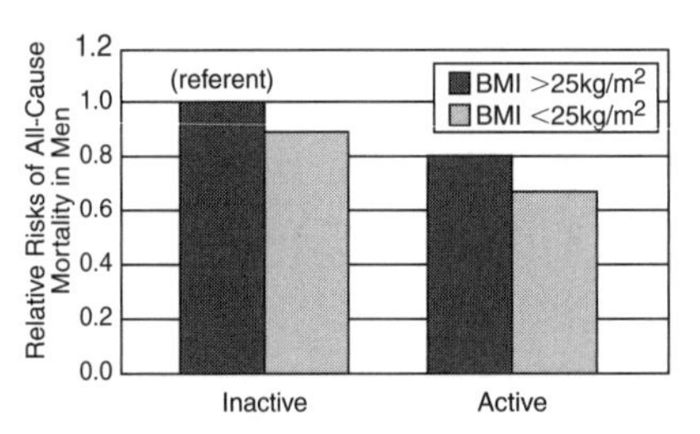

*Adjusted for age, smoking, alcohol, early parental mortality
(Based on data from the Harvard Alumni Health Study, Lee & Paffenbarger, 2000.)

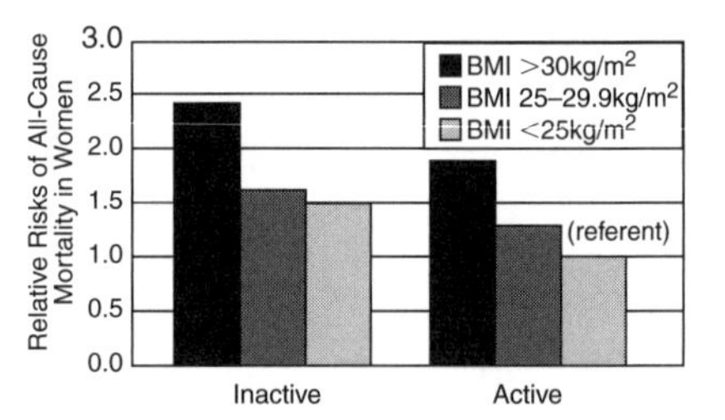

*Adjusted for age, smoking, alcohol, menopausal status/hormone use, parental history of coronary heart disease
(Based on data from the Nurses' Health Study, Hu et al., 2004.)

Figure 12.3 Independent effects of physical activity and body mass index on all-cause mortality.

were 1.00 (referent), 0.90 (0.79–1.02), 0.80 (0.71–0.91), and 0.67 (0.60–0.75), respectively. Similarly, in the Nurses' Health Study (Fig. 12.3), the RRs of all-cause mortality among active (≥3.5 hours/week of activity) normal-weight women, inactive (<1 hour/week) normal-weight women, active obese women, and inactive obese women were 1.00 (referent), 1.91 (1.60–2.30), 1.55 (1.42–1.70), and 2.42 (2.14–2.73), respectively.

A clinical endpoint for which BMI appears to be a stronger risk factor than cardiorespiratory fitness or physical activity is type 2 diabetes. In the ACLS (Wei et al., 1999), cardiorespiratory fitness was strongly and inversely related to the risk of developing this disease among men with BMI less than 27 kg/m^2 and also among men with BMI of 27 kg/m^2 or greater. However, rates of type 2 diabetes were far higher among the heavier men. Similarly, in the Nurses' Health Study as well as in the Women's Health Study, obesity was more strongly related to risk than physical inactivity. In the former study (Hu et al., 1999), the multivariate RR of developing type 2 diabetes among least active women with BMI of 25 kg/m^2 or greater was 1.00 (referent); for most active women with BMI 25 kg/m^2 or greater, the RR was 0.7; but the RRs were only 0.16 among least active women with BMI less than 25 kg/m^2 and 0.08 among most active women with BMI less than 25 kg/m^2. That is, risk for type 2 diabetes varied up to twofold between extreme groups of physical activity but up to more than eightfold between BMI groups of less than 25 and 25 kg/m^2 or greater. In the Women's Health Study (Weinstein et al., 2004), when examining the joint effects of physical activity and obesity on risk, inactivity (<1,000 vs. ≥1,000 kcal/week) was associated with only modest increases in risk (≤15%), whereas obesity (BMI ≥30 vs. <25 kg/m^2) was associated with more than an 11-fold increase in risk.

Gender Differences in the Effect of Physical Activity on Weight Control

There is evidence that men and women respond differently to interventions for weight control. An important factor to consider is whether differences in the effect of physical activity on weight control between men and women are the result of gender *per se* or whether the differences are the consequence of different amounts of energy expended by men and women. French et al. (1994) examined predictors of weight gain in the Healthy Worker Project, where 1,639 male and 1,913 female employees from 32 companies participated in a worksite intervention for smoking cessation and weight control. In observational analyses, the average weight gain over a 2-year period was 0.6 kg in women and 0.4 kg for men. An increase of one high-intensity exercise session per week was associated with 0.6-kg weight loss in women but a 1.6-kg weight loss in men. However, physical activity, dietary behaviors, and weight loss history accounted for only approximately 9% to 10% of the variation in weight loss observed. This suggests that additional behavioral, physiological, and metabolic factors may have contributed to the differences observed between men and women. Additionally, because physical activity was assessed via self-reporting using a 13-question exercise frequency recall, this may not have adequately captured differences in energy expenditure from lifestyle, occupational, or structured periods of leisure-time physical activity.

Gender differences have also been observed in randomized, controlled trials. For example, Wood et al. (1991) randomly assigned 132 men and 132 women, ages 25 to 49 years, to a control group, a diet group, or a diet plus exercise group for 1 year. In the combined diet plus exercise group (energy restricted diet and exercise that progressed to 45 minutes/day, 3 days/week), an average weight loss of 8.7 kg (approximately 9%) occurred in men vs. 5.1 kg (approximately 7%) in women. Some of this gender difference likely resulted from the amount of energy expended: Men in the study averaged 14.7 km of walking or running per week, whereas women averaged 12.5 km per week.

In a more recent exercise intervention study, Donnelly et al. (2003) randomly assigned 131 men and women, ages 17 to 35 years, who were overweight or had class I obesity to a control or exercise group for 16 months (74 completed the study). All exercise was supervised and energy expenditure was measured. The goal was 45 minutes/day of moderate-to-vigorous exercise, for 5 days/week, to expend 400 kcal/day for a total of 2,000 kcal/week. Diet remained unchanged throughout the study. Compared to baseline, men in the exercise group lost 5.2 kg, whereas men in the control group lost 0.5 kg, for a net difference of –4.8 kg. In contrast, exercise in women merely blunted weight gain over time: Women in the exercise group gained 0.6 kg, whereas women in the control group gained 2.9 kg, for a net difference of –2.3 kg. Further examination of this difference suggests that the observed results may have resulted from different energy expenditures in men and women. Donnelly and Smith (2005) calculated that the average energy expenditure for each exercise session was 667 kcal (6.7 kcal/kg of fat-free mass) in men vs. 438 kcal (5.4 kcal/kg fat-free mass) in women.

Additional support for the premise that observed gender differences result from different energy expenditures comes from two exercise intervention studies by Ross et al. One, described under "Methodologic Considerations," had men in one arm of the trial performing supervised exercise designed to expend 700 kcal/day, without changing their diet (Ross et al., 2000). As stated earlier, over the 12-week trial, this should have resulted in a 58,800-kcal ($700 \times 7 \times 12$) deficit, and a theoretical calculation states that a 7.6-kg weight loss (3,500-kcal energy deficit = 0.45 kg [1 1b]) should be attained. The observed weight loss for this arm in the trial was 7.6 kg (Fig. 12.2), equal to the calculated amount. In another exercise intervention study in women, supervised exercise in one arm of the trial was designed to expend 500 kcal/day, again with diet remaining constant (Ross et al., 2004). At the end of the 14-week study, the calculated caloric deficit should have been 49,000 kcal ($500 \times 7 \times 14$), resulting in a theoretical 6.3-kg weight loss. The observed weight loss was 6.2 kg, which was almost identical to what was expected.

To further clarify the issue of gender differences, it is important for future studies to examine if clamping energy expenditure—that is, ensuring that the energy deficit is the same in men and women, although this might result in exercise sessions of longer duration in women—will result in similar changes in body weight in men and women.

Physical Activity Recommendations for Weight Control

It is important for physical activity recommendations to be based on scientific evidence and for these recommendations to target desired health-related outcomes. Therefore, as data have emerged from new research studies, physical activity recommendations have been evolving over the past 10 to 15 years, particularly with regard to the minimum dose of physical activity necessary for sedentary adults (*see* Chapter 15 for detailed discussion). Three landmark publications (Department of Health and Human Services, 2005; Pate et al., 1995; U.S. Department of Health and Human Services, 1996) have consistently confirmed the consensus public health recommendation stating that at least 30 minutes of moderate-intensity physical activity most days of the week will reduce the risk of chronic diseases such as heart disease, certain cancers, and type 2 diabetes. ("Most days of the week" generally has been accepted as 5 days; thus, the recommendation is for a total of 150 minutes/week of activity.) Because data from several studies show that this level of physical activity is associated with decreased risk of chronic diseases and premature mortality, even in overweight and obese persons, initial physical activity goals for overweight and obese adults should be the consensus public health recommendation of 30 minutes/day of moderate-intensity physical activity on most days. However, if the desired goal is to achieve weight loss and further reduce the risk of developing chronic diseases, then 30 minutes/day of physical activity may not be sufficient.

In 2001, the American College of Sports Medicine published a position stand suggesting that 200 to 300 minutes/week of at least moderate-intensity physical activity is required to enhance long-term weight loss (Jakicic et al., 2001). At that time, the recommendation was based on a limited but convincing body of literature in this area. For example, as described earlier, observational data from the NWCR suggest that physical activity equivalent to approximately 2,800 kcal/week (brisk walking for some 5–6 hours/week or lesser amounts of vigorous exercise) contributes to sustaining a large weight loss (at least 13.6 kg or 30 lb). Although a potential limitation of NWCR is that the physical activity data are self-reported, Schoeller et al. (1997) confirmed the need for high levels of physical activity to maintain weight loss in a study that used doubly labeled water (DLW) to accurately measure total energy expenditure. Investigators recruited 32 women, ages 20 to 50 years, with average BMI of 20 to 30 kg/m^2 who had lost 12 kg or more and maintained this weight loss to within 1 kg in the previous 1 to 3 months. Over the next year, women were seen at baseline, 3, 6, 9, and 12 months, where DLW was administered and body weight and fat measured. Investigators analyzed weight change as a function of energy expended in physical activity and observed a threshold for weight maintenance at 47 kJ/kg body weight per day. This was estimated to correspond to 80 minutes/day of moderate-intensity physical activity or 35 minutes/day of vigorous activity, on top of a sedentary lifestyle. Thus, the level of physical activity needed to sustain long-term weight loss is more than twice the consensus public health recommendation for physical activity. To further confirm these findings, evidence from additional studies are required.

In two behavioral intervention trials, Jakicic et al. investigated the role of physical activity in weight loss among overweight and obese women (Jakicic et al., 2003; Jakicic et al., 1999). To provide data on the amount of physical activity needed to maintain weight loss over time, investigators carried out *post hoc* analyses of self-reported physical activity during the trial. Their findings revealed that 250 to 300 minutes/week of moderate- to vigorous-intensity physical activity was required to sustain a weight loss of 10% or greater for a period of 12 to 18 months. Recently, unpublished data from our laboratory have further indicated that a weight loss of 10% or greater can be sustained for as long as 24 months with leisure-time physical activity of 2,000 kcal/week or more (equivalent to 60–90 minutes/day of moderate-intensity activity). Jeffery et al. (2003) have also reported that prescribing physical activity of 2,500 kcal/week or more was associated with less weight re-gain following an 18-month intervention. Although the findings of these last three studies are based on physical activity assessed via self-reporting, their data are consistent with the findings of Schoeller et al. (1997), in which physical activity was assessed objectively using DLW. These higher doses of physical activity—more than 30 minutes/day and up to 90 minutes/day—to control body weight and enhance long-term weight loss maintenance have been endorsed by expert panels writing for the Institute of Medicine (2002), the International Association for the Study of Obesity (IASO; Saris et al., 2003), and the 2005 U.S. Dietary Guidelines for Americans (Department of Health and Human Services, 2005). In particular, both the IASO and the U.S. Dietary Guidelines concluded that at least 60 to 90 minutes/day of moderate-intensity physical activity is needed to sustain weight loss in adulthood and, although data are limited, that some 45 to 60 minutes/day of moderate-intensity physical activity appears needed to prevent weight gain in adults over time.

Daily Steps

Pedometers or step counters are increasingly used to promote physical activity. It has been suggested that the accumulation of at least 10,000 steps/day is necessary to improve health-related outcomes (Tudor-Locke and Bassett, 2004). This appears to be consistent with the consensus public health recommendation for physical activity, which requires the addition of 30 minutes of activity per day on top of the activities required for daily living. The average mobile, sedentary adult will take approximately 3,000 to 5,000 steps/day. Assuming 2,500 steps per 15 to 20 minutes of walking (a brisk pace of walking), this will result in approximately 8,000 to 10,000 steps/day with the addition of 30 minutes of moderate-intensity physical activity. However, as indicated earlier, this may not be sufficient for weight control. Therefore, daily steps in excess of 10,000/day may be required to adequately control body weight. This is supported by findings from Villanova et al. (2006), who reported that long-term weight loss of approximately 12.5 to 15.0 kg was associated with more than 12,000 steps/day.

Exercise Intensity

For the purpose of weight loss, it appears that the total volume of physical activity may be more important than the intensity of physical activity. For example, in a 24-week study, Duncan et al. (1991) reported that when energy expenditure was clamped for walking (i.e., all groups expended the same total amount of energy on walking, but the groups varied in their speed of walking), there was no improvement in weight loss or changes in body composition with increasing intensity (speed) of exercise. More recently, these findings were confirmed by Jakicic et al. (2003) in a 12-month study. Physical activity was prescribed at either 1,000 or 2,000 kcal/day, with intensity at either a moderate or vigorous intensity, with all exercise groups also following an energy-restricted diet (Fig. 12.4). Weight loss improved from approximately 8% to 10% with the higher volume of physical activity. However, for the same energy expenditure, there was no improvement in weight loss at either 6 or 12 months in the moderate-intensity group compared to the vigorous group. These results suggest that energy expenditure, rather than intensity of the activity performed, is important for weight control. These results have implications for prescribing physical activity to overweight adults, because some may be averse to higher intensity physical activity, which may result in poor adherence. This was seen in the exercise intervention study by Duncan et al. (2005) described earlier, where moderate-intensity prescriptions resulted in better compliance (65.8%) compared to vigorous-intensity prescriptions (57.8%).

Resistance Exercise

Studies examining the effect of physical activity on weight control have primarily focused on aerobic forms of physical activity. This may partly result from overweight adults tending to self-select this form of activity when given a preference (Jakicic et al., 2003). However, resistance exercise may provide a useful alternate form of exercise for the overweight or obese sedentary adult. For example, Jakicic (2005) has suggested that resistance exercise may improve physical function in these individuals. In fact, there is clear evidence that resistance exercise can increase muscular strength in overweight adults (Donnelly et al., 2004; Donnelly et al., 1991; Donnelly et al., 1993; Kraemer et al., 1997; Kraemer et al., 1999), and this can lead to improved function. Moreover, resistance exercise can result in favorable changes in body composition (Schmitz et al., 2003). However, although improved

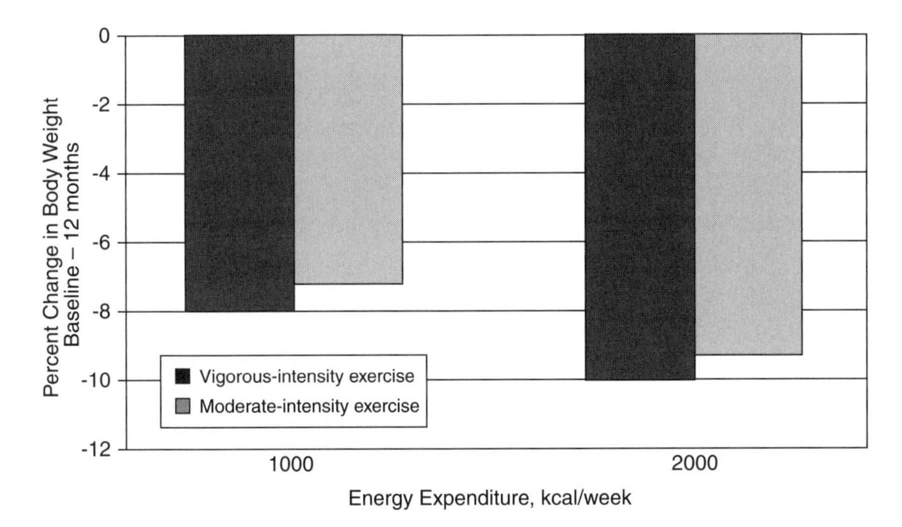

* Women were randomly assigned to these four groups; all were also asked to reduce intake to 1200 – 1500 kcal/day.

(Based on data from Jakicic et al., 2003.)

Figure 12.4 Effect of fixed energy expenditure, at different exercise intensities, on weight loss.*

muscular strength and body composition can occur, an extensive review of the literature suggests that resistance exercise has limited impact on enhancing weight loss based on short-term (weeks to months) studies, with few data available on resistance exercise and long-term (years) weight control (Donnelly et al., 2004). Thus, there is a need for additional research to examine the impact of resistance exercise on weight control, particularly over the long term.

Personal Perspective

Excess body weight is linked to increased risk of numerous chronic diseases, including heart disease, type 2 diabetes, and several forms of cancer. Based on the aforementioned review of the literature, physical activity is an important lifestyle behavior that can result in favorable changes to body weight, body composition, and related health risks. However, to achieve favorable changes in body weight, an adequate dose of physical activity is required. Of interest is the finding that the dose of physical activity required to control body weight in some individuals likely exceeds the dose required to reduce risk for developing chronic diseases. However, there remain gaps in the scientific literature that limit our understanding of the role of physical activity in weight control. Therefore, future research in this area should considering the following:

1. There remains a need to define the dose of exercise required for initial weight loss, maintenance of weight loss, and prevention of weight gain over time. Although several guidelines exist regarding doses for maintenance of weight loss and prevention of weight gain, the expert writing panels do acknowledge that the guidelines are based on limited data. When addressing this research need in the future, it will be

important to include an objective quantification of physical activity dose across studies that is consistent. Currently, the majority of studies continue to use self-reported physical activity in studies of weight control.

2. There is a need to understand "responders" and "non-responders" to physical activity interventions for weight control. Donnelly et al. (2003) report that there is wide variability to changes in body weight in response to supervised exercise. This may be a result of demographic, metabolic, behavioral, or genetic factors, and there is limited research examining the interaction of these parameters in the context of physical activity and weight control.
3. Despite the importance of physical activity for weight control, few studies have specifically developed interventions to address the barriers to physical activity experienced by overweight and obese adults. Thus, future studies need to examine how to better translate data from cross-sectional, observational, or efficacy studies (clinical trials) into effective interventions that will impact weight control.

References

Ball K, Brown W, Crawford D. 2002. Who does not gain weight? Prevalence and predictors of weight maintenance in young women. *Int J Obes* 26: 1570–8.

Barlow CE, H.W. K, Gibbons LW, Blair SN. 1995. Physical activity, mortality, and obesity. *Int J Obes* 19: S41-S4.

Blair SN, Kohl III H, Paffenbarger RS, Clark DG, Cooper KH, Gibbons LW. 1989. Physical fitness and all-cause mortality. A prospective study of healthy men and women. *JAMA* 262: 2395–401.

Bull FC, Armstrong TP, Dixon T, Ham SA, Neiman A, Pratt M. 2004. Physical inactivity. In CJL Murray (Ed.), *Comparative quantification of health risks. Global and regional burden of disease attributable to selected major risk factors*, Geneva, Switzerland: WHO, pp. 729–881.

Byrne NM, Meerkin JD, Laukkanen R, Ross R, Fogelholm M, Hills AP. 2006. Weight loss strategies for obese adults: personalized weight management program vs. standard care. *Obesity (Silver Spring)* 14: 1777–88.

Church TS, Earnest CP, Skinner JS, Blair SN. 2007. Effects of different doses of physical activity on cardiorespiratory fitness among sedentary, overweight or obese postmenopausal women with elevated blood pressure: a randomized controlled trial. *JAMA* 297: 2081–91.

Church TS, LaMonte MJ, Barlow CE, Blair SN. 2005. Cardiorespiratory fitness and body mass index as predictors of cardiovascular disease mortality among men with diabetes. *Arch Intern Med* 165: 2114–20.

Department of Health and Human Services and US Department of Agriculture. 2005. *Dietary Guidelines for Americans:* www.healthierus.gov/dietaryguidelines. Accessed 7 April 2008.

Diabetes Prevention Program Research Group. 2002. Reduction in the incidence of type 2 diabetes with lifestyle intervention or metformin. *N Engl J Med* 346: 393–403.

Di Pietro L, Dziura J, Blair SN. 2004. Estimated change in physical activity level (PAL) and prediction of 5-year weight change in men: the Aerobics Center Longitudinal Study. *Int J Obes Relat Metab Disord* 28: 1541–7.

DiPietro L, Kohl HW, Barlow CE, Blair SN. 1998. Improvements in cardiorespiratory fitness attenuate age-related weight gain in healthy men and women: the Aerobics Center Longitudinal Study. *Int J Obes* 22: 55–62.

Donnelly JE, Hill JO, Jacobsen DJ, et al. 2003. Effects of a 16-month randomized controlled exercise trial on body weight and composition in young, overweight men and women. *Arch Int Med* 163: 1343–50.

Donnelly JE, Jakicic JM, Pronk NP, et al. 2004. Is resistance exercise effective for weight management? *Evidenced Based Preventive Medicine* 1: 21–9.

Donnelly JE, Pronk NP, Jacobsen DJ, Pronk SJ, Jakicic JM. 1991. Effects of a very-low-calorie diet and physical-training regimens on body composition and resting metabolic rate in obese females. *Am J Clin Nutr* 54: 56–61.

Donnelly JE, Sharp T, Houmard J, et al. 1993. Muscle hypertrophy with large-scale weight loss and resistance training. *Am J Clin Nutr* 58: 561–5.

Donnelly JE, Smith BK. 2005. Is exercise effective for weight loss with ad libitum diet? Energy balance, compensation, and gender differences. *Exerc Sport Sci Rev* 33: 169–74.

Duncan GE, Anton SD, Sydeman SJ, et al. 2005. Prescribing exercise at varied levels of intensity and frequency: a randomized trial. *Arch Intern Med* 165: 2362–9.

Duncan JJ, Gordon NF, Scott CB. 1991. Women walking for health and fitness: how much is enough? *JAMA* 266: 3295–9.

Farrell SW, Braun L, Barlow CE, Cheng YJ, Blair SN. 2002. The relation of body mass index, cardiorespiratory fitness, and all-cause mortality in women. *Obes Res* 10: 417–23.

Fogelholm M, Kukkonen-Harjula K. 2000. Does physical activity prevent weight gain—a systematic review. *Obes Rev* 1: 95–111.

Foster JA, Gore SA, West DS. 2006. Altering TV viewing habits: an unexplored strategy for adult obesity intervention? *Am J Health Behav* 30: 3–14.

Fox CS, Massaro JM, Hoffmann U, et al. 2007. Abdominal visceral and subcutaneous adipose tissue compartments: association with metabolic risk factors in the Framingham Heart Study. *Circulation* 116: 39–48.

French SA, Jeffery RW, Forster JL, McGovern PG, Kelder SH, Baxter JE. 1994. Predictors of weight change over two years among a population of working adults: the Healthy Worker Project. *Int J Obes* 18: 145–54.

Hagan RD, Upton SJ, Wong L, Whittam J. 1986. The effects of aerobic conditioning and/or calorie restriction in overweight men and women. *Med Sci Sports Exerc* 18: 87–94.

He XZ, Baker DW. 2004. Changes in weight among a nationally representative cohort of adults aged 51 to 61, 1992 to 2000. *Am J Prev Med* 27: 8–15.

Hu FB, Li TY, Colditz GA, Willett WC, Manson JE. 2003. Television watching and other sedentary behaviors in relation to risk of obesity and type 2 diabetes mellitus in women. *JAMA* 289: 1785–91.

Hu FB, Sigal RJ, Rich-Edwards JW, et al. 1999. Walking compared with vigorous physical activity and risk of type 2 diabetes in women: a prospective study. *JAMA* 282: 1433–9.

Hu FB, Willett WC, Li T, Stampfer MJ, Colditz GA, Manson JE. 2004. Adiposity as compared with physical activity in predicting mortality among women. *N Engl J Med* 351: 2694–703.

Institute of Medicine. 2002. *Dietary Reference Intakes for Energy, Carbohydrates, Fiber, Fat, Protein and Amino Acids (Macronutrients)*. Washington, DC: The National Academies Press.

Irwin ML, Yasui Y, Ulrich CM, et al. 2003. Effect of exercise on total and intra-abdominal body fat in postmenopausal women: A randomized controlled trial. *JAMA* 289: 323–30.

Jakicic JM. 2005. Physical activity considerations for the treatment and prevention of obesity. *Am J Clin Nutr* 82: 226S-9S.

Jakicic JM, Clark K, Coleman E, et al. 2001. American College of Sports Medicine Position Stand: Appropriate Intervention Strategies for Weight Loss and Prevention of Weight Regain for Adults. *Med Sci Sports Exerc* 33: 2145–56.

Jakicic JM, Marcus BH, Gallagher KI, Napolitano M, Lang W. 2003. Effect of exercise duration and intensity on weight loss in overweight, sedentary women. A randomized trial. *JAMA* 290: 1323–30.

Jakicic JM, Winters C, Lang W, Wing RR. 1999. Effects of intermittent exercise and use of home exercise equipment on adherence, weight loss, and fitness in overweight women: a randomized trial. *JAMA* 282: 1554–60.

Jeffery RW, Wing RR, Sherwood NE, Tate DF. 2003. Physical activity and weight loss: Does prescribing higher physical activity goals improve outcome? *Am J Clin Nutr* 78: 684–9.

Kayman S, Bruvold W, Stern JS. 1990. Maintenance and relapse after weight loss in women: behavioral aspects. *Am J Clin Nutr* 52: 800–7.

Klein S, Sheard NF, Pi-Sunyer X, et al. 2004. Weight management through lifestyle modification for the prevention and management of type 2 diabetes: rationale and strategies: a statement of the American Diabetes Association, the North American Association for the Study of Obesity, and the American Society for Clinical Nutrition. *Diabetes Care* 27: 2067–73.

Klem ML, Wing RR, McGuire MT, Seagle HM, Hill JO. 1997. A descriptive study of individuals successful at long-term maintenance of substantial weight loss. *Am J Clin Nutr* 66: 239–46.

Kraemer WJ, Volek JS, Clark KL, et al. 1997. Physiological adaptations to a weight-loss dietary regimen and exercise programs in women. *J Appl Physiol* 83: 270–9.

Kraemer WJ, Volek JS, Clark KL, et al. 1999. Influence of exercise training on physiological and performance changes with weight loss in men. *Med Sci Sports Exer*. 31: 1320–9.

Lee CD, Blair SN, Jackson AS. 1999. Cardiorespiratory fitness, body composition, and all-cause and cardiovascular disease mortality in men. *Am J Clin Nutr* 69: 373–80.

Lee I-M, Paffenbarger R. 2000. Associations of Light, Moderate, and Vigorous Intensity Physical Activity with Longevity: The Harvard Alumni Health Study. *Am J Epidemiol* 151: 293–9.

Lee IM, Rexrode KM, Cook NR, Manson JE, Buring JE. 2001. Physical activity and coronary heart disease in women: is "no pain, no gain" passe? *JAMA* 285: 1447–54.

Lee S, Kuk JI, Katzmarzyk PT, Blair SN, Church TS, Ross R. 2005. Cardiorespiratory fitness attenuates metabolic risk independent of subcutaneous and visceral fat in men. *Diabetes Care* 28: 895–901.

Leser MS, Yanovski SZ, Yanovski JA. 2002. A low-fat intake and greater activity level are associated with lower weight regain 3 years after completing a very-low-calorie diet. *J Am Diet Assoc* 102: 1252–6.

Li TY, Rana JS, Manson JE, et al. 2006. Obesity as compared with physical activity in predicting risk of coronary heart disease in women. *Circulation* 113: 499–506.

Manson JE, Greenland P, LaCroix AZ, et al. 2002. Walking compared with vigorous exercise for the prevention of cardiovascular events in women. *N Engl J Med* 347: 716–25.

Manson JE, Hu FB, Rich-Edwards JW, et al. 1999. A prospective study of walking as compared with vigorous exercise in the prevention of coronary heart disease in women. *N Engl J Med* 341: 650–8.

McGuire MT, Wing RR, Klem ML, Lang W, Hill JO. 1999. What predicts weight regain in a group of successful weight losers? *J Consult Clin Psychol* 67: 177–85.

McTigue K, Larson JC, Valoski A, et al. 2006. Mortality and cardiac and vascular outcomes in extremely obese women. *JAMA* 296: 79–86.

National Institutes of Health. 1998. Clinical Guidelines on the Identification, Evaluation, and Treatment of Overweight and Obesity in Adults—The Evidence Report. *Obes Res* 6(Suppl 2): 51S–210S

Ogden CL, Carroll MD, Curtin LR, McDowell MA, Tabak CJ, Flegal KM. 2006. Prevalence of overweight and obesity in the United States, 1999–2004. *JAMA* 295: 1549–55.

Pate RR, Pratt M, Blair SN, et al. 1995. Physical activity and public health: a recommendation from the Centers for Disease and Prevention and the American College of Sports Medicine. *JAMA* 273: 402–7.

Ravussin E, Bogardus C. 1989. Relationship of genetics, age, and physical fitness to daily energy expenditure and fuel utilization. *Am J Clin Nutr* 49: 968–75.

Ross R, Dagnone D, Jones PJ, et al. 2000. Reduction in obesity and related comorbid conditions after diet-induced weight loss or exercise-induced weight loss in men. A randomized, controlled trial. *Ann Intern Med* 133: 92–103.

Ross R, Janssen I, Dawson J, et al. 2004. Exercise-induced reduction in obesity and insulin resistance in women: a randomized controlled trial. *Obes Res* 12: 789–98.

Saris WHM, Blair SN, van Baak MA, et al. 2003. How much physical activity is enough to prevent unhealthy weight gain? Outcome of the IASO 1st Stock Conference and consensus statement. *Obes Rev* 4: 101–14.

Schmitz KH, Jacobs DR, Jr., Leon AS, Schreiner PJ, Sternfeld B. 2000. Physical activity and body weight: associations over ten years in the CARDIA study. Coronary Artery Risk Development in Young Adults. *Int J Obes Relat Metab Disord* 24: 1475–87.

Schmitz KH, Jensen MD, Kugler KC, Jeffery RW, Leon AS. 2003. Strength training for obesity prevention in midlife women. *Int J Obes* 27: 326–33.

Schoeller DA, Shay K, Kushner RF. 1997. How much physical activity is needed to minimize weight gain in previously obese women. *Am J Clin Nutr* 66: 551–6.

Shaw K, Gennat H, O'Rourke P, Del Mar C. 2006. Exercise for overweight or obesity. *Cochrane Database Syst Rev:* CD003817.

Sherwood NE, Jeffery RW, French SA, Hannan PJ, Murray DM. 2000. Predictors of weight gain in the Pound of Prevention study. *Int J Obes* 24: 395–403.

Slentz CA, Duscha MS, Johnson JL, et al. 2004. Effects of the amount of exercise on body weight, body composition, and measures of central obesity. STRIDDE—a randomized controlled study. *Arch Int Med* 164: 31–9.

St Jeor ST, Brunner RL, Harrington ME, et al. 1997. A classification system to evaluate weight maintainers, gainers, and losers. *J Am Diet Assoc* 97: 481–8.

Tataranni PA, Harper IT, Snitker S, et al. 2003. Body weight gain in free-living Pima Indians: effect of energy intake vs expenditure. *Int J Obes Relat Metab Disord* 27: 1578–83.

Tudor-Locke C, Bassett DR. 2004. How many steps/day are enough? Preliminary pedometer indices for public health. *Sports Med* 34: 1–8.

US Department of Health and Human Services. 1996. *Physical Activity and Health: A Report of the Surgeon General*. Atlanta: GA: US Department of Health and Human Services, Centers for Disease Control and Prevention, National Center for Chronic Disease Prevention and Health Promotion.

van Baak MA, van Mil E, Astrup AV, et al. 2003. Leisure-time activity is an important determinant of long-term weight maintenance after weight loss in the sibutramine trial on obesity reduction and maintenance (STORM trial). *Am J Clin Nutr* 78: 209–14.

Villanova N, Pasqui F, Burzacchini S, et al. 2006. A physical activity program to reinforce weight maintenance following a behavior program in overweight/obese subjects. *Int J Obes* 30: 697–703.

Wadden TA, West DS, Delahanty L, et al. 2006. The Look AHEAD study: a description of the lifestyle intervention and the evidence supporting it. *Obesity (Silver Spring)* 14: 737–52.

Wareham NJ, van Sluijs EM, Ekelund U. 2005. Physical activity and obesity prevention: a review of the current evidence. *Proc Nutr Soc* 64: 229–47.

Wei M, Kampert J, Barlow CE, et al. 1999. Relationship between low cardiorespiratory fitness and mortality in normal-weight, overweight, and obese men. *JAMA* 282: 1547–53.

Wei M, Gibbons LW, Mitchell TL, Kampert JB, Lee CD, Blair SN. 1999. The association between cardiorespiratory fitness and impaired fasting glucose and type 2 diabetes mellitus in men. *Ann Intern Med* 130: 89–96.

Weinstein AR, Sesso HD, Lee IM, et al. 2004. Relationship of physical activity vs body mass index with type 2 diabetes in women. *JAMA* 292: 1188–94.

Wing RR. 2002. Behavioral Weight Control. In TA Wadden, AJ Stunkard (Eds.), *Handbook of Obesity Treatment*. New York: The Guilford Press, pp. 301–16.

Wing RR, Venditti EM, Jakicic JM, Polley BA, Lang W. 1998. Lifestyle intervention in overweight individuals with a family history of diabetes. *Diabetes Care* 21: 350–9.

Wood PD, Stephanick ML, Dreon DM, et al. 1988. Changes in plasma lipids and lipoproteins in overweight men during weight loss through dieting as compared with exercise. *N Engl J Med* 319: 1173–9.

Wood PD, Stephanick ML, Williams PT, Haskell WL. 1991. The effects of plasma lipoproteins of a prudent weight-reducing diet, with or without exercise, in overweight men and women. *N Engl J Med* 325: 461–6.

13

Risk of Acute Cardiac Events With Physical Activity

I-Min Lee and
Jacob Sattelmair

Regular physical activity is widely recommended as an essential component of a healthy lifestyle because it prevents the development of many chronic diseases, including cardiovascular disease, several cancers, and type 2 diabetes, and decreases the occurrence of premature mortality (*see* Chapters 8–11). However, physical activity can also have adverse effects that must not be overlooked. It is important to understand the balance between health benefits and risks to optimize the benefits while mitigating the potential risks associated with physical activity. This chapter and Chapter 14 discuss several adverse effects associated with physical activity, with this chapter reviewing the most severe adverse effects that can potentially be triggered by vigorous physical activity, that is, acute cardiac events, including acute myocardial infarction (MI), sudden cardiac death (SCD), and sudden death.

Exercise-related acute cardiac events generally occur in persons with structural cardiac disease, which may not have been previously diagnosed. The underlying cardiac disease differs according to the age of the individual. Among young individuals, defined as younger than 30 years or younger than 40 years in different studies (Thompson et al., 2007), congenital cardiovascular disease is the most common pathological finding in persons who die during exercise, although among older individuals (hereafter referred to as "adults") who experience exercise-related acute cardiac events, coronary artery disease is the most common pathology seen. This chapter discusses the two age groups separately, with the main focus on adults, among whom rates of exercise-related acute cardiac events are far higher. Additionally, because the emphasis of this book is on primary prevention, we concentrate on studies conducted in adults who are apparently healthy (as opposed to adults with documented coronary artery disease). The chapter first reviews studies in adults, examining the risk of acute cardiac events related to vigorous physical activity and discussing relevant methodological factors pertinent to the interpretation of data from these studies, before proceeding to studies of SCD among young athletes.

Exercise-Related Acute Cardiac Events in Adults

The incidence of exercise-related acute cardiac events in adults varies with the prevalence of cardiac disease in the population, with extremely low rates observed among apparently healthy adults (Table 13.1). Thompson et al. estimated a rate of 1 sudden death per year for every 7,620 male joggers (or 1/396,000 person-hours of jogging) among whom half had known or readily diagnosed coronary heart disease (Thompson et al., 1982), whereas Albert

Table 13.1 Incidence of Acute Cardiac Events in Adults

Reference	*Event*	*Incidence rate*
Thompson et al., 1982	Sudden death	1 per 396,000 person-hours of jogging (men)
Albert et al., 2000	Sudden death	0.7 per 1,000,000 person-hours of vigorous exercise (men)
Whang et al., 2006	Sudden cardiac death	0.03 per 1,000,000 person-hours of moderate-to-vigorous physical activity (women)
Hallqvist et al., 2000	Non-fatal myocardial infarction	1.8 per 1,000,000 person-hours of vigorous exercise (men and women)

et al. estimated 1 sudden death per 1.42 million person-hours (or 0.7 per million person-hours) at risk associated with vigorous exercise in apparently healthy men (Albert et al., 2000). In ostensibly healthy women, the rate of sudden cardiac death was estimated at 1 per 36.5 million person-hours (or 0.03 per million person-hours) of participation in moderate-to-vigorous physical activity (Whang et al., 2006). For acute MI, the rates are higher, with data from the Thompson et al. study used to extrapolate rates of exercise-related acute MI ranging from 1 per 593 to 1 per 3,852 apparently healthy, middle-age men per year (Thompson et al., 2007). In Sweden, the incidence rate of non-fatal, acute MI during vigorous exercise among men and women without a history of MI was estimated at 1.8 per million person-hours (Hallqvist et al., 2000).

Biological Plausibility for Physical Activity to Trigger Acute Cardiac Events

Physical activity can be regarded as a "two-edged sword": habitual physical activity reduces the *overall*, long-term risk of MI and SCD by improving blood pressure, lipid profiles, and insulin sensitivity; preventing the development of atherosclerotic coronary artery disease; and protecting against ventricular fibrillation by enhancing myocardial electrical stability (Maron, 2000). However, there is now clear evidence showing that in the short-term during and immediately following physical activity, vigorous exertion can trigger or cause a *transient* increase in the risk of acute cardiac events, especially in individuals who are not regularly active (Thompson et al., 2007).

As mentioned earlier, exercise-related acute cardiac events typically occur in adults with structural cardiac disease, whether they have been previously diagnosed or not. In previously asymptomatic adults, the predominant cause of exertion-related MI or SCD is occult coronary artery disease (Burke et al., 1999). An acute cardiac event occurs when there is atherosclerotic plaque rupture in the coronary arteries, with subsequent acute thrombosis (Davies and Thomas, 1985). Among asymptomatic adults, vigorous physical activity may acutely induce plaque injury, worsen an existing injury, or increase the risk of thrombosis in an already damaged coronary arterial segment. During vigorous exertion, it has been postulated that stress motions (twisting and bending) occur in the coronary arteries, exacerbated by increases in heart rate and myocardial contractility, increasing the frequency of plaque rupture (Black et al., 1975). Additionally, although healthy coronary arteries dilate with exercise, atherosclerotic segments vasoconstrict, and such spasms may induce plaque rupture in thickened, non-compliant atherosclerotic plaques (Hambrecht et al., 2000). Exercise also can have prothrombotic effects during a period of vigorous exertion, increasing platelet-to-platelet aggregation and platelet-to-leukocyte aggregation, which may facilitate leukocyte migration into the coronary vessel wall and contribute to plaque disruption (Li et al., 1999). Other contributing factors may be the rise in heart rate and systolic blood pressure during exercise, resulting in greater shear forces in the coronary arteries, which may deepen existing coronary fissures and exacerbate the damage in previously mildly damaged coronary plaques (Bartsch, 1999).

Among patients who already have coronary artery disease, SCD can result from plaque disruption as described earlier or from ischemia-induced ventricular fibrillation from an evolving infarction or previous ischemic tissue or scar (Cobb and Weaver, 1986). Vigorous physical activity increases myocardial oxygen demand; however, at the same time, it also shortens coronary perfusion time because of increased heart rate, potentially contributing to myocardial ischemia and malignant cardiac arrhythmias.

Epidemiologic Studies of Physical Activity and Acute Cardiac Events in Adults

Case Reports/Case Series

Early studies on this topic consist primarily of case reports or case series describing sudden deaths, almost exclusively in men, which occurred during or immediately following an episode of vigorous physical activity (e.g., Opie, 1975; Sadaniantz et al., 1989; Thompson et al., 1979; Waller and Roberts, 1980). However, because of the lack of a comparison group, we cannot attribute the sudden deaths to vigorous exertion based on these data.

The first detailed study that attempted to make some reasonable comparison of risks was conducted in Rhode Island (Thompson et al., 1982). As part of the protocol of the Office of the State Medical Examiner in this state, all sudden deaths were reviewed. Between 1975 and 1981, 12 men (ages 28–74 years) died while jogging or running; 11 deaths were attributed to coronary heart disease and 1 to gastrointestinal hemorrhage (10 deaths occurred among men ages 30–64 years). To estimate the incidence rate of sudden death during jogging, investigators used random-digit telephone dialing to inquire about jogging at least twice a week. Among men ages 30–64 years, the prevalence was found to be 7.4%. Investigators then assumed that each jogging episode lasted 30 minutes. This yielded an estimated incidence rate of 13 sudden deaths (95% confidence interval [CI], 7–46) per 100,000 joggers per year, and 1 sudden death per 396,000 hours of jogging (95% CI, 1 per 112,000 to 1 per 680,000) among men in this age group.

To place these estimated rates in perspective, investigators ascertained the number of deaths from acute or chronic coronary heart disease occurring among men ages 30 to 64 years in the state from 1975 to 1980, then subtracted the 10 deaths that occurred during jogging or running, as well as 38 other deaths documented to occur during vigorous sports (it is possible that there were additional men who died during vigorous activities that were not recorded). These numbers resulted in an estimate of 1 death from coronary heart disease per 3,000,000 person-hours engaged in non-vigorous activities. Investigators thus calculated that the sudden death rate during jogging or running was 7 times the death rate (95% CI, 4–26) from coronary heart disease occurring during non-vigorous activities.

Study limitations included the possibility of misclassification of coronary heart disease deaths as occurring during non-vigorous activity, because all such deaths were assumed to happen during non-vigorous activity unless there was documentation that the decedent was engaging in vigorous activity at the time of death, and it is unclear how complete this documentation might have been. Additionally, a true relative risk (RR) was not calculated: The rate of sudden death during jogging or running was compared to the rate of death from acute or chronic coronary heart disease that occurred during non-vigorous activities.

Table 13.2 Relative Risks of Acute Cardiac Events With Physical Activity

Study/Reference	*Exposure investigated*	*Event*	*Overall relative risk(95% confidence interval)*
Siscovick et al., 1984	Vigorous activity (≥6 kcal/minutes)	SCD	5 (2–14) to 56 (23–131), depending on usual activity level (no overall result provided)
Onset Study; Mittleman et al., 1993	Vigorous activity (≥6 METs)	Nonfatal MI	5.9 (4.6–7.7)
Willich et al., 1993	Vigorous activity (≥6 METs)	Nonfatal MI	2.1 (1.6–3.1)
Hartford Hospital Acute MI Study; Giri et al., 1999	Vigorous activity (≥6 METs)	Nonfatal MI	10.1 (1.56–65.63)
SHEEP Study; Hallqvist et al., 2000	Vigorous activity (≥6 METs)	Nonfatal MI	3.3 (2.4–4.5)
Physicians' Health Study; Albert et al., 2000	Vigorous activity (≥6 METs)	SD	16.9 (10.5–27.0)
Nurses' Health Study; Whang et al., 2006	Moderate-to-vigorous activity (≥5 METs)	SCD	2.38 (1.23–4.60)

MI: myocardial infarction; SCD: sudden cardiac death; SD: sudden death.

Case–Control and Case–Crossover Studies (Table 13.2)

Subsequently, Siscovick et al. conducted a population-based case–control study to assess the risk of SCD during vigorous exercise (Siscovick et al., 1984). Cases were 133 married men ages 25 to 75 years, apparently free of heart disease, suffering an out-of-hospital primary cardiac arrest between 1979 and 1981 in the Seattle area. Their wives were interviewed to obtain information regarding physical activity at the time of cardiac arrest, as well as habitual physical activity level. Nine men (6.8%) died during vigorous activity (requiring 6 kcal/minute or more), whereas 124 died during non-vigorous activity. Controls were 133 married men sampled from the community using random-digit telephone dialing who were ostensibly free from heart disease and matched to cases on age and residence. The wives of controls were interviewed to estimate the amount of time in the previous year that their husbands engaged in vigorous activities, with the remaining time presumed to be spent on non-vigorous activities. These data were then used to estimate the incidence of SCD during vigorous and non-vigorous activities.

The RR of SCD during vigorous activity varied by habitual physical activity level; among men who habitually exercised vigorously less than 20 minutes/week, the RR of cardiac arrest during vigorous exercise compared to non-vigorous activities was 56 (95% CI, 23–131), whereas among men who habitually engaged in vigorous exercise for 140 minutes/week or more, this RR fell to 5 (95% CI, 2–14). Distinguishing between the short- and long-term risks of physical activity, investigators estimated that among men who habitually engaged in vigorous physical activity for 20 minutes/week or more, the *overall*, long-term risk of cardiac arrest was 60% that of less active men (RR = 0.40; 95% CI, 0.23–0.67).

The next two case–control studies, in addition to using traditional case–control analytic methods, utilized a new epidemiologic technique to analyze their data. This new technique, the case–crossover design, was specifically developed for the Onset Study (*see* paragraph below) to assess the transient change in risk of an acute event during a defined hazard period following exposure to a trigger (Maclure, 1991). Its advantage over traditional study designs is that it utilizes each patient as his/her own control, minimizing several traditional sources of bias. With this method, the observed frequency of exposure to the risk factor, such as vigorous exercise, during a defined hazard window (e.g., 1 hour) immediately prior to the acute event is divided by the expected frequency of exposure to vigorous exercise (e.g., estimated based on usual frequency over the past year) to estimate the RR.

In the first of these investigations published in 1993 (Mittleman et al., 1993), the Determinants of Myocardial Infarction Onset Study ("Onset Study") enrolled 1,228 patients, ages 22 to 92 years, with non-fatal, acute MI from community hospitals and tertiary care centers throughout the United States, and 218 population-based controls matched on age, sex, and residence. The hazard period associated with vigorous exercise was defined to be the 1-hour time window prior to the acute MI. Of the 1,228 patients, 54 (4.4%) had engaged in vigorous exercise (requiring ≥6 metabolic equivalents [METs]) during the hazard period, as assessed by direct interview with the patients. Investigators estimated the RR of acute MI triggered by vigorous exercise by calculating the ratio of the observed frequency of vigorous exercise during the hazard period to the expected frequency of vigorous exercise, which was measured in three different ways: *(1)* according to the patient's usual annual frequency of vigorous physical activity (case–crossover analysis); *(2)* according to the frequency of vigorous physical activity in the same 1-hour time window, but on the day before the onset of symptoms (case–crossover analysis); and *(3)* according to the frequency of vigorous physical activity in the matched controls (traditional case–control analysis).

The overall RR of acute MI in the 1-hour hazard window following exposure to vigorous exertion, based on annual frequency data, was 5.9 (95% CI, 4.6–7.7). Investigators conducted sensitivity analyses, expanding the hazard window to additional periods beyond the 1-hour window, but concluded that the relevant hazard period for triggering of acute MI by vigorous exertion was limited only to the first hour. In additional analyses using data from the control period on the day before the acute MI, the estimated RR was similar (RR= 5.6; 95% CI, 2.7–12.8). Using controls as the referent, no controls reported vigorous physical activity in the designated analogous hazard period (1-hour time window prior to time of acute MI of their matched case), and so the RR was infinity (lower bound of 95% CI, 2.2). As noted previously by Siscovick et al., the estimated RR varied significantly according to level of habitual physical activity (Figure 13.1). Among those who usually exercised vigorously less than once, one to two, three to four, or five or more times per week, the RRs for acute MI associated with vigorous exertion were 107 (95% CI, 67–171), 19.4 (9.9–38.1), 8.6 (3.6–20.5), and 2.4 (1.5–3.7), respectively (p-trend < 0.001).

In the same year, Willich et al., published the findings from a similar study that included a case–crossover comparison as well as a traditional case–control analysis (Willich et al., 1993). Cases were 1,194 men (mean age: 61 years) from two cities in Germany with non-fatal, acute MI, and controls were 532 individuals selected from the general population, matched to cases on age, sex, and residence. For the case–crossover analysis, the hazard period was defined to be the 1 hour prior to the onset of acute MI, and the usual frequency of vigorous activity (≥6 METs) in the past year was used for comparison. Among cases, 7.1% had participated in vigorous exercise during the hazard period, as assessed by direct interview. Controls provided information via telephone interview.

The case–crossover analysis showed that those who engaged in vigorous physical activity (≥6 METs) in the 1 hour preceding MI had a RR of 2.1 (95% CI, 1.6–3.1). The traditional case–control analysis yielded a similar estimate, with RR of 2.1 (1.1–3.6). The RR was significantly modified by usual physical activity level; the RRs for patients whose frequency

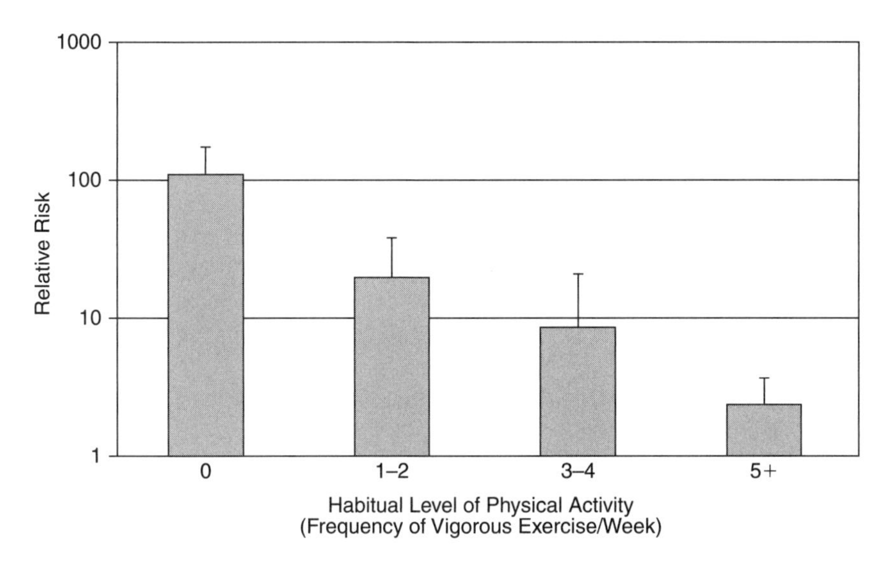

Figure 13.1 Risk of non-fatal myocardial infarction triggered by vigorous exercise, according to habitual level of physical activity, Onset Study.

of regular vigorous exercise was less than four and four or more times per week were 6.9 (4.1–12.2) and 1.3 (0.8–2.2), respectively. Although the magnitude of the RRs from this study differed from the U.S. study described earlier, both studies showed that the increased transient risk of MI from vigorous exercise was modified by habitual physical activity with the increased risk of lesser magnitude among regular exercisers.

The Hartford Hospital Acute MI study is a prospective cohort study designed to evaluate the clinical outcomes among patients with MI treated with primary angioplasty (Giri et al., 1999). Investigators were able to use the data from this study to conduct a case–crossover analysis of exercise-related MI, with data on usual physical activity patterns collected after the occurrence of MI, making the study design similar to the two case–control studies described earlier. Subjects for this analysis were 640 consecutive patients with non-fatal, acute MI who were hospitalized within 12 hours of their symptoms and selected for primary angioplasty. To determine the activities in which patients engaged at the time of MI or up to 1 hour prior, they were interviewed during their hospital stay, the information was determined from a spouse or family member, or there was a telephone interview after discharge. Usual physical activity patterns were ascertained using the Framingham Heart Study and Lipid Research Clinics physical activity questionnaires.

Sixty-four patients (10%) experienced acute MI during or within an hour of vigorous exercise (≥6 METs). Overall, the RR for acute MI associated with vigorous exercise was 10.1 (95% CI, 1.56–65.63). As in the previous studies, the magnitude of the increased risk was modified by usual physical activity level: among those who were usually very low active, low active, moderately active, and highly active, the corresponding RRs were 30.5 (4.4–209.9), 20.9 (3.1–142.1), 2.9 (0.5–15.9), and 1.2 (0.3–5.2), respectively.

Hallqvist et al. conducted a population-based case–control study in Sweden, the Stockholm Heart Epidemiology Program (the SHEEP Study) to assess vigorous physical activity as a trigger for acute MI (Hallqvist et al., 2000). Cases were 699 patients with a first non-fatal, acute MI (ages 45 to 70 years) in Stockholm County, Sweden, and controls were a random sample of the population in the same county, matched to cases on age, sex, and neighborhood (n = 369). The hazard period associated with vigorous exercise was defined as the 1-hour time window prior to the acute MI. A total of 42 patients with MI (6.4%) had engaged in vigorous exercise during the hazard period. The analyses in this study closely paralleled those in the Onset Study, with investigators estimating the expected frequency of vigorous exercise in three different ways: *(1)* according to the patient's usual annual frequency of vigorous physical activity (case–crossover analysis); *(2)* according to the frequency of vigorous physical activity in the same 1-hour time window, but on the day before the onset of symptoms (case–crossover analysis); and *(3)* according to the frequency of vigorous physical activity in the matched controls (traditional case–control analysis; controls provided information by telephone). The usual annual frequency of vigorous exercise in cases was inquired about twice, once during their hospital stay, and again via a mailed questionnaire.

The overall RR of acute MI in the 1-hour hazard window following vigorous exercise, based on annual frequency data assessed in the hospital interview, was 3.3 (95% CI, 2.4–4.5). Investigators conducted sensitivity analyses, examining the 1-hour hazard window in blocks of 15 minutes and reported that most of the increased risk appeared in the first 45 minutes following vigorous exercise. In analyses using data from the control period on the day before the acute MI, the estimated RR was similar (RR = 4.2; 95% CI, 2.0–8.7). With the traditional case–control analysis, the RR was 4.7; (0.9–23.6). The increased transient risk was modified by habitual physical activity. When habitual activity was assessed in the hospital interview, the transient increased RRs were 100.7, 6.9, 3.7, and 3.3, respectively (p-trend < 0.001), among those who exercised vigorously less than one, one to two, more than two to four, and more than four times/week. However, there appeared to be a U-shaped relationship according to habitual physical activity as assessed by mailed questionnaire, with RRs of 54.7, 4.6, 2.3, and 12.1, respectively (p-trend < 0.001), among patients whose typical exercise level was classified as "very little," "sporadic walks," "occasional exercise," and "regular exercise." There also appeared to be effect modification by socioeconomic status, with a smaller risk among those with higher socioeconomic status.

Prospective Cohort Studies Using Nested Case–Crossover Designs (Table 2)

Prospective cohort studies allow for the ascertainment of baseline physical activity levels prior to cardiac events, making it less likely for the activity assessment to be biased. In the Physicians' Health Study (Albert et al., 2000), investigators examined the risk of sudden death during and up to 30 minutes after an episode of vigorous exertion in men. Physical activity at the time of sudden death was determined from medical records or reported from next-of-kin. The usual annual frequency of physical activity was assessed via mailed questionnaires at baseline; these data were used to estimate the expected frequency of vigorous exercise in a nested case–crossover analysis.

During more than 12 years of follow-up from 1982, 122 sudden deaths occurred among over 21,000 male physicians, leading to an overall incidence of sudden death of 1 death per 19 million person-hours. Information on physical activity in the hour before sudden death was available in 80% of decedents; 17 (13.9%) occurred during and 6 (4.9%) occurred within 30 minutes of vigorous exercise. The absolute risk of sudden death associated with an episode of vigorous exercise was 1 per 1.42 million person-hours; for periods of lesser or no exertion, this was 1 per 23 million person-hours. The RR of sudden death during and up to 30 minutes after vigorous exertion, compared to periods of lighter or no exertion, was estimated at 16.9 (95% CI, 10.5–27.0). Supporting previous studies, in stratified analysis, habitual physical activity attenuated the RR of sudden death associated with vigorous exertion. Men who engaged in vigorous exercise less than once per week, one to four times per week,

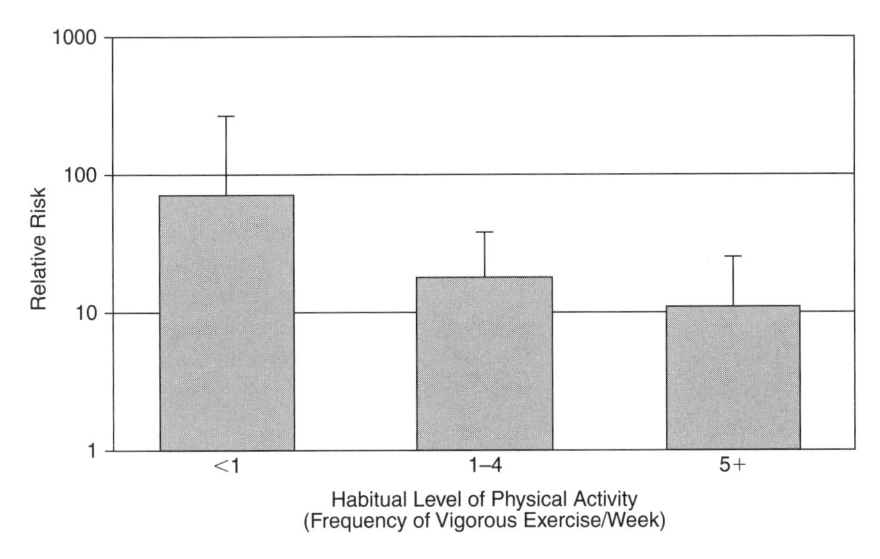

Figure 13.2 Risk of sudden death triggered by vigorous exercise, according to habitual level of physical activity, Physicians' Health Study.

and five or more times per week had RRs of 74.1 (22.0–24.9), 18.9 (10.2–35.1), and 10.9 (4.5–26.2), respectively (*p*-trend = 0.006; Fig. 13.2).

A similar study was conducted among women in the Nurses' Health Study (Whang et al., 2006), where investigators assessed the risk of SCD during moderate-to-vigorous exercise (activities typically requiring ≥5 METs, as contrasted with ≥6 METs in the previous studies described) compared to no to lighter exertion, using both traditional prospective cohort analysis and nested case–crossover analysis. Physical activity at the time of SCD was ascertained from medical records or next-of-kin. The usual annual frequency of physical activity was assessed via mailed questionnaires at baseline and updated every 2 years; the data closest to the time of death were used to estimate the expected frequency of vigorous exercise in a case–crossover analysis.

Among more than 84,000 women followed from 1986 to 2004, 288 SCD cases occurred. Only 9 deaths (3.1%) occurred during an episode of moderate-to-vigorous exercise. The overall risk of SCD with moderate-to-vigorous exercise was very low (1 per 36.5 million hours of exertion) compared to 1 SCD per 59.4 million hours of activity at lesser or no exertion, yielding an unadjusted RR of 1.63 for the traditional prospective cohort analysis. Case–crossover analysis estimated the RR of SCD during moderate-to-vigorous exertion to be 2.38 (95% CI, 1.23–4.60). Again, habitual physical activity attenuated this transient elevated risk, such that those women who typically participated in moderate-to-vigorous physical activity 2 hours/week or more did not have a significantly elevated transient risk with these activities (RR = 1.49; 95% CI, 0.61–3.61) compared to women who reported less than 2 hours/week (RR = 8.98; 95% CI, 3.32–24.3).

Methodological Considerations

Study Design

The study designs described earlier each had particular advantages and limitations. In case–control studies, incidence rates for the outcome of interest (e.g., SCD) typically cannot be determined among study subjects, whereas they can be determined in prospective cohort studies. Ascertainment of incidence rates can be relevant, because the exercise-related RR of acute cardiac events may vary, depending on the baseline incidence rate in the population (e.g., the RRs may be different in populations with higher baseline incidence rates, such as men or individuals with documented coronary heart disease, than in populations with lower baseline rates).

Case–control studies also may yield biased results if the response rate is low and/or differential between cases and controls. Generally, the aforementioned studies all had good response rates (in excess of 70% for both cases and controls), with the exception of the SHEEP study, where the response rate was 47% for cases and 96% in controls (Hallqvist et al., 2000). However, with the use of the case–crossover design, the control response rate is irrelevant, because each case acts as his/her control, essentially ensuring 100% "control response" among participating cases.

This case–crossover method of analysis was developed in the early 1990s specifically to investigate the transient risk of an acute event following exposure to a trigger (Maclure, 1991). Several studies that used this new analytic design also simultaneously employed traditional analytic methods to compare their results, and in all these studies, the findings from case–crossover analyses corresponded well with those from traditional case–control (Hallqvist et al., 2000; Mittleman et al., 1993; Willich et al., 1993) and prospective cohort analyses (Whang et al., 2006), supporting the validity of the new design. A particular advantage of the case–crossover design is its ability to control for confounding by traditional cardiovascular risk factors, because each case subject acts as his/her own control subject. However, there is a possibility of confounding by other triggers that may have coincided with vigorous physical activity, such as coffee intake or stress (Baylin et al., 2006; Siscovick, 2006). Nevertheless, it is unlikely that these other triggers are closely associated with vigorous exercise, nor are they likely to account for the strong associations observed between an episode of vigorous exercise and acute cardiac events.

Because of the rarity of exercise-related acute cardiac events, limited statistical power is an issue. The proportion of patients engaged in vigorous exercise during the defined hazard period generally ranged from 4% to 10%, with a high of 18.8% in the Physicians' Health Study (Albert et al., 2000). Thus, imprecise estimates of RR with wide CIs typically were reported. Therefore, small changes in the number of events classified as acute cardiac events or not (*see* Misclassification) have the potential to make a large impact on the estimates of RR.

Recall Bias

An important consideration with regard to the aforementioned case–control studies (whether using traditional or case–crossover analytic techniques) is the potential for recall bias. Patients may overestimate vigorous physical activity immediately prior to an acute cardiac event and underestimate their usual frequency of vigorous exercise (whether assessed over the past year or during the specified control period 24 hours before their cardiac event), partly because of the common awareness of an association between vigorous physical activity and sudden death. For example, in parts of the country with winter weather, deaths during snow shovelling make the news every year (Hammoudeh and Haft, 1996). Additionally, if patients are queried some time after the acute cardiac events, recall about physical activities at the time of the cardiac event may be further limited. This was less likely to occur in the Onset Study because patient interviews occurred soon after MI (mean: 4 days) (Mittleman et al., 1993) and was more likely in some of the other studies where there was a longer time between the acute event and patient interviews (Hallqvist et al., 2000; Willich et al., 1993).

To further minimize recall bias in the Onset Study and maintain comparability of the reporting of activities during the hazard and control time periods, interviewers asked patients about their activities in 26 hours prior to MI, which was treated as one long hazard period (instead of just asking about activities in the 1-hour period before MI and the 1-hour period in the control period on the day before).

However, recall bias is unlikely to explain the results of the case–control studies because the findings from these studies concurred with the findings from prospective cohort studies with nested case–crossover design, where reporting of physical activity occurred prior to the acute cardiac event (Albert et al., 2000; Whang et al., 2006). Further evidence to suggest minimal impact of recall bias includes the observed effect modification of the association between vigorous exertion and acute cardiac events by habitual physical exertion, again in agreement with the prospective cohort studies.

Misclassification of Exposure and Outcome

Misclassification can occur on several levels in the studies discussed earlier. In the prospective cohort studies with nested case–crossover design, physical activity was assessed by questionnaire prior to the acute cardiac event. Although the questionnaires used have reasonable reliability and validity, they are subject to misclassification (*see* Chapters 2 and 3) that is likely to be random, because the physical activity information was collected before the occurrence of the outcomes of interest. Because random misclassification tends to bias findings toward the null, the results from these studies are likely to be of larger magnitude than those observed. Additionally, physical activity levels change over time, so if this information is not updated over a long period of time, further misclassification may occur. For example, in the Physicians' Health Study, usual frequency of vigorous physical activity was estimated from a questionnaire at baseline, but this was not updated over the more than 12 years of follow-up during which SCD was ascertained, potentially adding to the misclassification of the frequency of vigorous exercise (Albert et al., 2000).

Misclassification of activities at the time of sudden death was less likely in the two prospective cohort studies with nested case–crossover design, because the physical activity information was obtained from medical records or from direct observations of persons (e.g., next-of-kin) witnessing the event (Albert et al., 2000; Whang et al., 2006).

Another area in which misclassification may occur is in the definition of SCD. In the Nurses' Health Study, the strictest definition was limited to cases where the witnessed death or cardiac arrest occurred within 1 hour of symptom onset or, if the death was not witnessed, where autopsy findings were consistent with SCD (Whang et al., 2006). In additional analyses, deaths occurring during sleep also were included, with similar findings observed. However, even with the strict definition, not all these cases may have been SCD because the clinical perception of SCD is frequently not supported by autopsy findings—even in groups of patients at high risk of SCD—with the autopsy indicating sudden death of non-cardiac origin (Pratt et al., 1996). Because exertion-related acute cardiac events are rare, small changes in the number of events classified as SCD can make a large difference to the estimates of RR if the misclassification is differential (e.g., if deaths occurring during exertion are more likely to be diagnosed as SCD because of an awareness of an association between vigorous physical activity and sudden death).

Intensity of Physical Activity

In most of the studies described earlier, acute cardiac events were related to "vigorous/strenuous physical exertion" vs. "less or no exertion." By convention, vigorous physical activity is defined as any activity requiring 6 METs or higher—that is, six times resting metabolic rate or more (Pate et al., 1995). A slow jog, for example, may require 6 METs. However, this is an arbitrary threshold, and it is not clear that 6 METs is the level beyond which physical activity elicits the pathophysiologic processes leading to an acute cardiac event.

Additionally, the use of METs measures the intensity of physical activity on an absolute scale, regardless of the physical conditioning of the individual. For example, brisk walking at 4 mph is typically regarded as a moderate-intensity activity that requires 4 METs (Ainsworth et al., 1993). However, among older women, who are less physically fit than their younger peers, this walking may actually require vigorous effort relative to their maximal capacity (Kline et al., 1987). Thus, for poorly conditioned or older individuals, activities requiring less than 6 METs may still stress the cardiovascular system, potentially causing exercise-related cardiac events. The only study to assess activities requiring less than 6 METs as a trigger for acute cardiac events was the Nurses' Health Study (Whang et al., 2006), where "moderate-to-vigorous" activity (5 or more METs) was investigated. Interestingly, although there was an overall transiently elevated risk of SCD in women engaging in such activities, this transient risk disappeared among women who regularly exercised 2 hours/week or more.

Hazard Window

The "hazard window"—the relevant exposure period—within which acute cardiac events were designated to be exertion-related in the studies described earlier is another arbitrary measure that may influence RR estimates. Three studies (Siscovick et al., 1984; Thompson et al., 1979; Whang et al., 2006) included only cardiac events that occurred during the time of vigorous physical activity (or moderate-to-vigorous activity in the Nurses' Health Study), whereas the remaining studies considered a hazard window that included the time spent on physical activity and a short time (30–60 minutes) following physical activity (Albert et al., 2000; Giri et al., 1999; Hallqvist et al., 2000; Mittleman et al., 1993; Willich et al., 1993).

It is unclear what the relevant exposure period is—that is, at what time during and/or after physical activity do the pathophysiologic processes causing acute cardiac events occur? Using a hazard window that is wider than biologically relevant can lead to an underestimate of the RRs. In the Onset Study (Mittleman et al., 1993), investigators attempted to clarify the hazard window by examining incremental 1-hour periods for hours two through five. They concluded that the transient risk of MI associated with vigorous exercise was limited only to the first hour immediately following vigorous exertion. Similarly, in the SHEEP study, investigators examined time blocks of 15 minutes within the hour following vigorous activity and concluded that most of the risk appeared to be within the first 45 minutes (Hallqvist et al., 2000).

Effect Modification

Perhaps the most important effect modifier of the transient, increased risk of acute cardiac events associated with vigorous exercise is the frequency of habitual physical activity, with all of the studies describing an attenuation of the elevated risk with regular physical activity. For example, in the Onset Study (Mittleman et al., 1993), the RR of exertion-related non-fatal, acute MI was 107 (95% CI, 67–171) among those who rarely exercised vigorously but 2.4 (1.5–3.7) among those who exercised vigorously at least five times a week (Fig. 13.1). In the Physicians' Health Study (Albert et al., 2000), the RR of exertion-related SCD was 74.1 (22.0–249) among men who exercised vigorously less than once per week but 10.9 (4.5–26.2) among those exercising vigorously five or more times per week (Fig. 13.2).

In most studies, the transient risk remained significantly elevated even for those in the highest category of habitual physical activity. One exception was the Nurses' Health

Study (Whang et al., 2006), where the transient risk of exertion-related SCD among women who reported exercising at moderate-to-vigorous intensity for 2 hours/week or more was no longer statistically significant (RR = 1.49; 95% CI, 0.61–3.61). It is unclear why the results from this study differed from the majority; it may have resulted from the fact that the physical activity trigger in this study required a lesser threshold—the exposure of interest in this study was any physical activity requiring 5 METs or more, as contrasted to all the other studies where the exposure was any activity requiring 6 METs or more.

The results from the Nurses' Health Study are contrasted to those from most of the other studies where even among habitual exercisers the transient risk of acute cardiac events following vigorous exertion (≥6METs) was still significantly elevated, albeit at far lesser magnitude than among non-habitual exercisers (Albert et al., 2000; Hallqvist et al., 2000; Mittleman et al., 1993; Siscovick et al., 1984).

Other potential effect modifiers that have been investigated include age, sex, socioeconomic status, history of heart disease, and traditional cardiovascular risk factors (smoking, obesity, hypertension, high cholesterol, diabetes, family history), as well as medication use. However, none of these factors were consistently observed to modify the relationship between vigorous activity and transient risk of acute cardiac events. Although acute MI and SCD are more likely to occur in the early morning hours than at other times of the day (Muller et al., 1987), the Physicians' Health Study investigators did not observe time of day to significantly modify the transient elevated risk with exertion (Albert et al., 2000).

Sex Differences

As stated in the preceding paragraph, there has not been clear indication of any differences between men and women with regard to the triggering of acute cardiac events by physical activity. However, most studies have included only men (Albert et al., 2000; Siscovick et al., 1984; Thompson et al., 1982) or primarily men (well over half the study participants were men in several studies; Giri et al., 1999; Hallqvist et al., 2000; Mittleman et al., 1993; Willich et al., 1993), with the Nurses' Health Study being the only study comprised entirely of women (Whang et al., 2006). Thus, statistical power likely was limited to detect any differences between the sexes in the studies that included both men and women. Power is likely to be further limited because more men participate in vigorous activities than women and thus are more likely to suffer exertion-related events. For example, in the Onset Study, 32% of the 1,228 participants were women; however, among the 54 patients with exertion-related MI, only 4 (7.4%) were women (Mittleman et al., 1993). Similarly, in the Hartford Hospital Acute MI study, among the 64 cases of exertion-related MI, 86% were men, whereas among the 576 cases of MI that were not related to exertion, 68% were men ($p < 0.05$) (Giri et al., 1999). With regard to the magnitude of the RRs observed for men and women, the Nurses' Health Study of women reported an overall RR of 2.38 (95% CI, 1.23–4.60) for SCD (Whang et al., 2006) compared to 16.8 (10.5–27.0) for sudden death in men in the Physician's Health Study (Albert et al., 2000) and between 5 (2–14) and 56 (23–131) for SCD, depending on usual activity level (no overall result was provided; Siscovick, 2006). Although the magnitude appears smaller for women than men, this comparison is limited, because the exposure of interest was moderate-to-vigorous physical activity in the Nurses' Health Study but vigorous exercise in both of the men's studies.

Risk–Benefit Assessment

In the context of evaluating physical activity as a trigger for acute cardiac events, it is essential to differentiate between relative and absolute risks. The data are clear in showing that vigorous physical activity triggers acute cardiac events in susceptible individuals and that the increased risk with vigorous exertion can be very large compared to lesser degrees of exertion (i.e., large increases in *relative* risks). However, if the occurrence of the event is rare, as in the case of acute cardiac events (Table 13.1), then this may still translate to a low *absolute* risk. For example, in the Physicians' Health Study, the risk of SCD during vigorous physical activity was 1 per 1.42 million person-hours; during periods of lesser exertion, this was 1 per 23 million person-hours (Albert et al., 2000). These rates translate to an unadjusted RR of more than 16— that is, a more than 16-fold increase in risk of SCD during vigorous exertion among these men. Although the increase in RR was large, the absolute risk of SCD during vigorous exertion was still very low in the physicians, at 1 for every 1.42 million person-hours of vigorous exercise. For acute MI, the Onset Study (Mittleman et al., 1993) showed a transient increased RR of 107 among habitually sedentary individuals—a huge increase in RR. However, using data from the Framingham Heart Study, the absolute risk of a 50-year-old non-smoking, non-diabetic man suffering an acute MI in any 1-hour period is about 1 in 1 million, a very small absolute risk, such that even if this absolute risk were increased by 100-fold, the new absolute risk would still only be 1 in 10,000. (Because the Onset Study was a case–control study using case–crossover analyses of data, rates of acute MI could not be calculated directly from the study.)

Weighed against the transient increase in risk of acute cardiac events associated with vigorous physical activity is the large body of evidence showing that over the long term, higher levels of physical activity or fitness are associated with decreased risks of cardiovascular disease and premature mortality (Pate et al., 1995). Thus, on balance, regular physical activity should still be considered beneficial for health. A panel of experts recently reviewed the risks of acute cardiac events with vigorous exercise and concluded that: "Ostensibly healthy adults without known cardiac disease should be encouraged to develop gradually progressive exercise regimens. Because the least fit individuals are at greatest risk for exercise-related events, gradually progressive programs should theoretically increase fitness and reduce acute (cardiac) events without excessive risk" (Thompson et al., 2007). Furthermore, the American College of Cardiology, the American Heart Association, and the American College of Sports Medicine recommend that individuals who are at greater risk of underlying coronary heart disease should be considered for exercise testing before embarking on a vigorous exercise program (American College of Sports Medicine, 2005; Thompson et al., 2007).

Sudden Cardiac Death in Young Athletes

SCD among young individuals tends to occur either during or immediately following athletic activity, suggesting that participation in competitive sports may increase the risk (Corrado et al., 2003; Corrado et al., 2005a; Maron et al., 1980). The most frequent pathological findings at autopsy are hereditary or congenital cardiovascular abnormalities, such as hypertrophic cardiomyopathy, coronary artery anomalies, aortic stenosis, aortic dissection associated with connective tissue defects (e.g., Marfan's syndrome), mitral valve prolapse, arrythmogenic right ventricular cardiomyopathy, and arrhythmias (Corrado et al., 2003; Corrado et al., 1990; Maron et al., 1996a; Van Camp et al., 1995). The immediate cause of death tends to be ventricular arrhythmias—with the exception of Marfan's syndrome, where aortic rupture often is the immediate cause.

The incidence of SCD in young athletes is extremely low. Based on a retrospective review of competitive high school athletes in Minnesota (ages 13–19 years), Maron et al. identified three cases of SCD between 1985 and 1997, all male, leading to an estimated rate of 0.46 per 100,000 per year (Maron et al., 1998a). Another retrospective review of high school and college athletes (ages 13–24 years) identified 126 high school and 34 college athletes who suffered non-traumatic deaths (not just SCD) between 1983 and 1993 nationally (Van Camp et al., 1995). Estimated death rates were 0.66 and 1.45 per 100,000 male athletes per year for high school and college athletes, respectively. Rates were lower for female athletes, with corresponding figures of 0.12 and 0.28 per 100,000 per year, respectively. The most common causes of death were hypertrophic cardiomyopathy and congenital coronary artery anomalies.

To assess the increased risk of sudden death with sports participation and whether male athletes had a higher risk, Corrado et al. conducted a prospective cohort study of adolescents and young adults (ages 12–35 years) in the Veneto Region of Italy, who were followed for 21 years between 1979 and 1999 (Corrado et al., 2003). A total of 300 sudden death cases were identified, for an overall incidence of 1 per 100,000 per year. Of these sudden deaths, 55 (50 male and 5 female) occurred in competitive athletes (2.3 of 100,000 per year), and 245 occurred in non-athletes (0.9 of 100,000 per year). In analyses that adjusted for athletic/non-athletic status and sex, the RR for sudden death associated with being an athlete was 1.95 (95% CI, 1.4–2.6); for SCD, this was 2.1 (1.5–2.8). Being male was associated with increased risks of 2.5 (1.9–3.2) and 2.8 (2.1–3.7) for sudden death and SCD, respectively. At autopsy, the majority of sudden death cases (259 of 300) were found to have an underlying cardiovascular abnormality, leading the investigators to conclude that sports participation itself was not the cause of the sudden death, but rather, the sports activity triggered cardiac arrest among those susceptible because of their underlying cardiovascular conditions.

The authors attributed the observed higher rates of sudden death compared to U.S. rates to several factors, including the prospective study design that may have resulted in more complete case ascertainment. Additionally, the age range was wider in the Italian study, including subjects up to age 35 years; in fact, 10 athletes and 48 non-athletes were found to have atherosclerotic coronary artery disease at autopsy. With pre-participation screening of athletes required by law in Italy since 1982, the distribution of the underlying causes of sudden death differed from those seen in the U.S. studies. In particular, there were no sudden deaths resulting from hypertrophic cardiomyopathy, which was specifically screened for. Genetic and ethnic differences also may have played a role. Finally, the authors postulated that the sports participation level may have been more intense in Italy compared with the United States.

There continues to be debate regarding pre-participation screening of young athletes. In the United States, the American Heart Association recommends taking a personal and family medical history and a physical examination that focuses on detecting the cardiovascular conditions most commonly associated with sudden death in young athletes (*see* earlier discussion), with no additional non-invasive testing such as routine electrocardiogram (ECG) (Maron et al., 1998b; Maron et al., 1996b). In contrast, in Europe, a routine ECG is included as well (Corrado et al., 2005b). The European recommendation is based largely on the Italian experience (based on data collected from the Veneto Region, discussed earlier), where pre-participation screening of athletes, including an ECG, has been mandated since 1982. The incidence of sudden death decreased 89% among athletes ages 12 to 35 years with screening, whereas no change was seen in non-athletes, suggesting that the screening was responsible for the decreased rates of sudden death. However, there was no comparison of screening without, and with, a routine ECG. In the United States, with its large numbers of high school and college athletes, the cost of a routine ECG also has to be balanced against the very small numbers of sudden death occurring in the group and the lack of clear evidence that an ECG adds to the history taking and medical examination screening process.

Future Research

To date, all studies of adults investigating the risk of acute cardiac events triggered by physical activity have used the absolute scale to classify the intensity of physical activity. As discussed previously, under this classification scheme, vigorous activities are those requiring 6 METs or more (Pate et al., 1995). However, this may not accurately reflect activities that require vigorous effort in a particular individual, because for older and/or more unfit persons with lower maximal cardiorespiratory capacity, even activities requiring less than 6 METs may require vigorous effort for that individual. Future studies that classify the intensity of physical activity according to both absolute and relative scales will be helpful in providing information on how much misclassification occurs when using the absolute, rather than relative, scale to assess intensity and whether one scale may be preferable to use over another.

Additionally, all studies except the Nurses' Health Study (Whang et al., 2006) have used 6 METs as the cutpoint to define exposure to "high-risk" physical activity. The choice of this cutpoint is arbitrary; it will be informative for investigators to conduct sensitivity analyses, setting the cutpoint at different MET levels (in addition to 6 METs) to examine whether this is truly the intensity level beyond which activities can be considered high risk. Using the relative intensity scale, investigators can also vary the definition of high-risk activity using different thresholds (e.g., vigorous, moderate-to-vigorous, moderate, etc.).

Among young athletes, findings from additional studies can inform the debate regarding the value of ECG screening in preventing SCD. Such investigations can compare SCD rates among young athletes screened by means of a personal and family medical history and a physical examination vs. SCD rates among young athletes undergoing pre-participation screening that also includes a routine ECG.

Finally, current studies of acute cardiac events triggered by physical activity have been conducted primarily in Caucasian populations. Although it is unlikely that the underlying pathological processes leading to acute cardiac events differ among persons of different racial or ethnic groups, the baseline incidence rate of such events can differ, which may affect the magnitude of the excess RR. Additionally, the most common pathology observed for SCD in young athletes are hereditary or congenital cardiovascular abnormalities, and the prevalence of these conditions can vary by race/ethnic group. Thus, studies conducted among other race/ethnic groups will contribute further information.

Personal Perspective

Jim Fixx, author of the best-seller "The Complete Book of Running" (1977), is equally well-known for the fact that he suffered sudden cardiac death while running at age 52 years. Those loath to engage in physical activity may point to him as an illustration of the dangers of exercising, and they would be correct—to an extent. This chapter clearly shows that acute cardiac events in adults can be triggered by vigorous physical activity, particularly among those who are not regularly physically active. However, it is also clear that these risks operate during a small window of time—during and immediately after vigorous physical activity—and that during other times (the vast majority of time for most individuals), the risks of cardiovascular disease and all-cause mortality is *lower*, leading to an overall benefit associated with being physically active. Additionally, to further balance the perspective (*see* Risk–Benefit Assessment), the absolute risk of suffering an acute cardiac event, even during vigorous exercise, is very low (e.g., 1 case of SCD per 1.42 million person-hours in the Physicians' Health Study; Albert et al., 2000).

Thus, physical activity must still be considered essential for health and must continue to be promoted by health professionals because on balance, its numerous benefits clearly outweigh its risks. As for Jim Fixx, running may indeed have extended his life—he was overweight and a heavy smoker when he started running at age 35 years; also, his father died of an acute MI at age 43years, 9 years earlier than did Jim.

References

Ainsworth BE, Haskell WL, Leon AS, et al. 1993. Compendium of physical activities: classification of energy costs of human physical activities. *Med Sci Sports Exerc* 25: 71–80.

Albert CM, Mittleman MA, Chae CU, Lee IM, Hennekens CH, Manson JE. 2000. Triggering of sudden death from cardiac causes by vigorous exertion. *N Engl J Med* 343: 1355–61.

American College of Sports Medicine. 2005. *Guidelines for exercise testing and prescription*. Baltimore, MD: Lippincott Williams & Wilkins.

Bartsch P. 1999. Platelet activation with exercise and risk of cardiac events. *Lancet* 354: 1747–8.

Baylin A, Hernandez-Diaz S, Kabagambe EK, Siles X, Campos H. 2006. Transient exposure to coffee as a trigger of a first nonfatal myocardial infarction. *Epidemiology* 17: 506–11.

Black A, Black MM, Gensini G. 1975. Exertion and acute coronary artery injury. *Angiology* 26: 759–83.

Burke AP, Farb A, Malcom GT, Liang Y, Smialek JE, Virmani R. 1999. Plaque rupture and sudden death related to exertion in men with coronary artery disease. *JAMA* 281: 921–6.

Cobb LA, Weaver WD. 1986. Exercise: a risk for sudden death in patients with coronary heart disease. *J Am Coll Cardiol* 7: 215–9.

Corrado D, Basso C, Rizzoli G, Schiavon M, Thiene G. 2003. Does sports activity enhance the risk of sudden death in adolescents and young adults? *J Am Coll Cardiol* 42: 1959–63.

Corrado D, Basso C, Thiene G. 2005a. Essay: Sudden death in young athletes. *Lancet* 366 (Suppl 1): S47–8.

Corrado D, Pelliccia A, Bjornstad HH, et al. 2005b. Cardiovascular pre-participation screening of young competitive athletes for prevention of sudden death: proposal for a common European protocol. Consensus Statement of the Study Group of Sport Cardiology of the Working Group of Cardiac Rehabilitation and Exercise Physiology and the Working Group of Myocardial and Pericardial Diseases of the European Society of Cardiology. *Eur Heart J* 26: 516–24.

Corrado D, Thiene G, Nava A, Rossi L, Pennelli N. 1990. Sudden death in young competitive athletes: clinicopathologic correlations in 22 cases. *Am J Med* 89: 588–96.

Davies MJ, Thomas AC. 1985. Plaque fissuring—the cause of acute myocardial infarction, sudden ischaemic death, and crescendo angina. *Br Heart J* 53: 363–73.

Fixx J. 1977. *The complete book of running*. New York: Random House

Giri S, Thompson PD, Kiernan FJ, et al. 1999. Clinical and angiographic characteristics of exertion-related acute myocardial infarction. *JAMA* 282: 1731–6.

Hallqvist J, Moller J, Ahlbom A, Diderichsen F, Reuterwall C, de Faire U. 2000. Does heavy physical exertion trigger myocardial infarction? A case-crossover analysis nested in a population-based case-referent study. *Am J Epidemiol* 151: 459–67.

Hambrecht R, Wolf A, Gielen S, et al. 2000. Effect of exercise on coronary endothelial function in patients with coronary artery disease. *N Engl J Med* 342: 454–60.

Hammoudeh AJ, Haft JI. 1996. Coronary-plaque rupture in acute coronary syndromes triggered by snow shoveling. *N Engl J Med* 335: 2001.

Kline GM, Porcari JP, Hintermeister R, et al. 1987. Estimation of V02max from a one-mile track walk, gender, age, and body weight. *Med Sci Sports Exerc* 19: 253–9.

Li N, Wallen NH, Hjemdahl P. 1999. Evidence for prothrombotic effects of exercise and limited protection by aspirin. *Circulation* 100: 1374–9.

Maclure M. 1991. The case-crossover design: a method for studying transient effects on the risk of acute events. *Am J Epidemiol* 133: 144–53.

Maron BJ. 2000. The paradox of exercise. *N Engl J Med* 343: 1409–11.

Maron BJ, Gohman TE, Aeppli D. 1998a. Prevalence of sudden cardiac death during competitive sports activities in Minnesota high school athletes. *J Am Coll Cardiol* 32: 1881–4.

Maron BJ, Roberts WC, McAllister HA, Rosing DR, Epstein SE. 1980. Sudden death in young athletes. *Circulation* 62: 218–29.

Maron BJ, Shirani J, Poliac LC, Mathenge R, Roberts WC, Mueller FO. 1996a. Sudden death in young competitive athletes. Clinical, demographic, and pathological profiles. *JAMA* 276: 199–204.

Maron BJ, Thompson PD, Puffer JC, et al. 1998b. Cardiovascular preparticipation screening of competitive athletes: addendum: an addendum to a statement for health professionals from the Sudden Death Committee (Council on Clinical Cardiology) and the Congenital Cardiac Defects Committee (Council on Cardiovascular Disease in the Young), American Heart Association. *Circulation* 97: 2294.

Maron BJ, Thompson PD, Puffer JC, et al. 1996b. Cardiovascular preparticipation screening of competitive athletes. A statement for health professionals from the Sudden Death Committee (clinical cardiology) and Congenital Cardiac Defects Committee (cardiovascular disease in the young), American Heart Association. *Circulation* 94: 850–6.

Mittleman MA, Maclure M, Tofler GH, Sherwood JB, Goldberg RJ, Muller JE. 1993. Triggering of acute myocardial infarction by heavy physical exertion. Protection against triggering by regular exertion. Determinants of Myocardial Infarction Onset Study Investigators. *N Engl J Med* 329: 1677–83.

Muller JE, Ludmer PL, Willich SN, et al. 1987. Circadian variation in the frequency of sudden cardiac death. *Circulation* 75: 131–8.

Opie LH. 1975. Sudden death and sport. *Lancet* 1: 263–6.

Pate RR, Pratt M, Blair SN, et al. 1995. Physical activity and public health. A recommendation from the Centers for Disease Control and Prevention and the American College of Sports Medicine. *JAMA* 273: 402–7.

Pratt CM, Greenway PS, Schoenfeld MH, Hibben ML, Reiffel JA. 1996. Exploration of the precision of classifying sudden cardiac death. Implications for the interpretation of clinical trials. *Circulation* 93: 519–24.

Sadaniantz A, Clayton MA, Sturner WQ, Thompson PD. 1989. Sudden death immediately after a record-setting athletic performance. *Am J Cardiol* 63: 375.

Siscovick DS. 2006. Triggers of clinical coronary heart disease. *Epidemiology* 17: 495–7.

Siscovick DS, Weiss NS, Fletcher RH, Lasky T. 1984. The incidence of primary cardiac arrest during vigorous exercise. *N Engl J Med* 311: 874–7.

Thompson PD, Franklin BA, Balady GJ, et al. 2007. Exercise and acute cardiovascular events placing the risks into perspective: a scientific statement from the American Heart Association Council on Nutrition, Physical Activity, and Metabolism and the Council on Clinical Cardiology. *Circulation* 115: 2358–68.

Thompson PD, Funk EJ, Carleton RA, Sturner WQ. 1982. Incidence of death during jogging in Rhode Island from 1975 through 1980. *JAMA* 247: 2535–8.

Thompson PD, Stern MP, Williams P, Duncan K, Haskell WL, Wood PD. 1979. Death during jogging or running. A study of 18 cases. *JAMA* 242: 1265–7.

Van Camp SP, Bloor CM, Mueller FO, Cantu RC, Olson HG. 1995. Nontraumatic sports death in high school and college athletes. *Med Sci Sports Exerc* 27: 641–7.

Waller BF, Roberts WC. 1980. Sudden death while running in conditioned runners aged 40 years or over. *Am J Cardiol* 45: 1292–300.

Whang W, Manson JE, Hu FB, et al. 2006. Physical exertion, exercise, and sudden cardiac death in women. *JAMA* 295: 1399–403.

Willich SN, Lewis M, Lowel H, Arntz HR, Schubert F, Schroder R. 1993. Physical exertion as a trigger of acute myocardial infarction. Triggers and Mechanisms of Myocardial Infarction Study Group. *N Engl J Med* 329: 1684–90.

14 Physical Activity, Fitness, and Musculoskeletal Injury

Jennifer M. Hootman and
Kenneth E. Powell

In Chapters 8 through 12, a clear case has been made for the benefits of a physically active lifestyle. Given the interest in promoting increased physical activity levels among the general population, the potential adverse events associated with increased activity should also be discussed, especially in relation to potential mediating factors (Finch et al., 2001). Injuries to the musculoskeletal system and degenerative joint disease are the most commonly reported complications associated with physical activity and exercise, whereas other rare events such as sudden cardiac arrest, hematological and metabolic disorders, and heat stroke can also occur (U.S. Department of Health and Human Services, 1996). (For additional discussion on sudden death, please refer to Chapter 13.) Musculoskeletal injuries are important because they can have severe short- and long-term effects such as pain, temporary and permanent loss of function, increased health-care costs, as well as negative effects on physical activity participation. For example, fear of injury has been associated with inactivity, and injury is one of the most common reasons people relapse from an exercise program (King et al., 2000; Finch et al., 2001). Because of the overwhelming benefits of physical activity and exercise in terms of mortality reduction and morbidity prevention, identifying factors that will mitigate the potential risks associated with activity is an important public health goal.

Injury experiences, including types and magnitude of exposures, as well as potential risk factors may be vastly different for specific groups of physically active people, such as competitive athletes (youth, high school, and collegiate athletes), elite athletes (Olympic and professional athletes), and military recruits. Therefore, we focus our discussion here on population-based studies of sports and recreation injuries from around the world. In some instances, we use examples from studies of competitive athletes, or military recruits to illustrate select concepts because there may be limited scientific literature pertaining to the general population. Specifically in this chapter, we cover the epidemiology of sports- and recreation-related injury and discuss the dose–response relationship between physical activity and activity-related injuries, focusing on the issues surrounding measurement and definitions used in epidemiologic studies of physical activity and injury.

Descriptive Epidemiology of Sports and Recreation-Related Injuries

Factors affecting injury rates are often related to differing rates and characteristics of participation in various sports and recreation activities. Many population-based studies do not adequately capture activity participation and thus are constrained to report injury rates based on the total population, including those persons who do not participate in sports and recreation activities. This is an important issue to remember while reading this chapter and is discussed further in the section on Exposure Measurement.

Overall Population Burden

The incidence of sports- and recreation-related injuries varies markedly according to the definition of injury. Deaths and severe injuries are fortunately rare, with population-based incidence rates in Australia of 0.0006% and 0.002%, respectively (Gabbe et al., 2005; Table 14.1). The incidence of hospitalization for sports and related injuries is around 0.1%, and estimates for injuries requiring a medical visit are generally 1% to 2% (Dempsey et al., 2005; Cassell et al., 2003; Burt and Overpeck, 2001; Centers for Disease Control, 2002; Gerson and Stevens, 2004; Ni et al., 2002; Conn et al., 2003) In contrast, estimates that include less severe injuries, such as those that require a reduction in activity but not a visit to a health-care professional, are 10% to 20%. (Mummery et al., 1998; Uitenbrook, 1996).

These incidence estimates, although seemingly low, indicate that large numbers of people suffer sports- and recreation-related injuries every year. National health surveys in the United States indicate that 4 to 7 million people are medically treated in emergency departments each year for sports- and recreation-related injuries (Centers for Disease Control and Prevention, 2002; Conn et al., 2003; Burt and Overpeck, 2001.

Person, Place, and Time Factors

In population-based studies, males have two to four times higher rates of sports- and recreation-related injury than females, and this seems to hold true across all age groups (Burt and Overpeck, 2001; Cassell et al., 2003; Centers for Disease Control and Prevention, 2002; Conn et al., 2003; Dempsey et al., 2005; Gabbe et al., 2005; Uitenbroek, 1996). However, in certain sports, women may have higher rates of select types of injuries (e.g., stress fractures in runners, or anterior cruciate ligament injuries in soccer). We discuss this further later in the chapter. Younger persons, especially 10- to 19-year olds, have the highest injury rates (Burt and Overpeck, 2001; Centers for Disease Control and Prevention, 2002; Conn et al., 2003; Dempsey et al., 2005; Ni et al., 2002), although older adults (age 65 years and older) have recently been identified as a potential high-risk group for sports- and recreation-related injuries (Gerson and Stevens, 2004). In general, few studies have investigated racial/ethnic disparities in sports- and recreation-related injury rates. However, two reports have suggested that Caucasians have 1.5 to 2 times higher rates than African-Americans. (Conn et al., 2003; Ni et al., 2002) Not unexpectedly, the most common places where sports- and recreation-related injuries occur are sports or recreation facilities, schools, and in and around the home (Conn et al., 2003; Ni et al., 2002; Finch et al., 1998). Information about the time of injuries (e.g., season, day of week, time of day) has been infrequently reported, although higher rates of sports injuries in the colder months in Sweden have been reported (Lindquist et al., 1996).

Injury Cause, Type, and Site Distribution

Activities reported as the most common cause of sports- and recreation-related injuries vary by gender and age. Among children, the leading cause of sports- and recreation-related injuries and hospitalizations are bicycling, team sports, and scooter and skateboarding injuries (Centers for Disease Control and Prevention, 2002; Conn et al., 2003; Burt and Overpeck, 2001; Ni et al., 2002; Dempsey et al., 2005). Among all adults, the leading causes

Table 14.1 Annual Injury Incidence Rates From Selected Population-Based Studies of Sports and Recreation-Related Injuries

Study	*Data source*	*Population*	*Injury severity indicator*	*Annual injury incidence estimate*
Gabbe et al., 2005	Trauma Registry and Coroner's records	Victoria, Australia ≥15 years	(1) death, or (2) serious injury events (requiring ICU admission, surgery within 24 hours, or injury severity score >15 upon admission) caused by sports or recreation	1) 0.0006% 2) 0.002%
Dempsey et al., 2005	Hospital discharge records	Wisconsin, United States All ages	Inpatient hospitalizations using sports and recreation ICD injury E-codes	0.032%
Cassell et al., 2003	Medical records	Victoria, Australia All ages	Medically attended injury events: (1) Hospitalizations (2) Emergency Department (3) General Practitioner	(1) 0.16% (2) 1.7% (3) 1.9%
Burt and Overpeck, 2001	Medical records (NHAMCS*)	U.S. civilian, non-institutionalized 5–24 years	Emergency Department visits using text description for injury events	0.34%
Centers for Disease Control, 2002	Medical records (NEISS-AIP*)	U.S. civilian, non-institutionalized All ages	Emergency Department visits using consumer product codes and text description for injury events	1.6%
Gerson and Stevens, 2004	Medical records (NEISS-AIP*)	U.S. civilian, non-institutionalized ≥65 years	Emergency Department visits using consumer product codes and text description for injury events	0.18%
Ni et al., 2002	Personal interview (NHIS*)	U.S. civilian, non-institutionalized 6–17 years	Verbatim text description for self-reported injury events translated to ICD injury E-codes	0.91%
Conn et al., 2003	Personal interview (NHIS*)	U.S. civilian, non-institutionalized ≥18 years	Verbatim text description for self-reported, medically treated injury events translated to ICD injury E-codes	0.26%
Mummery et al., 1998	Telephone interview (ASRIS*)	Alberta, Canada 6–93 years	Self-reported, medically attended sports and recreation-related injuries	11%
Uitenbroek, 1996	Telephone interview	Glascow and Edinburgh Scotland, United Kingdom 18–60 years	Self-reported, activity-limiting injury caused by sports or exercise during the past month	20%**

*NHAMCS: National Hospital Ambulatory Medical Care Survey; NEISS-AIP: National Electronic Injury Surveillance System All Injury Program; NHIS: National Health Interview Survey; ASRIS: Alberta Sport and Recreation Injury Survey; ICU: intensive care unit.

**Monthly incidence multiplied by 12 for annualized estimate; estimate may be inflated, interpret with caution.

of sports- and recreation-related injuries are team and recreational sports and general exercise (Conn et al., 2003; Dempsey et al., 2005), whereas adults over age 65 years also report cycling and golfing as common causes of injury (Gerson and Stevens, 2004). Males tend to sustain injuries while participating in team sports such as football, basketball, soccer, and baseball and while skateboarding or riding scooters. Females tend to report injuries from a wider variety of activities such as sports (basketball, soccer, gymnastics, and softball), bicycling, playground activities, and general exercise (Burt and Overpeck, 2001; Centers for Disease Control and Prevention, 2002; Conn et al., 2003; Ni et al., 2002).

In general, most sports and recreation injuries are classified as sprains, strains, contusions, and open wounds (Burt and Overpeck, 2001; Conn et al., 2003; Gerson and Stevens, 2004; Ni et al., 2002). Among older adults, fractures are common, especially among women (Gerson and Stevens, 2004). About two-thirds of injuries occur to the extremities: 20% to 30% to the upper extremity and 35% to 75% to the lower extremity. The most common extremity sites injured are the ankle, knee, and foot (Conn et al., 2003; Ni et al., 2002; Hootman et al., 2002a). Head and neck injuries may account for up to 25% of all sports- and recreation-related injuries, equating to more than 1 million injuries annually (Conn et al., 2003). These injuries can not only be severe but sometimes catastrophic, resulting in death, hospitalization, and morbidity more often than injuries to other body sites (Cassell et al., 2003; Mueller, 2001).

Injury Severity and Impact

Because they are usually self-limiting and rarely require hospitalization, most sports- and recreation-related injuries are considered minor in terms of severity (Centers for Disease Control and Prevention, 2002; Ni et al., 2002; Conn et al., 2003). Despite this, some injuries such as anterior cruciate ligament tears are serious, requiring expensive surgical treatment and long-term rehabilitation and potentially may lead to early onset degenerative joint disease (Nebelung and Wuschech, 2005; Roos, 2005). Even ankle sprains that do not require surgery have been associated with long-term disability and activity limitation (Marchi et al., 1999). Fatal and catastrophic activity-related injuries do happen, usually in collision and contact sports such as football, track and field, baseball, and cheerleading, although rarely (Mueller, 2001; Boden et al., 2003). The good news is that because of changes in rules, improved equipment design and usage, facility management, and coaching and technological advances, fatalities in football have declined in the past two decades.

In addition, some injuries may have significant impact on individuals and society in terms of lost school and workdays. About 20% to 25% of children with sports and recreation injuries miss 1 to 5 days of school (Ni et al., 2002; Conn et al., 2003), and one-third of parents may have to take time off work because of their child's injury (Abernethy and McAuley, 2003). Among adults, 17% to 28% report missing at least 1 day of work because of a sport- or recreation-related injury (Conn et al., 2002; Hootman et al., 2002a).

Dose–Response Relationships

Physical Activity Dose and Musculoskeletal Injury

Common sense suggests that to be at risk for an activity-related injury, one must first be physically active. This is generally true, because the probability of sustaining an activity-related injury does increase with increasing dose of activity. However, data from a retrospective cohort study of adults enrolled in the Aerobics Center Longitudinal Study (Hootman et al., 2002a) has suggested that there may be a baseline risk of activity-related injuries even among those who classify themselves as sedentary: As many as 16% of inactive adults sustained an

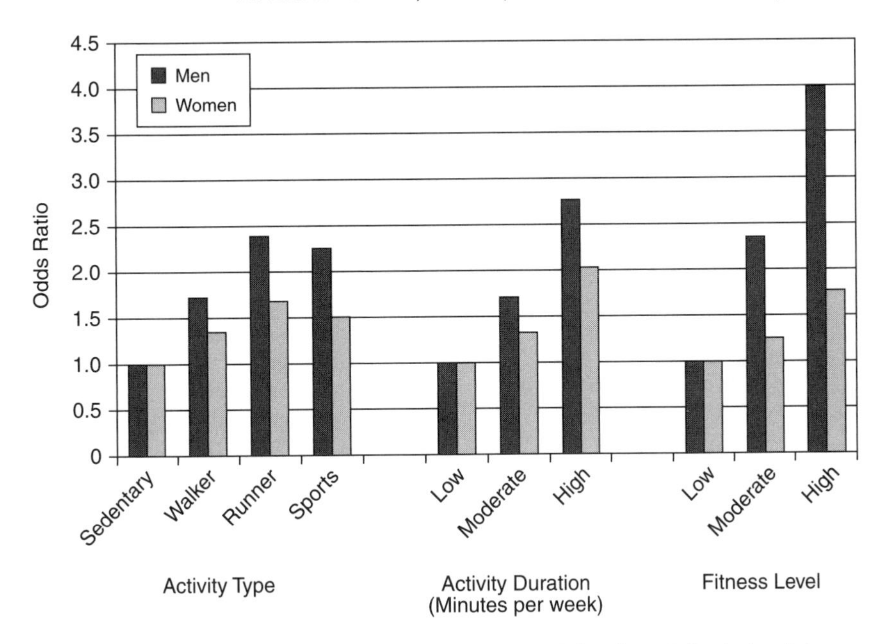

Figure 14.1 The dose–response relationship between type and duration of physical activity, cardiorespiratory fitness, and activity-related musculoskeletal injuries among adult men and women. All odds ratios are adjusted for age, body mass index, previous injury, and participation in weight training, stretching, and calisthenic exercises at least twice a week. (Adapted from Hootman et al., 2000.)

activity-related injury in a 12-month period. At first glance, this may seem counterintuitive. But most likely, this means that persons who classify their "usual" activity level as inactive or sedentary may on limited occasions actually engage in sports or exercise, such as on weekends, at church, or at social gatherings, and so forth. This interesting finding suggests that there may not be a completely linear relationship between physical activity and exercise dose and risk of injury.

Figure 14.1 shows the dose relationship for cardiorespiratory fitness and several "dose" measures of physical activity and the likelihood of reporting an activity-related injury. Compared to those classified as sedentary, adults who engage in running and vigorous sports have two to three times higher risk of injury than their sedentary peers (Hootman et al., 2000), and the odds of injury increase with increased duration (minutes per week) of activity. In contrast, the same phenomenon has not been consistently demonstrated among walkers. Several studies have reported that walking is a lower injury-risk activity, especially compared to running and sports participation (Macera et al., 1989; Macera, 1992; van Mechelen, 1992; Jones et al., 1994; Colbert et al., 2000; Hootman et al., 2000; Hootman et al., 2002b), and injury risk does not seem to increase among walkers who walked at levels (at least 30 minutes/day) recommended by public health agencies (Colbert et al., 2000).

One additional issue to consider is the possibility that persons with high cardiorespiratory and muscular fitness may be somewhat protected from injuries because of the fact that their musculoskeletal systems are stronger and more efficient. One way to examine this is to examine the probability of injury with different activity levels while simultaneously adjusting for fitness level. Data from the Aerobics Center Longitudinal Study depicted in Figure 14.2 indicate that the probability of injury may actually be lower per unit of exposure among those with higher levels of exposure. To illustrate this concept we can look at two hypothetical subjects, one who is "low active" and one who is "high active," and calculate their probability of injury adjusted for age, sex, body mass index, previous injury history, and fitness level. The low-active person expends about 2,000 kcal/week in exercise, and their

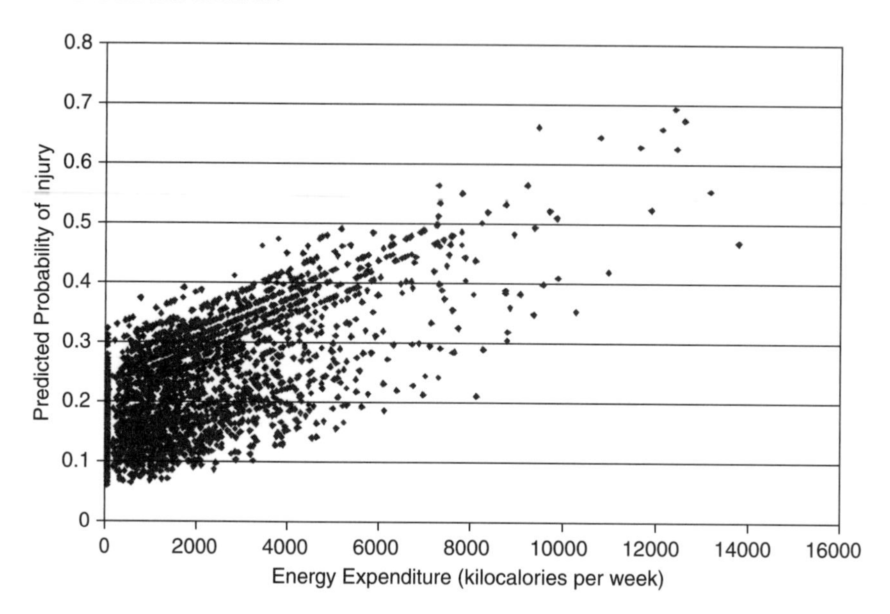

Figure 14.2 Adjusted predicted probability of activity-related musculoskeletal injury per level of energy expenditure spent in leisure-time physical activity per week.*
* Unpublished data from 6311 men and women subjects in the Aerobics Center Longitudinal Study, Dallas, TX. Predicted probability of injury adjusted for age, gender, body mass index, previous injury status, and fitness level.

overall probability of injury is 0.22. The high-active person expends about 10,000 kcal/week, and their probability of injury is 0.65. The probability of injury per 1,000 kcal/week of energy expenditure for the low-active person is 0.11 and for the high-active person is 0.065. So, the high-active person actually has a lower probability of injury per unit of energy expenditure than the less active person.

Cardiorespiratory Fitness Levels and Musculoskeletal Injury

Few studies in the general population have investigated the relationship between cardiorespiratory fitness levels and the occurrence of activity-related injuries. Looking again at the data depicted in Figure 14.2, higher fitness levels (measured here by energy expenditure in kilocalories per week) are associated with an increased likelihood of activity-related injury. This makes intuitive sense, because to gain cardiorespiratory fitness beyond a genetically determined baseline, one must engage in exercise with sufficient intensity and duration to elicit a physiological adaptation response (American College of Sports Medicine, 1998). The more one is exposed to physical activity or exercise, the greater one's chance of sustaining an activity-related injury (Macera et al., 1989; van Mechelen et al., 1992; Brill and Macera, 1995; Hootman et al., 2000; Hootman et al., 2002b).

Thus, a related question of interest is: When undertaking the same amount of physical activity or exercise, does the level of physical fitness influence the incidence of activity-related injury? Among military recruits entering basic training, those with a low fitness level at entry are two to three times more likely to sustain a training-related injury during basic training (Jones and Knapik, 1999; Centers for Disease Control and Prevention, 2000; Knapik et al., 2001). This suggests that higher fitness mitigates the risk of injury among individuals who are exposed to an identical amount of physical activity, as is the case in military recruits.

In summary, for the general population, persons with high fitness levels are more likely to sustain an activity-related injury because they are exposed to more opportunities for potential injury, in the course of achieving and maintaining their fitness level. However, highly active persons may have a lower risk of injury per unit of exposure, suggesting that fitness may act as a potential protective factor for injury.

Risk Factors for Activity-Related Injuries

In the next section, we discuss risk factors for activity-related injuries. We focus on potentially modifiable risk factors—that is, factors that may be manipulated to reduce one's risk of activity-related injury while allowing them to participate in sufficient exercise to gain fitness and health benefits.

Non-Modifiable Risk Factors

For select sporting activities, males have higher overall sports- and recreation-related injury rates, but in the general population, no consistent gender differences have been reported (Macera, 1992; van Mechelen et al., 1992; van Mechelen et al., 1996; Dane et al., 1997; Hootman et al., 2002a; Tauton et al., 2003). However, select types of sports injuries, such as anterior cruciate ligament knee injuries and stress fractures, are more commonly reported among high school and collegiate female athletes (Arendt and Dick, 1995; Nattiv, 2000; Agel et al., 2005), and the distribution of injuries by body site may differ between genders (van Mechelen, 1992; Hootman et al., 2002a). Race and ethnicity has been inadequately studied in regard to activity-related injuries. Cross-sectional studies have reported higher injury rates for Caucasians compared to African-Americans, but this has not been validated in a prospective study design (Conn et al., 2003; Ni et al., 2002). Most studies have suggested that age is not consistently associated with activity-related injuries; however, some studies have only studied adults within a limited age range and, subsequently, may not be able to definitively examine the age–injury relationship. One explanation for this may be that age can modify the effect of physical activity on the risk of injury. Colbert et al. (2000) reported that the risk of injury was somewhat attenuated among younger men in their study of runners and walkers. Male walkers less than age 45 years had a 25% reduced risk of injury compared to male runners of the same age, whereas older male walkers (ages 45 years and older) had a 36% reduced risk. No similar trend was noted among women.

Modifiable Risk Factors

Age, gender, and race/ethnicity, although important risk factors for many diseases as well as injury, are non-modifiable risk factors. In contrast, the most commonly identified modifiable risk factors for activity-related injury include previous injury, excess body mass, and training-related factors (activity type, dose, terrain, etc.).

Having a history of a previous musculoskeletal injury is one of the strongest and most consistently reported risk factors for future injuries. Persons who report a positive injury history are three to five times more likely to have a subsequent musculoskeletal injury (Macera et al., 1989; van Mechelen, 1992; Colbert et al., 2000; Hootman et al., 2000; Hootman et al., 2002b). Although an individual cannot change the fact of a previous injury, what can be done is to ensure that one has adequately recovered, including ensuring no pain or swelling is present and the individual has returned to full function (range-of-motion, strength, endurance, etc.), and that one slowly progresses back to normal activity. In a large study, only 25% of persons who reported an activity-related injury stated performing rehabilitation exercises post-injury, (Hootman et al., 2002a), and in another study, 42% of those who reported a previous injury stated they were not completely rehabilitated upon starting a 13-week training program (Tauton et al., 2003), despite the fact that therapeutic rehabilitation has shown to be effective for a variety of musculoskeletal injuries and conditions.

Excess body mass may interfere with the normal center of gravity, proprioception, and neuromuscular processing during human movement and, thus, may play a role in activity-related injuries (Spyropoulos et al., 1991; McGraw et al., 2000; Whitting and Zernicke, 1998). In addition, having higher body mass may generate higher forces that may lead to more frequent—and possibly more severe—injuries to joints and other soft tissue during falls. Overweight and obese persons may also have lower fitness levels and, therefore, may not be able to respond to potential injurious events quickly enough to prevent or mitigate an injury (Whitting and Zernicke, 1998).

Body size has been inconsistently associated with activity-related injury. Both low and high body mass have been related to injury among men and women (Macera et al., 1989; Colbert et al., 2000; Hootman et al., 2002b; Tauton et al., 2003). One explanation of this phenomenon is that the distribution of body fat mass is gender-dependent and, coupled with the biomechanical alignment differences between males and females (females have wider hip/pelvis, greater genu valgum, and tibial torsion, etc.), may effectively cause excess body mass to differentially affect injury risk among women (Whitting and Zernicke, 1998). High body mass is expected to produce a proportional increase in impact and joint loading forces, possibly resulting in injury. Low body mass may be associated with hypocaloric intake, excessive energy expenditure, or both, which may adversely affect bone and soft tissue resistance to injurious forces and subsequent ability to repair.

The factors associated with increased risk of activity-related injuries that may be the most modifiable are primarily related to exercise training parameters or "activity dose." Later in this chapter, we discuss factors that are related to the measurement of exposure in epidemiological studies of activity-related injuries in more detail. With regard to modifiable risk factors for injury, several dose-related issues are important to discuss. Looking back at Figure 14.1, we can see that an increasing total dose of activity, as measured by kilocalorie per week of energy expenditure in leisure-time physical activity, is associated with an increased probability of injury. This phenomenon has been consistently reported using various measures of exposure time, such as total running or walking mileage per week, minutes per week of activity, frequency of activity, pace or speed, and so forth, in both the military and civilian populations (Macera, 1992; van Mechelen 1992; Brill et al., 1995; Centers for Disease Control and Prevention, 2000; Colbert et al., 2000; Hootman et al., 2000; Hootman et al., 2002b).

Figure 14.3 illustrates injury incidence data from a classic exercise training study conducted about 25 years ago. Here, a clear increased incidence of injury occurred with both increasing frequency (1, 3, or 5 days/week) and increasing duration (15, 30, or 45 minutes/session) of exercise training (Pollock et al., 1977). This study was conducted in a restricted population of prison inmates and may not be generalizable to the typical adult. However, it is of historical importance because it illustrates the importance of balancing exercise benefits (e.g., gains in cardiorespiratory health) with exercise risks (e.g., incidence of injuries).

The same concept of risk–benefit has been illustrated in other studies of community-dwelling adults who engage in habitual physical activity. Adults who accumulate more than 20 miles/week of walking, jogging, or running are twice as likely to report a musculoskeletal injury over 12 months compared to those who accumulate a moderate "dose" of activity (less than 20 miles/week) (Macera et al., 1989; Macera, 1992; Hootman et al., 2002b). Not only does the total dose of activity relate to injury risk but the type and intensity of activity also may play a role. Walkers have a 50% reduced risk of activity-related injury compared to runners, and those

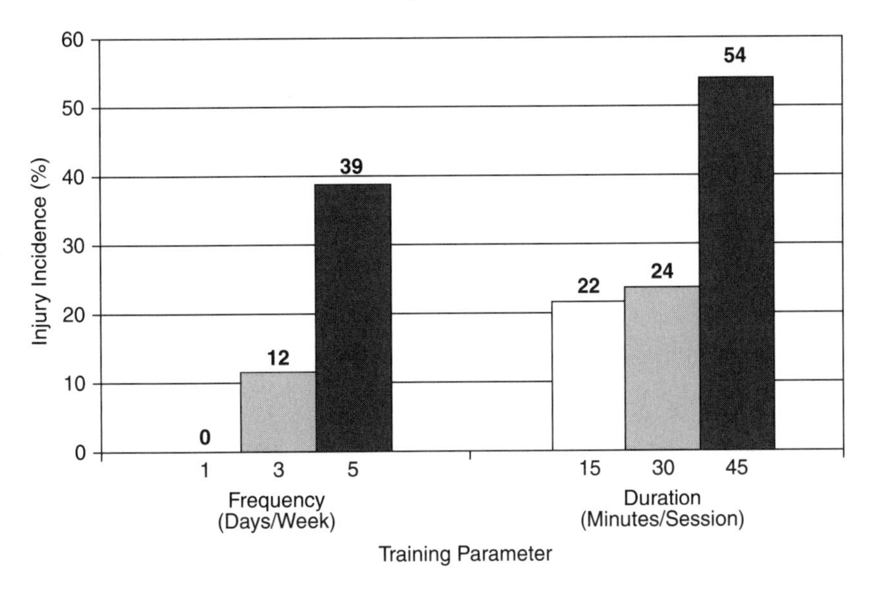

Figure 14.3 Injury incidence by training frequency and duration among inmates participating in an exercise training study. (From Pollock et al., 1977.)

who run or walk at a faster pace (<15 minutes/mile) have a higher risk of injury (Colbert et al., 2000; Hootman et al., 2002b) To date, no prospective, community-based injury prevention studies have been conducted to evaluate whether modifying activity dose parameters can impact the overall injury rate. However, studies in the military population have reported significant reductions in the risk of stress fractures with injury prevention programs aimed at limiting running distance during basic training (Jones and Knapik, 1999).

Methodological Issues to Consider in Studies of Physical Activity and Injury

Unlike other diseases such as diabetes or heart disease, there are no standardized measures of outcome in studies of musculoskeletal injury. Equally difficult is defining, collecting, and measuring the relevant information needed to classify exposure in epidemiological studies of physical activity and exercise. Despite the fact that experts have cited the need for standardized definitions in injury research for over a decade (van Mechelen et al., 1992; van Mechelen, 1997; Meeuwisse and Love, 1997; Finch, 1997; Wills and Leathem, 2001), there is still a considerable amount of heterogeneity in outcome and exposure definitions used in the published literature, and subsequently, the results from different studies cannot be directly compared. In this next section, we discuss some of the issues associated with defining outcomes and exposures in epidemiologic studies of physical activity and injury.

Definition of Outcome: Injury

The definition of injury used may vary by the source of the data (e.g., medical system encounters), the activity at the time of the injury (e.g., running), the place the injury occurred (e.g., playground), the cause of injury (e.g., fall), the severity (e.g., time lost from participation), and a whole host of other variables. One size may not fit all when it comes to injury definitions. For example, in studies of high school and collegiate athletic populations, many feel it is most important to capture injuries that result in time lost from competition or practice, because this captures an aspect of injury severity. As such, the National Collegiate Athletic Association and the National Athletic Trainers Association have traditionally used a "time-loss"-based definition in their injury surveillance programs (Arendt and Dick, 1995; Powell and Barber-Foss, 1999; Powell and Barber-Foss, 2000; Agel et al., 2005).

These organized sports injury surveillance systems, as well as those in the military, depend on trained medical personnel and/or medical records to capture injury events and record injury data. This would be almost impossible to do in the general population because many injury events are never brought to the attention of a health-care provider. Therefore, injury surveillance studies in the general population usually define injuries based on: *(1)* documented contact with the medical system (emergency room visits, insurance claims, etc.) or *(2)* self-reported events (*see* Tables 14.1 and 14.2 for examples of data sources and definitions of injury outcomes and exposure reported in the literature).

Injury definitions based on medical encounters usually capture only the most severe injuries and cannot be linked to exposure data. Self-reported injuries have the added benefit that different levels of severity can be used (stopped or changed activity level, required medical treatment, missed work or school because of injury, etc.) to create operational definitions of an injury event, and the event can then be linked with the exposure of interest (e.g., hours of exercise or physical activity participation per week). The drawback to self-reported injury definitions, as with any self-reported condition, is that they may be prone to recall bias. In the sports community, research suggests that recall of the occurrence of injury events over a 12-month period is relatively accurate, although details of the injury (i.e., number, site, diagnosis, etc.) may not be as accurately recalled (Junge and Dvorak, 2000; Grimmer et al., 2000; Wills and Leathem, 2001; Gabbe et al., 2003; Valuri et al., 2005). The accuracy of activity-related injury recall among the general population is generally unknown. However, some research has suggested the accuracy of recall of other acute musculoskeletal events, such as fractures and motor vehicle crash-related injuries, in the general adult population is moderate to good (78%–86% agreement) (Begg et al., 1999; Ivers et al., 2002; Chen et al., 2004). Gathering information on the relative "severity" of an injury (limited activity >7 days, required medical attention and/or treatment, etc.) as well as using shorter recall periods may assist in reducing recall bias (Mock et al., 1999; Petridou et al., 2004).

It is very important to gather adequate information to be able to operationally define an injury event. One simple definition of injury is any "damage, caused by physical trauma, sustained by tissues of the body" (Whitting and Zernicke, 1998). If the goal is to capture "activity-related" injuries, then a clear definition of what is considered "activity-related" is a critical part of the injury definition. Because more serious events are better recalled, it may be helpful to include a minimum level of injury severity within the case definition. Severity may be determined in various ways, including pain level, the need for or type of medical care, injury severity indices used in trauma care, and level of activity limitation and/or disability.

Definition of Exposure: Physical Activity

As you have learned in previous chapters, in epidemiological studies, physical activity is often measured using self-reporting instruments, activity logs, or motion sensors. To create summary measures from self-reporting and exercise log data, standard intensity values (such as metabolic equivalents) are often assigned to each activity and, together with information on the frequency and duration of the activity, are mathematically combined to provide a quantitative score of the amount of energy expended. This method of calculation has its basis on the theory behind the cardiorespiratory, metabolic, and/or physiological effects

Table 14.2 Select Injury (Outcome) and Physical Activity (Exposure) Definitions Used in Sports and Recreation Injury Research

Study	*Population*	*Outcome definition*	*Exposure definition*
Special population studies			
Agel et al., 2005	Collegiate soccer and basketball athletes, national sample	Any event that required medical attention from a Certified Athletic Trainer or physician that resulted in restriction of participation for 1 day or more	One athlete participating in one game or practice where there is an opportunity for injury. Rates calculated using athlete-exposures as the denominator.
Powell and Barber-Foss, 2000	High school athletes, national sample of high schools	Any injury that resulted in loss of participation on that day or the next; all fractures, dental injuries, and mild traumatic brain injury	One coach-directed session that involves physical activity equals one athlete-exposure (opportunity for injury). Rates calculated using athlete-exposures as the denominator.
Beachy et al., 1987	High school athletes, one school in Hawaii	Any complaint that required the attention of a Certified Athletic Trainer	No exposure reported. Rates were calculated using the number of athletes as the denominator.
Knapik et al., 2001	U.S. Army recruits in basic training	Any event that resulted in damage to the body and required a visit to a medical provider	One soldier participating in 1 day of training. Rates were calculated using person-days as the denominator.
Community-based studies			
Hootman et al., 2000; Hootman et al., 2002a; Hootman et al., 2002b	Community-dwelling adults participating in a longitudinal study of health in Dallas, TX	(1) All-cause = any self-reported muscle, tendon, bone, joint or ligament injury; (2) any injury (as defined above) attributed to participation in physical activity and caused the participant to take medication, see a physician, or stop/change their exercise program	(1) Self-reported primary type of physical activity in past 12 months, categorized as sedentary, walkers, runners, or sports participants; (2) duration (hours per week of activity), frequency per week and intensity (pace); (3) weekly mileage (among runners and walkers).
Colbert et al., 2000	Community-dwelling adults participating in a longitudinal study of health in Dallas, TX	Any activity-related injury during past 12 months that required a physician visit	Self-reported running or walking during the past 3 months (dichotomized as walkers vs. runners).
Powell et al., 1998	National sample of community-dwelling U.S. adults with a telephone	Any self-reported injury occurring in the past 30 days while participating in selected physical activities	No specific exposure information. Incidence rates were calculated per 100 respondents.

Continued

Table 14.2 Select Injury (Outcome) and Physical Activity (Exposure) Definitions Used in Sports and Recreation Injury Research *(continued)*

Study	*Population*	*Outcome definition*	*Exposure definition*
van Mechelen et al., 1996	Community-dwelling adolescents participating in a longitudinal study in the Netherlands	Any injury occurring as a result of sports activity and caused at least one of the following consequences: (1) stopped sports activity; (2) could not fully participate in the next planned sports activity; (3) missed work the next day; (4) required medical attention	Hours of self-reported participation in sports activities (of ≥4 MET intensity) during a 12-month period.

of physical activity on the human body. In the case of musculoskeletal outcomes such as injury, such measures may not adequately capture the "dose" of activity delivered to the musculoskeletal system. Many different factors besides frequency, intensity, and duration of activity influence how a specific activity will affect an individual's risk of musculoskeletal injury and include type of activity (weight-bearing vs. non-weight-bearing, collision/contact vs. non-contact sports, etc.), biomechanical factors (torsional stress, compression forces, acceleration/deceleration, etc.), environmental factors (heat, playing surface, etc.), anatomic factors (pes planus, femoral anteversion, etc.), among others.

No standard measures of exposure have been adopted, despite the critical need advocated by experts in injury epidemiology (de Loes, 1997; Finch, 1997; van Mechelen, 1997) Researchers have begun, however, to develop scoring algorithms for self-reported physical activity epidemiological data in an attempt to capture a more accurate measure of the "dose" of activity delivered to the musculoskeletal system (Ainsworth et al., 2002; Kemper et al., 2002; Hootman et al., 2003).

Selected measures of exposure that have been used in epidemiological studies of activity-related injury are presented in Table 14.1. In studies of competitive athletics, the unit of exposure most often used is the athlete-exposure (AE). This unit of measurement is equivalent to one athlete participating in one session (game, practice, or training session) where there is an opportunity for injury. The drawback to using the AE measure is that it is a crude measure of time at risk for injury, because one athlete may participate in an entire football game, whereas another athlete may only participate in two to three individual plays during the game. These two athletes will have very different total time at risk for injury, but using the AE measurement unit, they both would be classified as having 1 AE unit for that game. The benefits to using the AE unit of measurement are: *(1)* it has been used in several sports injury surveillance systems, allowing for comparison of injury rates per AE unit across various studies, and *(2)* the data collection procedure is relatively easy and can likely be collected accurately by minimally trained personnel, such as coaches, parents, and team managers.

In studies of the general population, the concept of the AE can be measured by frequency or "bouts" of participation in various activities. For example, let's say in the past week an individual walked on the treadmill 5 days (five exposures), played softball 1 day (one exposure), rode a bike to class and back 3 days (six exposures), and went bowling once (one exposure). At the end of the week, the person would have had 13 opportunities to sustain an activity-related injury and thus would be considered to have accumulated 13 AE units. (However, in this instance, a better term to use may be "activity-exposure" instead of athlete-exposure.) As you can see, the AE measure is a simple concept and has been historically used to capture time at risk for injury. But the AE unit of measurement may not capture enough detail regarding an individual's true exposure status. Other units of measurement that can be used to capture more detailed levels of exposure include time (seconds, minutes, or hours) per week, days or sessions, kilocalories of energy expenditure, and activity counts from motion sensors. However, as noted earlier, these measures still do not incorporate other factors that may be important for injury (type of activity, biomechanical factors, environmental factors, etc.).

Confounding By Other Factors

In addition to the methodological issues discussed earlier, several factors may confound the activity–injury relationship:

- **Exposure to multiple activities.** Athletes and persons engaging in recreational or leisure-time physical activities may be participating in a variety (more than one sport/activity) of activities during a given time period. Most current research has classified subjects either by the activity considered to be their "primary" activity or by the activity in which the most time is spent. This may not adequately capture the differing exposures: one activity may have a higher risk for injury than another—for example, football vs. walking for exercise. Thus, injury attributed to the "primary" activity may, in fact, have resulted from other activities.
- **Time trends.** Because of changes in sports rules and regulations, advances in equipment design and technology, introduction of advanced physical training techniques, as well as the proliferation and change in intensity and level of play of women's sports, activity-related injury rates over time may not be directly comparable. For example, the rates of deaths and catastrophic head and neck injuries in football have declined significantly since the 1970s, which is mostly attributed to changes in rules (e.g., no spearing) and improvements in helmet design. More noticeably, over the past 20 years, women's sports have significantly changed to include more contact, higher levels of competition, as well as entry into traditionally male sports, such as wrestling.
- **Fitness vs. physical activity.** The current literature still has not resolved the concomitant roles of fitness and physical activity in the risk of activity-related injuries. Few studies have simultaneously measured both variables and, therefore, were unable to control for potential confounding. In addition, more work needs to be done to investigate how other risk factors (gender, age, excess body mass, etc.) influence fitness, physical activity, and injury risk.

Strategies to Reduce the Risk of Activity-Related Injuries

Earlier we identified some potentially modifiable risk factors for activity-related injuries. To date, no body of literature has clearly indicated "best practices" for injury prevention among the physically active; however, a few potential strategies have been studied. In the next section, we discuss two strategies for possible injury prevention initiatives: protection for persons with a history of previous injury and modification of training-related factors.

Previous Injury

Because a history of previous injury is the most often reported risk factor for sustaining a subsequent injury, targeting injury prevention interventions to those persons with a positive injury history can result in a reduction of the injury burden. For example, persons with a history of ankle sprains have been identified as a high-risk group for future sprains (Thacker et al., 1999). Interventions aimed at reducing the risk and severity of ankle injuries (ankle taping and bracing, therapeutic exercise, neuromuscular and balance training, etc.) have been shown to be most effective (approximately 50% reduced risk) among those with previous ankle injuries (Thacker et al., 1999; Handoll et al., 2001), suggesting the need for comprehensive dissemination of evidence-based interventions in this population.

Training Factors

Accumulation of more miles per week in training has been associated with increased injury incidence among runners (Yeung and Yeung, 2001). Few studies have prospectively intervened on this factor; however, data from community-based epidemiological studies and military studies suggest that modifying the amount of weekly training can effectively reduce the risk of activity-related injury (Yeung and Yeung, 2001). For example, several observational studies have reported that the risk of activity-related injury increases significantly for those who accumulate more than 20 miles/week of running mileage (Macera et al., 1989; Hootman et al., 2002b). In addition, Jones and Knapik (1999) reported that modification of the basic physical exercise training program, specifically limiting the running distance, resulted in a lower incidence of training-related injuries.

It is worth noting that the risk–benefit relationships for health-related physical activity and competition- or performance-related activity are not equivalent. Health benefits accrue at more modest levels of physical activity, such as the recommended 30 minutes of moderate-intensity activity on most days of the week (Pate et al., 2005; U.S. Department of Health and Human Services, 1995). Top-level performance by competitive athletes, however, requires much greater time and intensity of activity. Therefore, when health is the intended goal, somewhat less physical activity may be preferable because the risk of injury is less. The quantitative aspects of this trade-off, however, are poorly understood, and the interface among health, performance, and injuries deserves more attention.

Stretching immediately before engaging in activity is a common practice and is believed to protect against injury. Recently, however, this claim has been challenged in the scientific literature. A considerable body of evidence now suggests that pre-activity stretching provides no protection against an activity-related injury (Shrier, 1999; Yeung and Yeung, 2001; Herbert and Gabriel, 2002; Weldon and Hill, 2003; Thacker et al., 2004; Witvrouw et al., 2004). However, current studies on this topic have significant methodological weaknesses, including the lack of focused and well-controlled interventions and outcomes, and small sample sizes. Pre-activity stretching may have other benefits, such as serving as a "psychological warm-up" prior to activity or competition and reducing the pain threshold during muscle lengthening activities (Shrier, 1999; Yeung and Yeung, 2001; Herbert and Gabriel, 2002). In addition, evidence is still inconclusive about whether stretching at other times, besides prior to activity, is beneficial in terms of reducing injury risk (Shrier, 1999; Yeung and Yeung, 2001; Herbert and Gabriel, 2002).

Currently there is limited, but promising, evidence that suggests there is value in select strategies for reducing activity-related injuries:

- Screening for previous injury history and targeting those with positive histories for neuromuscular and balance exercise training programs and/or supportive devices or equipment may reduce the risk and severity of future injuries.
- Modifying training dose parameters (frequency, intensity, and/or duration), selecting appropriate activities (low-impact, non-contact or collision sports, etc.),

and maintaining adequate levels of neuromuscular and cardiorespiratory fitness may provide protection from activity-related injury.
- Pre-activity stretching does not likely protect against risk of activity-related injury.

Future Research Directions

Published studies on the topic of activity-related injuries basically fall into two categories: *(1)* "burden" estimates or injury surveillance studies and *(2)* etiologic studies or studies that are designed to elucidate risk factors for various types of injuries in special populations. Few studies have been published that address the development and evaluation of injury prevention interventions in both the general community and in specific sports and recreation settings. Three critical areas need to be addressed in future population-based research on activity-related injuries:

- Development and infusion of standardized methodological procedures into injury research field
  - Develop and implement methods to collect exposure information on large national health surveys.
  - Use consistent case definitions of injury and exposure, as well collect information on potential risk factors, across studies so that direct comparisons can be made.
- Conduct ongoing, population-based, activity-related injury research studies
  - Monitor injury trends and the prevalence of risk factors for activity-related injuries.
  - Identify potential high-risk groups to target for intervention.
  - Define the relationship between physical activity for health vs. physical activity for performance and the incidence of related injuries.
  - Determine and monitor long-term consequences of activity-related injuries.
  - Estimate the costs (direct and indirect) of activity-related injuries.
- Develop, test, and implement interventions that address activity-related injury prevention in the community
  - Disseminate targeted health promotion messages.
  - Develop methods to use surveillance data to evaluate prevention initiatives.
  - Monitor prevention effectiveness.

Personal Perspective

The Surgeon General's Report (U. S. Department of Health and Human Services, 1996) and the Centers for Disease Control and Prevention/American College of Sports Medicine (Pate et al., 2005) physical activity recommendations have been promoted now for about a decade. The benefits of physical activity and exercise for the prevention and treatment of a variety of health conditions and overall mortality reduction are well-known. Less research has investigated the risks of physical activity, including injury (as discussed in this chapter), and exercise. Current knowledge suggests the risk–benefit ratio sides heavily in favor of the health benefits of physical activity. However, without adequate information on specific high-risk populations and associated factors, it is impossible to assess the balance between risks and benefits. The good news is that the data suggest it is possible to choose types and amounts of physical activity that will lessen one's risk of injury. Therefore, it is crucial for health practitioners, exercise specialists, and public health personnel to work together to provide the general public with evidence-based information to help them become physically active at levels that benefit health, while staying injury-free.

References

Abernethy L, McAuley D. 2003. Impact of school sports injury. *Br J Sports Med* 37(4): 354–55.

American College of Sports Medicine. 1998. The recommended quantity and quality of exercise for developing and maintaining cardiorespiratory and muscular fitness, and flexibility in healthy adults. *Med Sci Sports Exerc* 30(6): 975–91.

Agel J, Arendt EA, Bershadsky B. 2005. Anterior cruciate ligament injury in national collegiate athletic association basketball and soccer: a 13-year review. *Am J Sports Med* 33(4): 524–30.

Ainsworth BE, Shaw JM, Hueglin S. 2002. Methodology of activity surveys to estimate mechanical loading on bones in humans. *Bone* 30(5): 787–91.

Arendt EA, Dick R. 1995. Knee injury patterns among men and women in collegiate basketball and soccer: NCAA data and review of literature. *Am J Sports Med* 23(6): 694–701.

Beachy G, Akau CK, Martinson M, Olderr TF. 1987. High school sports injuries: A longitudinal study at Punahou School, 1988–1996. *Am J Sports Med* 25(5): 675–81.

Begg DJ, Langley JD, Williams SM. 1999. Validity of self-reported crashes and injuries in a longitudinal study of young adults. *Injury Prevention* 5(2): 142–44.

Boden BP, Tacchetti R, Mueller FO. 2003. Catastrophic cheerleading injuries. American Journal of Sports Medicine 31(6): 881–88.

Brill PA, Macera CA. 1995. The influence of running patterns on running injuries. *Sports Medicine* 20(6): 365–68.

Burt CW, Overpeck MD. 2001. Emergency visits for sports-related injuries. *Ann Emerg Med* 37(3): 301–8.

Cassell EP, Finch CF, Stathakis VZ. 2003. Epidemiology of medically treated sports and active recreation injuries in Latrobe Valley, Victoria, Australia. *Br J Sports Med* 37: 405–9.

Centers for Disease Control and Prevention. 2000. Exercise-related injuries among women: Strategies for prevention from civilian and military studies. *MMWR* 49(RR02): 13–33.

Centers for Disease Control and Prevention. 2002. Nonfatal sports- and recreation-related injuries treated in emergency departments -- United States, July 2000–June 2001. *MMWR* 51(33): 736–40.

Chen Z, Kooperberg C, Pettinger MB, et al. 2004. Validity of self-report for fractures among a multiethnic cohort of postmenopausal women: results from the Women's Health Initiative observational study and clinical trials. *Menopause* 11(3): 264–74.

Colbert LH, Hootman JM, Macera CA. 2000. Physical activity-related injuries in walkers and runnes in the Aerobics Center Longitudinal Study. *Clin J Sports Med* 10: 259–63.

Conn JM, Annest JL, Gilchrist J. 2003. Sports and recreation-related injuries episodes in the U.S. population, 1997-99. *Injury Prevention* 9: 117–23.

Dane S, Can S, Gursoy R, and Ezirmik N. 2004. Sport injuries: relations to sex, sport, injured body region. *Perception Motor Skills* 98(2): 519–24.

de Loes M. Exposure data: Why are they needed? 1997. *Sports Med* 24(3): 172–75.

Dempsey Rl, Layde PM, Laud PW, Guse CE, Hargarten SW. 2005. Incidence of sports and recreation related injuries resulting in hospitalization in Wisconsin in 2000. *Injury Prevention* 11: 91–6.

Finch C. An overview of some definitional issues for sports injury surveillance. 1997. *Sports Med* 24(3): 157–63.

Finch C, Owen, N, Price R. 2001. Current injury or disability as a barrier to being more physically active. *Med Sci Sports Exerc* 33(5): 778–82.

Gabbe BJ, Finch CF, Bennell KL, Wajswelner H. 2003. How valid is a self reported 12 month sports injury history? *Br J Sports Med* 37(6): 545–47.

Gabbe BJ, Finch CF, Cameron PA, Williamson OD. 2005. Incidence of serious injury and death during sport and recreation activities in Victoria, Australia. *Br J Sports Med* 39: 573–7.

Gerson LW, Stevens JA. 2004. Recreational injuries among older Americans, 2001. *Injury Prev* 10: 134–8.
Grimmer K, Williams J, Pitt M. 2000. Reliability of adolescents' self-report of recent recreational injury. *J Adolesc Health* 27(4): 273–5.
Herbert RD, Gabriel M. 2002. Effects of stretching before and after exercising on muscle soreness and risk of injury: systematic review. *Br Med J* 325(7362): 468.
Hootman, JM, Macera CA, Ainsworth BE, Martin M, Addy CL, Blair SN. 2000. Association among physical activity level, cardiorespiratory fitness and risk of musculoskeletal injury. *Am J Epidemiol* 154(3): 251–8.
Hootman, JM, Macera CA, Ainsworth BE, Martin M, Addy CL, Blair SN. 2002a. Epidemiology of musculoskeletal injuries among sedentary and physically active adults. *Med Sci Sports Exerc* 34(5): 838–44.
Hootman, JM, Macera CA, Ainsworth BE, Martin M, Addy CL, Blair SN. 2002b. Predictors of lower extremity injury among recreationally active adults. *Clin J Sports Med* 12: 99–106.
Hootman JM, Macera CA, Helmick CG, Blair SN. 2003. Influence of physical activity-related joint stress on the risk of self-reported hip/knee osteoarthritis: a new method to quantify physical activity. *Prev Med* 36(5): 636–44.
Ivers RQ, Cumming RG, Mitchell P, Peduto AJ. 2002. The accuracy of self-reported fractures in older people. *J Clin Epidemiol* 55(5): 452–7.
Jones BH, Cowan DN, Knapik JJ. 1994. Exercise, training and injuries. *Sports Med*18(3): 202–14.
Jones BH Knapik JJ. 1999. Physical training and exercise-related injuries. Surveillance, research and injury prevention in military populations. *Sports Med* 27(2): 111–25.
Junge A Dvorak J. 2000. Influence of definition and data collection on the incidence of injuries in football. *Am J Sports Med* 28(5 Suppl): S40–6.
Kemper HCG, Bakker I, Twisk J, van Mechelen W. 2002. Validation of a physical activity questionnaire to measure the effect of mechanical strain on bone mass. *Bone* 30(5): 799–804.
King AC, Castro C, Wilcox S, Eyeler AA, Sallis JF, Brownson RC. 2000. Personal and environmental factors associated with physical inactivity among different racial-ethnic groups of U. S. middle-aged and older aged women. *Health Psychology* 19(4): 354–64.
Knapik JJ, Sharp MA, Canham-Chervak M, Hauret K, Patton JF, Jones BH. 2001. Risk factors for training-related injuries among men and women in basic combat training. *Med Sci Sports Exerc* 33(6): 946–54.
Macera C. 1992.Lower extremity injuries in runners: Advances in prediction. *Sports Med* 13(1): 50–7.
Macera CA, Jackson KL, Hagenmaier GW, Kronefeld JJ, Kohl HW, Blair SN. 1989. Age, physical activity, physical fitness, body composition, and incidence of orthopedic problems. *Res. Quarter Exerc Sport* 60(3): 225–33.
Macera CA, Pate RR, Powell KE, Jackson KL, Kendrick JS, Craven TE. 1989. Predicting lower-extremity injuries among habitual runners. *Arch Intern Med* 149: 2565–8.
Marchi AG, Di Bello D, Messi G, Gazzola G. 1999. Permanent sequelae in sports injuries: a population based study. *Arch Dis Children* 81(4): 324–8.
McGraw B, McClenaghan BA, Williams HG, Dickerson J, Ward DS. 2000. Gait and postural stability in obese and nonobese prepubertal boys. *Arch Phys Med Rehab* 81(4): 484–9.
Meeuwisse WH, Love EJ. Athletic injury reporting: Development of universal systems. 1997. *Sports Med.* 24(3): 184–204.
Mock C, Acheampong F, Adjei S, Koepsell T. 1999. The effect of recall on estimation of incidence rates for injury in Ghana. *Intern J Epidemiol* 28(4): 750–5.
Mueller FO. 2001. Catastrophic head injuries in high school and collegiate sports. *J Athl Train* 36(3): 312–5.
Nattiv A. Stress fractures and bone health in track and field athletes. 2000. *J Sci Med Sport* 3(3): 268–79.
Nebelung W, Wuschech H. 2005. Thirty-five years of follow-up of anterior cruciate ligament-deficient knees in high-level athletes. *Arthroscopy* 21(6): 696–702.
Ni H, Barnes P, Hardy AM. 2002. Recreational injury and its relation to socioeconomic status among school aged children in the US. *Injury Prev* 8(1): 60–5.
Pate RR, Pratt M, Blair SN, et al. 1995. Physical activity and public health: A recommendation from the Centers for Disease Control and Prevention and the American College of Sports Medicine. *JAMA* 273(5): 402–07.

Petridou E, Dessypris N, Frangakis CE, Belechri M, Mavrou A, Trichopoulos D. 2004. Estimating the population burden of injuries: a comparison of household surveys and emergency department surveillance. *Epidemiology* 15(4): 428–32.

Pollock ML, Gettman LR, Milesis CA, Bah MD, Durstine L, Johnson, RB. 1977. Effects of frequency and duration of training on attrition and incidence of injury. *Med Sci Sports Exerc* 9(1): 31–6.

Powell JW, Barber-Foss KD. 2000. Sex-related injury patterns among selected high school sports. *Am J Sports Med* 28(3): 385–91.

Powell JW, Barber-Foss KD. 1999. Traumatic brain injury in high school athletes. *JAMA* 282(10): 958–63.

Powell KE, Heath GW, Kresnow MJ, Sacks JJ, Branche CM. 1998. Injury rates from walking, gardening, weightlifting, outdoor bicycling and aerobics. *Med Sci Sports Exerc* 30(8): 1246–9.

Roos EM. Joint injury causes knee osteoarthritis in young adults. 2005. *Curr Opin Rheumatol* 17(2): 195–200.

Shrier I. 1999. Stretching before exercise does not reduce the risk of local muscle injury: a critical review of the clinical and basic science literature. *Clin J Sports Med* 9(4): 221–7.

Spyropoulos P, Pisciotta JC, Pavlou KN, Cairns MA, Simon, SR. 1991. Biomechanical gait analysis in obese men. *Arch Phys Med Rehab* 72(13): 1065–70.

Tauton JE, Ryan MB, Clement DB, McKenzie DC, Lloyd-Smith DR, Zumbo BD. 2003. A prospective study of running injuries: the Vancoucer Sun Run "In Training" clinics. *Br J Sports Med* 37(3): 239–44.

Thacker SB, Gilchrist J, Stroup DF, Kimsey CD Jr. 2004. The impact os stretching on sports injury risk: a systematic review of the literature. *Med Sci Sports Exerc* 36(3): 371–8.

Uitenbroek DG. 1996. Sports, exercise and other causes of injuries: Results of a population study. *Res Quarter Exerc Sport* 67(4): 380–5.

U.S. Department of Health and Human Services. 1996. Centers for Disease Control and Prevention, National Center for Chronic Disease Prevention and Health Promotion. *Physical Activity and Health: A Report of the Surgeon General*. Atlanta, GA: U. S. Department of Health and Human Services.

Valuri G, Stevenson M, Finch C, Hamer P, Elliott B. 2005. The validity of a four week self-recall of sports injuries. *Injury Prev* 11(3): 135–7.

van Mechelen W. 1997. Sports injury surveillance systems: 'One size fits all?'. *Sports Medicine* 24(3): 164–8.

van Mechelen W. 1992. Running injuries: A review of the epidemiological literature. *Sports Med* 14(5): 320–35.

van Mechelen W, Hlobil H, Kemper HCG. 1992. Incidence, severity, aetiology and prevention of sports injuries: a review of concepts. *Sports Med* 14(2): 82–99.

van Mechelen W, Twisk J, Molendijk A, Blom B, Snel J, Kemper HC. 1996. Subject-related risk factors for sports injuries: A 1-year prospective study in young adults. *Med Science Sports Exerc* 28(9): 1171–9.

Weldon SM, HIll RH. 2003. The efficacy of stretching for prevention of exercise-related injury: a systematic review of the literature. *Man Ther* 8(3): 141–50.

Whitting WC, Zernicke RF. 1998. *Biomechanics of Musculoskeletal Injury*. Champaign, IL: Human Kinetics.

Wills SM, Leathem JM. 2001. Sports-related brain injury research: Methodological difficulties associated with ambiguous terminology. *Brain Injury* 15(7): 645–8.

Witvrouw E, Mahieu N, Danneels L, McNair P. 2004. Stretching and injury prevention: an obscure relationship. *Sports Med* 34(7): 443–9.

Yeung EW, Yeung SS. 2001. A systematic review of interventions to prevent lower limb soft tissue running injuries. Cochrane Database of Systematic Reviews 3:CD001256.

III

Promoting Physical Activity

15 Evolution of Physical Activity Recommendations

William L. Haskell

Throughout much of recorded history, various physicians, healers, philosophers, educators, and scientists promoted the idea that leading a sedentary life contributed to disease and disability, whereas being physically active contributed to improved health, better physical and mental function, and increased longevity. These recommendations were not based on scientific study as we know it but, at least in some cases, on systematic observation and good clinical judgment. For example, in 1569 Hieronymus Mercurialis published the text, *The Art of Gymnastics Among the Ancients*, where he established the following exercise principles based on nearly 200 published works by Greek and Roman authors: People who are ill should not be given exercise that might aggravate existing conditions; special exercise should be prescribed on an individual basis for convalescence, and for weak and older patients; people who lead sedentary lives need exercise urgently, and each exercise should preserve the existing healthy state; exercise should not disturb the harmony among the principal humors; exercise should be suited to each part of the body; and all healthy people should exercise regularly (Mercurialis, 1569).

It was not until the eighteenth century that the quantitative measurements of simple biological responses to exercise, such as heart rate, were technologically possible (Gibbs, 1969) and not until the latter half of the nineteenth century that quantitative measurements of various physiological responses to exercise were published (Byford, 1855; Smith, 1861). During the middle of the nineteenth century, quantitative observational studies were first conducted evaluating the health effects of vigorous occupational exercise (Guy, 1843) and comparing college oarsmen with their sedentary counterparts (Morgan, 1873), demonstrating favorable mortality outcomes for the more physically active men. Thus, by the start of the twentieth century, very preliminary scientific data were available indicating that moderate- or vigorous-intensity exercise resulted in a number of physiological changes and that frequent participation in physical activity might reduce morbidity and mortality caused by various diseases.

This chapter focuses on the scientific rationale and evolution of guidelines and recommendations made by various government agencies or professional organizations regarding the role of physical activity or physical fitness in promoting good health. Emphasis is given to the development of guidelines in the United States between 1970 and 2005. Also provided is a brief overview of the rapidly evolving science of physical activity and health—especially in the United States—during the 1900s that preceded and supported the development of guidelines by major organizations.

The Developing Scientific Basis for Relating Physical Activity to Health: United States 1900–1950

Our current understanding of the health benefits of a physically active lifestyle has been derived from a number of sources but especially from the sciences of exercise physiology and the epidemiology of physical activity and physical fitness. More recently other sciences, ranging from molecular biology to psychology, have made significant contributions to this understanding. Interestingly, exercise physiology and physical activity epidemiology developed quite independently during much of the twentieth century, with a more prolific development of exercise physiology during the first half of the century. It was only during the second half of the century that data from these two key sources began to be integrated into the science of "physical activity and health."

Starting in the late nineteenth and early in the twentieth centuries, substantial research was initiated on the physiological responses to exercise—especially of the muscular, respiratory, cardiovascular, and metabolic systems, with a focus on regulatory mechanisms (Franz, 1900; McCurdy, 1901). Initially much of the research was on the acute responses to walking, running, and cycling, but as the research progressed, the effects of exercise training on physical performance and various physiological responses were investigated, initially in athletes (Buchanan, 1909) and later in healthy men (Schneider and Ring, 1941). Along with the increasing volume of research in exercise physiology during 1900 to 1950, data, although somewhat more limited, continued to be published in the field of physical activity epidemiology. Such reports demonstrated the health benefits of being physically active primarily at work (Silversten, 1922; Headley, 1939) but also at play (Hartley, 1939). This early research on the physiology and epidemiology of physical activity provided the scientific basis for evolving hypotheses regarding the potential health benefits of remaining physical active.

Research Conducted During 1950 to 1960s, Prior to National Recommendations

During the 1950s and 1960s, research in both exercise physiology—particularly the health-related effects of exercise—and physical activity epidemiology continued to expand and improve in quality along with new study designs, technology, and statistical methods. In exercise physiology, studies were conducted evaluating the effects of exercise training on such outcomes as blood lipids (Holloszy, 1964), blood pressure (Mann, 1969), body composition (Pollock, 1969), and cardiorespiratory function (Saltin, 1968).

It was during this time that research was initiated addressing the dose of exercise required for specific biological outcomes. Karvonen (1957) in Finland presented data supporting the idea that for young men to improve their response to submaximal exercise (running speed to produce a specific heart rate), they needed to exercise at an intensity that produced an increase in their heart rate reserve of at least 66%. In addition to comparing exercise training regimens used by high-performance athletes, studies were conducted looking at the benefits of moderate-intensity activity such as walking (Pollock, 1969).

A seminal event in physical activity epidemiology occurred in 1953 when Professor Jeremy Morris and colleagues first presented their hypothesis that vigorous exercise helped to protect against coronary heart disease (CHD; Morris, 1953) (*see* additional discussion in Chapter 1). They published data demonstrating that men in occupations that routinely required them to be physically active (double-decker bus conductors and postmen) developed less CHD than more sedentary men (bus drivers and postal clerks). Later, Morris and colleagues extended this hypothesis to include leisure-time physical activity (Morris, 1973). This hypothesis provided the framework for a rapid increase in the number of reports during the next two decades demonstrating that men in more physically demanding occupations generally had lower CHD and all-cause mortality rates (Breslow, 1960; Karvonen, 1961; Taylor, 1962; Kahn, 1963; Paffenbarger, 1970). Fox and Skinner published an early review of this research relating physical activity to CHD morbidity and mortality in 1964 (Fox and Skinner, 1964). It is interesting to note that in the summary of this review, the authors stated that although much more research was needed, the preliminary data suggested a protective effect of exercise and that "even light or a moderate amount of physical activity may have significance."

Stimulus for the Development of Physical Activity Guidelines in the United States in the 1970s

By the late 1960s in the United States, a substantial number of individuals and organizations had recognized the increasingly sedentary nature of the population and the negative health and fitness consequences of this decline in activity and were promoting their own interpretations of a good or best physical activity program. Substantial data from both observational and experimental studies supported the value of being more physically active throughout the lifespan, but no consensus existed on what programs were most effective and safe. Also, during the early 1960s, death rates from CHD were still on the rise in the United States and most technologically developed countries. There were few effective treatments for preventing sudden cardiac death, and it was well-established that the increased work of the heart during vigorous exercise could trigger cardiac arrest or myocardial infarction in persons with underlying coronary atherosclerosis. Because of a lack of understanding about the etiology of the atherothrombotic disease process, how to detect it in at-risk populations, and what types and intensities of exercise were safe, many people, including physicians, were very concerned about adults over age 45 years significantly increasing their physical activity, especially starting a vigorous exercise program or participating in athletic competition. It was this combined concern regarding the need for much of the population to increase their activity, but at the same time a fear that promoting such a program, if not carefully done, would cause many people to experience sudden cardiac death that precipitated the development of the initial guidelines and recommendations by various national organizations. As we will see, with the evolution of the guideline process over a 35-year period, the approach to reducing risk while maximizing benefit has been to develop clinically oriented recommendations for patients or "at-risk" populations and public health-oriented recommendations for the general public.

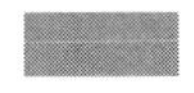

Recommendations for General Use Versus Guidelines for Use by Physical Activity and Fitness Specialists

Starting in the early 1970s, various professional organizations and government agencies began to issue recommendations, guidelines, and position stands on the importance of being physically active, how much of what types of activity should be performed, and how best to implement a safe activity plan for increasing health and fitness. Some of these recommendations have been relatively brief statements directed at health-care providers, health-care administrators and policymakers, and the public. These documents generally provided an overview of what needed to be done and why. Examples of such documents include the "Position Stands" by the American College of Sports Medicine (ACSM) (American College of Sports Medicine, 1978, 1990, 1998) and the Centers for Disease Control and Prevention (CDC)/ACSM report published in 1995 (Pate, 1995). Other publications have more detailed guidelines intended for the use of specialists such as physicians, exercise scientists, physical educators, physical therapists, coaches, and nurses who provide exercise and fitness evaluations, develop physical activity prescriptions or plans for individuals or groups, and provide exercise instruction or leadership for patients and healthy persons. Included in these documents are the seven editions of "Guidelines for Exercise Testing and Exercise Prescription" published by the ACSM between 1978 and 2005 (ACSM, 1975, 1980, 1986, 1991, 1995, 2000, 2005; *see* Table 15.1) and "Exercise Standards: A Statement for Healthcare Professionals from the American Heart Association" (Fletcher, 1990; *see* Figure 15.1).

Also during this same period, various organizations published recommendations or guidelines dealing with issues of exercise for specific patient populations, including, but not limited to, patients with coronary artery disease, hypertension, diabetes, osteoporosis, and arthritis. Many of these are important documents, but a discussion of their development and evolution is outside the scope of this chapter. Good examples of such guidelines are the various documents published by the American Heart Association (AHA) on exercise for patients with various forms of cardiovascular disease (CVD). Most of these documents can be accessed at www.americanheart.org. Additional guidelines for the use of exercise in cardiac rehabilitation and secondary prevention have been published by the American Association of Cardiovascular and Pulmonary Rehabilitation (1995). Additionally, ACSM has developed recommendations for exercise programs dealing with issues such as hypertension, osteoporosis, arthritis, and obesity; these can be obtained at www.acsm.org.

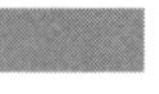

Initial Clinically Oriented Guidelines/Recommendations With a Focus on Safe Exercise to Promote Physical Fitness and Good Health

By the early 1970s, the leaders in various medical/health organizations began to recognize the need for evidence-based guidelines or recommendations regarding the health benefits and risks of exercise as well as how best a person should proceed with implementing an individualized exercise program. Over the prior two decades, data from several epidemiological and experimental studies demonstrated that more physically active persons, including patients with CHD, had better health outcomes than their less active counterparts. Of major concern in

Table 15.1 Exercise Dose Recommendations in the ACSM Guidelines for Exercise Testing and Exercise Prescription (Editions 1, 3, 5, 7).

Component	*1975 (1st)*	*1986 (3rd)*	*1995 (5th)*	*2005 (7th)*
Type	Aerobic Endurance	Aerobic Endurance	Aerobic Endurance	Aerobic Endurance
Intensity	60%–90% VO_{2max} 60%–90%	55%–80% VO_{2max} 60%–80%	40%–85% VO_{2max} or HRR HRR	40%–85% VO_{2max} or HRR HRR
Session Duration	20–60 minutes	15–60 minutes	20–60 minutes	20–60 minutes
Session Frequency	3–5 days/week	3–5 days/week	3–5 days/week	3–5 days/week
Total Activity	800–2000 kcal/week		1000–2000 kcal/week	

VO_{2max} = maximal oxygen uptake; HRR = heart rate reserve; kcal/week = kilocalories expended during physical activity per week.

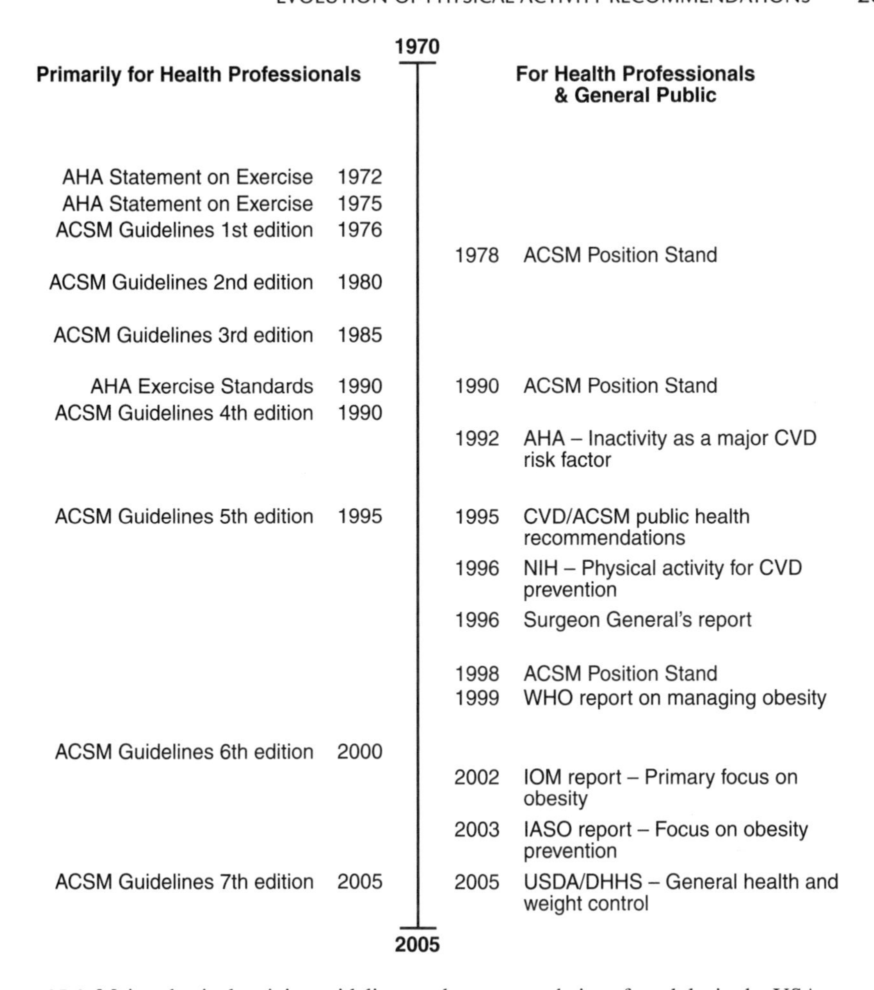

Figure 15.1 Major physical activity guidelines and recommendations for adults in the USA.

the preparation of these guidelines was how to minimize risk while achieving health benefits. The earliest of such guidelines were two publications by the AHA in 1972 and 1975.

The first of these was "Exercise Testing and Training of Apparently Healthy Individuals: A Handbook for Physicians" (AHA, 1972). These guidelines were more directed at how to reduce the cardiovascular risk from performing moderate- to vigorous-intensity exercise, including exercise testing for the "coronary prone," than at providing information on how to help patients become more physically active. The authors indicated that the available data supported exercise in the rehabilitation of patients with CHD but that data were still inadequate to support widespread promotion of exercise for the prevention of CHD. It was advised that exercise recommendations for the healthy but sedentary person—particularly the middle-aged male—"not be arbitrarily formulated" and that "exercise intensity must be adjusted to individual capacity at the beginning of the program and regulated periodically during the succeeding stages." A target heart rate of 75% of tested maximum rate or of age-corrected maximum heart rate could be used as long as this was at least 10 beats/minute below the highest tested rate.

The second publication, "Exercise Testing and Training of Individuals with Heart Disease or at High Risk for its Development: A Handbook for Physicians," again focused more on assessment of exercise capacity and issues of risk than on details of program implementation and focused more on rehabilitation than on secondary prevention (AHA, 1975). The following quote is an indication of the clinical approach taken by exercise prescription in the 1970s: "Exercise is a therapeutic agent designed to promote a beneficial clinical effect and, as such, has specific indications and contraindications and possible toxic or adverse reactions" (page 24). This booklet included sections on "Principals of Physical Conditioning," "Prescription of Exercise Training," and "Physical Conditioning Program Development," which provided information quite similar to that used today in guiding cardiac rehabilitation and secondary prevention programs for patients with documented CVD.

In 1973, a review of published research on endurance exercise training and cardiorespiratory fitness titled "The Quantification of Exercise Training Programs" was published by Michael Pollock in Exercise and Sport Sciences Reviews (Pollock, 1973). Much of the information developed during this review was used by Pollock and colleagues as the scientific basis for the first ACSM Position Statement on "The Recommended Quantity and Quality of Exercise for Developing and Maintaining Fitness in Healthy Adults" in 1978 (ACSM, 1978). The recommendations were for "developing and maintaining cardiorespiratory fitness and body composition in healthy adults." The key recommendations were to perform an endurance-type activity of 15 to 60 minutes in duration, 3 to 5 days/week at 60% to 90% of heart rate reserve or 50% to 85% of maximal oxygen uptake. Although reasonably brief (1.5 pages of text and 90 references), the recommendations in this document became the mantra for most exercise professionals and much of the public who wanted to know, "How much exercise is enough?" It is worth noting that all the references cited in this document were from the field of exercise physiology, with none from physical activity or behavioral epidemiology.

The ACSM reissued this Position Stand in 1990 and again in 1998. In 1990, its title was changed to "The Recommended Quantity and Quality of Exercise for Developing and Maintaining Cardioprespiratory and Muscular Fitness in Healthy Adults" (ACSM, 1990). The dose of exercise recommended was quite similar to the 1978 recommendation, with exercise mode and frequency remaining the same, session duration changing from 15 to 60 minutes to 20 to 60 minutes, and intensity changing from 60% to 90% of heart rate reserve or 50% to 85% of maximal oxygen uptake to 60% to 90% maximum heart rate or 50% to 85% of maximal oxygen uptake or heart rate reserve. A specific recommendation for enhancing muscle strength was added: one set of 8 to 12 repetitions of eight exercises 2 days/week. That less intensive exercise might provide health benefits was indicated by the statement "ACSM recognizes the potential health benefits of regular exercise performed more frequently and for a longer duration, but at lower intensities than presented in this position statement." (page 266).

In 1998, the third edition of the ACSM Position Stand was published, "Quantity and Quality of Exercise for Developing and Maintaining Cardiorespiratory and Muscular Fitness, and Flexibility in Healthy Adults" (ACSM, 1998). The primary recommendations for exercise to enhance cardiorespiratory fitness and body composition remained similar to the 1978 and 1990 recommendations, with the exception of a small reduction at the low end of the intensity range; 55% to 90% of maximum heart rate rather than 60% to 90% or 40% to 85% of maximal oxygen uptake reserve or heart rate reserve rather than 50% to 85% (*see* Table 15.2). Additionally, this most recent document included recommendations for flexibility and the concept of accumulation adopted from the CDC/ACSM public health recommendations published in 1995: "duration of training: 20–60 minutes of continuous or intermittent (minimum of 10-minute bouts accumulated throughout the day) of aerobic activity." (Pate, 1995). This version of the ACSM Position Stand expanded to 10+ pages and 292 references and included substantial detail on rational and background literature supporting the recommendations and information on program implementation and individualization.

Table 15.2 ACSM Position Stands on Physical Activity and Health

Component	*1978 (1st)*	*1990 (2nd)*	*1998 (3rd)*
Type	Aerobic Endurance	Aerobic Endurance	Aerobic Endurance
Mode	Large muscle, dynamic	Large muscle, dynamic	Large muscle dynamic
Intensity	60%–90% HRR 50%– 85% $V0_2$ max	60%–90% MHR 50%–85% VO_2 max or HRR	55%–90% MHR 40%–80% $V0_2R$ or HRR
Session Duration	15–60 minutes*	20–60 minutes*	20–60 minutes*
Session frequency	3–5 days/week	3–5 days/week	3–5 days/week
Resistance exercise	No specific recommendation	8–10 exer (1 set of 8–12 reps., two times/week)	8–10 exer (1 set of 8–12 reps., two times/week)

MHR = maximum heart rate; HRR = heart rate reserve; $V0_2$ max = maximum oxygen uptake; $V0_2R$ = oxygen uptake reserve; exer = exercises; reps = repetitions.
*Duration inversely related to intensity.

A Paradigm Shift to Public Health-Oriented Guidelines

Starting in the mid-1980s, discussions were held by various medical and public health organizations, and manuscripts were published, dealing with public health rather than clinical approaches to physical activity for achieving improved health outcomes (Haskell, 1984). The Behavioral Epidemiology and Evaluation Branch, CDC organized a meeting (Workshop on the Epidemiological and Public Health Aspects of Physical Activity and Exercise) of experts in 1984 to review the current knowledge base relating physical activity to health status and to discuss actions to be taken to increase the activity status of Americans (Mason and Powell, 1985). For the use by conference participants as a basis of discussion, 10 manuscripts were prepared and published along with a conference overview (Powell and Paffenbarger, 1985). This meeting played a significant role in setting the stage for the evolution of public health-oriented guidelines over the next decade, culminating in the publication of the first public health guidelines for physical activity and health by the CDC and ACSM in 1995 (Pate, 1995).

Between the CDC meeting in 1985 and the publication of the public health guidelines in 1995, a public health paradigm of physical activity evolved. The goal of this effort was to augment or supplement—but not necessarily replace—the existing exercise-for-fitness paradigm promoted by the ACSM and other organizations that had a primary focus of enhancing physical fitness or working capacity, either among healthy persons or in the physical rehabilitation of various patient populations (Haskell, 1993; *see* Fig. 15.2).

During this decade, substantial new data were published—especially from exercise epidemiology—relating inactivity to increased risk for several chronic diseases and documenting the potential protective effects of moderate-intensity as well as more vigorous-intensity activity in women and men. Additionally, there was rethinking of some of the prior epidemiological data with regard to what the most likely activity profile was among the more active people who comprised some of the lower risk groups (i.e., What kinds and patterns of physical activity were likely carried out by subjects?).

The Exercise Training – Performance Paradigm

Guidelines pre-1995 were based primarily on endurance exercise to enhance performance – especially aerobic power or endurance and muscular strength. Focus was on higher intensity exercise, such as jogging and running, since aerobic power most rapidly increases by increasing the intensity of the exercise.

The Physical Activity – Health Paradigm

Public health oriented guidelines since 1995 include the accumulation of ≥30 minutes of moderate-intensity physical activity on most days, preferably daily. Data from experimental and observational studies demonstrate health related benefits from moderate-intensity physical activity accumulated throughout the day.

Note: Current guidelines recognize both paradigms as being effective for promoting health and performance.

Figure 15.2 The shift from an exercise training to a physical activity paradigm in public health oriented physical activity guidelines to promote good health.

The tentative conclusion was that much of this activity was of moderate intensity (usually considered 3–6 metabolic equivalents [METS]) and that it was frequently performed in repeated bouts of no more than a few minutes each. Thus, there seemed to be somewhat of a disconnect between the existing exercise-fitness paradigm that emphasized more vigorous activity performed in bouts of at least 20 minutes' duration and epidemiologic data on the intensity and bout duration that appeared to provide some protection against selected chronic diseases and all-cause mortality.

For example, the results of some studies indicated that walking or other moderate-intensity activity on a regular basis, or moderate levels of cardiorespiratory fitness, were associated with lower rates of CVD and all-cause mortality (Leon, 1987; Shaper, 1991; Blair, 1989). Also, an increasing number of experimental studies were published showing disease risk factors or health-related fitness measures to be significantly improved in sedentary adults as a result of adherence to a program of regular walking or other moderate-intensity activity (Gossard, 1986; Duncan, 1991; Marceau, 1993). During this time, a team of Canadian exercise scientists organized two major international conferences on Exercise, Fitness, and Health (Bouchard, 1988) and Physical Activity, Fitness, and Health (Bouchard, 1992). For both conferences, the goal was to understand the relationship of physical activity and fitness to major health outcomes, develop a conceptual model for these relationships, and formulate a consensus statement. These conferences and publications provided an excellent background for the developing consensus that a physically inactive lifestyle is a major contributor to poor health outcomes throughout the lifespan.

In 1992, in light of the mounting evidence that a sedentary lifestyle significantly increased the risk or CHD morbidity and mortality, the AHA made sedentary lifestyle its fourth major CHD risk factor, joining cigarette smoking, hypertension, and hypercholesterolemia (Fletcher, 1992). This statement was the first formal recognition by the AHA that physical inactivity was a major independent risk factor for atherosclerotic heart disease and played a role in both the primary and secondary prevention of CHD. This document went beyond recognizing just the benefits of exercise for heart disease, also stating that people of all ages could benefit from a regular exercise program; that activities such as walking, hiking, swimming, cycling, tennis, and basketball were especially beneficial if performed at 50% or more of a person's work capacity; and that even low-intensity activities performed daily could have some long-term health benefits. This statement has been updated over the years by the AHA, but there have been no major changes in the key statements made in 1992, and the most recent update was published in 2003 (Thompson, 2003).

Given the influential nature of official position statements or recommendations by the AHA on heart disease prevention and treatment practices by the medical community in the United States, the elevation of inactivity to a major CHD risk factor brought substantial attention to the importance of a physically active lifestyle. Although this statement indicated the general nature of the activity that should be performed to help maintain good health, it lacked specific details regarding program design and implementation. However, it did indicate that intensities lower than that generally promoted in the past could provide health benefits.

In 1993 (the year following the AHA statement recognizing inactivity to be a major CHD risk factor), the CDC, in collaboration with the ACSM, initiated the development of a document that would provide specific recommendations about the profile of physical activity that should be performed to promote good health. To develop this statement, an expert panel was appointed that consisted of epidemiologists, exercise physiologists, public health professionals, and health psychologists. The panel was charged to develop a statement grounded in solid science, clearly communicate its key messages to the public, and provide a program that could be performed by a large segment of the general public with a minimal increase in risk. It took 2 years of work by the panel before the recommendations, "Physical Activity and Health," were released to the public in 1995 (Pate, 1995).

The approach to physical activity for health taken by these "public health" guidelines was quite different than prior guidelines primarily based on the "exercise training" or "clinical" paradigm. The primary recommendation was, "Every US adult should accumulate 30 minutes or more of moderate-intensity physical activity on most, preferably all, days of the week." Because many of the prior recommendations primarily advocated vigorous-intensity activity, having moderate-intensity activity as the key recommendation (although prior guidelines based on vigorous-intensity exercise were recognized as still effective) raised many questions by exercise scientists and practitioners. The idea that substantial health benefits could be derived from brisk walking was not appreciated by many fitness advocates, although this recommendation was based on data from a substantial number of epidemiological and experimental studies. Even more of a controversy was the idea that the activity each day did not need to be performed continuously for 30 minutes or more but could be accumulated throughout the day in bouts of 8 to 10 minutes. For many years, the idea that the activity needed to be continuous to be effective had been promoted in programs such as "Aerobics" (Cooper, 1968) but had no scientific evaluation. Although in retrospect the recommendation for accumulated bouts appears to have been correct, in 1995 the published scientific data supporting this concept was quite limited. Only a few experimental studies had directly compared the effects of continuous exercise bouts to accumulated exercise bouts of 8 to 10 minutes (Ebisu, 1985; DeBusk, 1990; Jakicic, 1992), and the nature of data collection in observational epidemiological studies made the evaluation of the accumulation concept difficult to assess, at best (*see* Chapter 4 for further discussion of these limitations).

Following close on the heels of the CDC/ACSM report, the National Institutes of Health (NIH) convened a consensus conference on "Physical Activity and Cardiovascular Health" (NIH Consensus Development Panel on Physical Activity and Cardiovascular Health, 1996). A non-federal, non-advocate, 13-member panel representing cardiology, psychology, exercise physiology, nutrition, pediatrics, public health, and epidemiology had as an objective "to provide physicians and the general public with a responsible assessment of the relationship between physical activity and cardiovascular health." During a 3-day conference, the panel listened to reports from 27 scientists on the relationship between physical activity and cardiovascular health, had open discussions with the presenting scientists and others in attendance, and then held closed deliberations to formulate their recommendations. The draft recommendations were shared with conference participants, conflicting views were resolved, and a final document was produced.

The panel concluded that: *(1)* most Americans have little or no physical activity in their daily lives; *(2)* accumulating evidence indicates that physical inactivity is a major risk factor for CVD; *(3)* moderate levels of physical activity confer significant health benefits; *(4)* all Americans should engage in regular physical activity at a level appropriate to their capacity, needs, and interests; and *(5)* children and adults should set a goal of accumulating at least 30 minutes of moderate-intensity physical activity on most, and preferably all, days of the week. The panel also recognized that a greater amount and/or intensity of activity than the recommended minimum would provide greater health benefits for most people and that cardiac patients should integrate increased physical activity into a comprehensive program of risk reduction. Thus, this panel made recommendations highly consistent with the CDC/ACSM working group in that it emphasized performing moderate-intensity physical activity (using brisk walking as a benchmark) on most or all days for 30 minutes/day or more and agreed that the activity could be accumulated in bouts of at least 8 to 10 minutes' duration. The panel also recognized that this was a minimal recommendation and that greater health benefits were achievable by performing greater amounts of activity or "vigorous exercise"—that is, the prior recommendations of vigorous exercise performed for 20 to 30 minutes on 3 days/week still applied.

At the same time that the NIH was producing its consensus panel report, the World Health Organization (WHO) also issued a report on the health benefits of regular activity (WHO/FIMS, 1995). The major recommendations in this document were very consistent with recommendations made by the CDC/ACSM working group and the NIH consensus panel: A target for all adults should be 30 minutes or more of moderate-intensity physical activity on most days. The WHO report also stated that daily physical activity should be the cornerstone for a healthy lifestyle throughout the lifespan; that more vigorous exercise, such as slow jogging, cycling, field and court games, and swimming can provide additional health benefits; and that people with disabilities or chronic disease have a great deal to benefit from an individualized activity program. Although recognizing that the responsibility for personal health decisions ultimately lies with the individual and family, policy recommendations for increasing physical activity were included in the report as well for major government organizations.

The CDC/ACSM, NIH, and WHO reports on physical activity and health, all published between 1995 and 1996, set the stage for the publication of *Physical Activity and Health: A Report of the Surgeon General* in 1996 (U.S. Department of Health and Human Services [USDHHS], 1996). This report was commissioned in 1994 by the Secretary of Health and Human Services, who authorized the CDC to be the lead agency for the development of the report, with collaboration from a number of federal organizations, especially the President's Council on Physical Fitness and Sports and the NIH. Non-government collaborating organizations included the ACSM, AHA, and the American Association of Health, Physical Education, Recreation, and Dance. The report was an extensive undertaking, with approximately 195 people listed as contributing to the writing, editing, review, and publication. The stated goal of the Surgeon General's report was to summarize the existing literature on the role of physical activity in preventing disease and on the status of interventions to increase physical activity. It provided a historical background on the relationship of physical activity to health, including the evolution of physical activity guidelines, a summary of acute and chronic physiological responses to exercise, a systematic review of the effects of physical activity on major health outcomes; patterns and trends of physical activity among different populations in the United States, and an overview of projects implemented to promote an increase physical activity in youth and adults. The report grew out of an emerging consensus among investigators and individuals working in exercise science, epidemiology, public health, clinical medicine, health psychology, and education that the high prevalence of sedentary behavior among the American population had a significant negative health impact, that a moderate amount and intensity of physical activity in this sedentary population could provide important health benefits, and that innovative, long-term programs were needed to reverse the continuing downward trend in physical activity.

The key recommendation from the Surgeon General's report was that people of all ages could improve the quality of their lives through a lifelong practice of moderate-intensity exercise. "A regular, preferably daily, regimen of at least 30–45 minutes of brisk walking, bicycling, or even working around the house or yard will reduce the risk of coronary heart disease, hypertension, colon cancer and diabetes." The report also stated that more activity is better: People who already perform this level of activity will benefit even more if they increased the intensity and/or duration of their activity.

The initial promotion of this report took place in conjunction with the Summer Olympic Games held in Atlanta in the fall of 1996. To bring attention to the document and its key messages to the general public and health professionals, the CDC and its collaborators implemented a promotion program. Because the core messages from this report and the 1995 ACSM/CDC and 1996 NIH reports were very similar, it is not possible to determine how much effect any individual report had in communicating the revised recommendations to the public. Both the CDC/ACSM report and the Surgeon General's report have frequently been cited in the professional literature on physical activity and health, and the key recommendations, usually with no or only minor modifications, have been adopted by national agencies in a number of other countries, including Canada, England, Australia, and Japan.

Scientific Support of the Public Health Guidelines and Controversy Regarding Physical Activity and Obesity

In the decade since the publication of the first public health-oriented recommendations in 1995, numerous studies have been published supporting the inclusion of brisk walking as a health-promoting activity (Hu, 1999; Lee, 2001; Tanasescu, 2002; Manson, 2002), supporting a duration of 30 minutes on most days (or 150 minutes/week) as a sufficient amount to provide a variety of health benefits (Manson, 2002; Lee, 2001) and supporting the notion that accumulating activity minutes over the day in bouts of 10 minutes or so is an acceptable alternative to performing continuous bouts of 30 minutes or longer (Lee, 2000; Hardman, 2001). The results of some studies have suggested that little, if any, benefit is derived from activity that is less than vigorous (Yu, 2003), but such studies have been in the minority. Additionally, methodological issues could have accounted for such findings; these are discussed in Chapter 4.

To help assess the information available on the dose of physical activity needed for specific health outcomes, an international "consensus symposium" was held at Hockley Valley, Ontario, Canada, in 2000 (Bouchard, 2001). The goal of this evidence-based symposium was to provide a comprehensive review of the existing science relating physical activity dose to health and to make specific recommendations regarding physical activity dose.

The major conclusion regarding the dose–response relationship for specific outcomes was that the available data were still inadequate to define any precise relationships. However, the consensus panel did endorse the recommendations made in the CDC/ACSM report (Pate, 1995) and the Surgeon General's report (USDHHS, 1996).

In 2002, the Institute of Medicine (IOM), National Academy of Sciences published a report primarily focusing on macronutrient intake and energy intake/expenditure and developing estimates of daily intake that are compatible with good nutrition throughout the lifespan that may decrease the risk for chronic disease (IOM, 2002). The preparation of this report by the IOM, a private nonprofit organization, was supported financially by the USDHHS, U.S. Department of Agriculture(USDA), and U.S. Department of Defense and Health Canada. The panel considered the level of macronutrients, and thus caloric intake, consistent with good health and the caloric expenditure needed to keep people in a healthy weight range—defined as a body mass index (BMI) of 18.5 to 25.0 kg/m^2. To achieve these goals the panel concluded the following regarding physical activity.

> "Physical activity and exercise promote health and vigor. As identified previously by other groups (DHHS, 1996), some benefits can be achieved with a minimum of 30 minutes of moderate-intensity physical activity most days of the week. However, 30 minutes per day of regular activity is insufficient to maintain body weight in adults in the recommended body mass index range from 18.5 to 25 kg/m^2 and achieve all the identified health benefits fully. Hence, to prevent weight gain as well as accrue additional weight-independent benefits of physical activity, 60 minutes of daily moderate-intensity physical activity (e.g., walking/jogging at 4 to 5 mph) is recommended, in addition to the activities required by a sedentary lifestyle. This amount of activity leads to an 'active' lifestyle, corresponds to physical activity levels (PAL) greater than 1.6, consistent with those observed in the doubly labeled water database utilized to derive the energy requirements in Chapter 5."

Upon the release of this report, many in the press, general public, and health professions considered there to be a very significant change in physical activity recommendations for health—with the target of 60 minutes of moderate-intensity activity daily rather than the 30 minutes or more that had been promoted since 1995. It is very important to understand that the prior guidelines/recommendations by CDC, ACSM, and NIH were based primarily on the amount of physical activity shown to be consistent with lower morbidity and mortality rates from selected chronic diseases and all-cause mortality and not on the amount for achieving an optimal BMI of 18.5 to 25.0 kg/m^2, in contrast to the major goal of the IOM report. Also, in the IOM report, the 60-minute recommendation was made to achieve *all* the identified health benefits fully, whereas in the other reports, the 30-minute or greater recommendation was considered a minimum, recognizing that more exercise brings additional benefits. (As an aside, it is not clear from existing research that 60 minutes/day will achieve *all* identified health benefits fully or will result in achieving an optimal BMI for all.) As with the prior reports, the IOM document indicated that the activity can be accumulated throughout the day and not just performed in a single session.

A key difference in the data considered during the formulation of the IOM recommendation vs. other previous physical activity recommendations was the emphasis on doubly labeled water (DLW) studies by the IOM panel. Combining data from available DLW studies worldwide, the panel estimated the total daily energy expenditure of men and women who had a BMI in the range of 18.5 to 25.0 kg/m^2 to be an average of about 1.75. Because the physical activity level (PAL) of people considered to be sedentary is about 1.25, the difference (1.75–1.25) when converted to minutes of moderate-intensity activity was considered to equate to approximately 60 minutes/day. However, the fact that the PAL for subjects in the DLW studies who were overweight or obese was not 1.25 but, rather, was in the range of 1.59 to 1.85 was not taken into consideration by the IOM panel (Blair, 2004). Thus, the data from the DLW studies did not fully support the conclusion by the IOM panel that 60 minutes/day of moderate-intensity activity is needed to maintain normal weight. Additionally, the cross-sectional data from the DLW studies cannot answer the question of how much added exercise will produce a meaningful change in body weight.

The IOM selection of a target activity level of 60 minutes/day, or a PAL of 1.6 or greater, to maintain optimal body weight is somewhat less than the target PAL of 1.75 in the report by the WHO published in 1998, "Obesity: Preventing and Managing the Global Epidemic" (WHO, 1998). In this extensive report, the authors stated that analyses of over 40 national physical activity studies worldwide showed that there was a significant relationship between the average BMI of adult men and their PAL, with the likelihood of becoming overweight being substantially reduced at PALs of 1.8 or above. For women, the PAL associated with a healthy weight is approximately 1.6. Therefore, the WHO report suggested "that people should remain physically active throughout life and sustain a PAL of 1.75 or more in order to avoid excessive weight gain" (page 124).

In 2002, an international group of scientists with expertise in physical activity, nutrition, energy balance, and obesity held a consensus meeting convened by the International Association for the Study of Obesity to assess "how much physical activity is enough to prevent unhealthy weight gain" (Saris, 2003). Part of their conclusion was: "The current physical activity guideline for adults of 30 minutes of moderate-intensity activity daily, preferably all days of the week, is of importance for limiting health risks for a number of chronic diseases, including coronary heart disease and diabetes. However, for the prevention of weight gain or regain this guideline is likely to be insufficient for many individuals in the current environment. There is compelling evidence that prevention of weight regain in formally obese individuals requires 60–90 minutes of moderate-intensity activity or lesser amounts of vigorous activity. Although definitive data are lacking, it seems likely that moderate-intensity activity of approximately 45 to 60 minutes per day or 1.7 PAL is required to prevent the transition to overweight or obesity." This consensus statement recognized that the amount of physical activity associated with lower chronic disease and mortality rates was very likely less than that needed in the current environment to prevent unhealthy weight gain or regain in many adults.

Every 5 years, the USDA and USDHHS are required by the U.S. Congress to prepare a set of dietary guidelines for Americans. In the guidelines published from 1995 onward and prior to 2005, there was a recognition that a physically active lifestyle should be maintained for optimal health, but no specific guidelines focused on prevention of weight gain or weight loss. For example, in 2000 the recommendations were highly consistent with the 1995 CDC/ACSM report directed to improving general health status: "Aim to accumulate at least 30 minutes (adults) or 60 minutes (children) of moderate-intensity activity on most days of the week, preferably daily. If you already get 30 minutes of physical activity daily, you can gain even more health benefits by increasing the amount of time you are physically active or by taking part in more vigorous activities. No matter what activity you choose, you can do it all at once, or spread it out over two or three times per day" (USDA, 2000).

In the 2005 Dietary Guidelines for Americans, the physical activity recommendations were structured to separate advice about chronic disease prevention from advice about the amount of physical activity required for prevention of unhealthy weight gain or re-gain in adults (USDA, 2005). The key physical activity recommendations included in the executive summary are provided in Table 15.3.

Table 15.3 Dietary Guidelines for Americans—2005: Physical Activity Recommendations*

Summary of recommendations for achieving good health and optimal weight in adults

- To reduce the risk of chronic disease in adulthood: Engage in at least 30 minutes of moderate-intensity physical activity, above usual activity, at work or home on most days of the week.
- For most people, greater health benefits can be obtained by engaging in physical activity of more vigorous intensity or longer duration.
- To help manage body weight and prevent gradual, unhealthy body weight gain in adulthood: Engage in approximately 60 minutes of moderate- to vigorous-intensity activity on most days of the week while not exceeding caloric intake requirements.
- To sustain weight loss in adulthood: Participate in at least 60 to 90 minutes of daily moderate-intensity physical activity while not exceeding caloric intake requirements. Some people may need to consult with a healthcare provider before participating in this level of activity.
- Achieve physical fitness by including cardiovascular conditioning, stretching exercises for flexibility, and resistance exercises or calisthenics for muscle strength and endurance.

* Published by the U.S. Departments of Agriculture and Health and Human Services, 2005.

These 2005 Dietary Guidelines take advantage of the very large amounts of experimental and observational data supporting the generally accepted position that a variety of health benefits are derived from 30 minutes or more of moderate-intensity exercise on most days and separate this recommendation from the less well-documented and more controversial recommendations regarding the amount of physical activity required for the prevention of unhealthy weight gain or regain and weight loss. The physical activity recommendations needed to help manage body weight were adopted in large part from the 2002 IOM report (IOM, 2002), which as discussed earlier, primarily considered cross-sectional data from DLW studies of energy expenditure (Brooks, 2005).

Difficult to reconcile with a target PAL of 1.6 or greater to maintain optimal body weight is the calculation in a commentary by Hill and colleagues (Hill et al., 2003) that "affecting energy balance by 100 kilocalories per day (by a combination of reducing energy intake and increases in physical activity) could prevent weight gain in most of the population." Even if all of the 100-kcal/day deficit were created by an increase in physical activity, this would only increase PAL in an inactive person from approximately 1.25 to 1.30, far from the target of 1.6 set by the IOM report to prevent obesity. In contrast, somewhat consistently with the IOM recommendation, Williams recently reported an average BMI of 29.1 kg/m^2 in women who reported walking less than 2 km/week compared to a BMI of 25.5 kg/m^2 in women who reported walking 10.0 to 19.9 km/week or 2 to 3 miles/day (about 30–60 minutes/day at 3.0–3.5 mph) (Williams, 2005). The PAL recommendations from the recent obesity prevention guidelines, together with their equivalent minutes/day, are summarized in Table 15.4.

Physical Activity and Health Guidelines: Where Do We Stand?

Since 1978, there have been a substantial number of guidelines or recommendations published in the United States, with significant evolution of selected aspects as more data have become available and a more comprehensive syntheses of existing data has occurred. In some public and professional venues, the focus has been on how dramatic the changes have been or on the major inconsistencies that exist among the various guidelines. Key issues that have stimulated discussion and debate have been the inclusion of moderate-intensity

Table 15.4. Guidelines Specifically Directed at Achieving or Maintaining Optimal Body Weight – Amount of Physical Activity Recommended

	PAL	Walking time daily
WHO (1997)		
Maintain BMI 18.5–25.0	1.75	—
IOM (2002)		
Maintain BMI 18.5–25.0	1.6–1.7	60 minutes
IASO (2003)		
Prevent unhealthy weight gain	1.7	45–60 minutes
DHHS (2005)		
Prevent unhealthy weight gain		60 minutes
Prevent weight regain after large weight loss		60–90 minutes

PAL = physical activity level (total daily energy expenditure/energy expenditure at rest)

activities as a major focus rather than vigorous-intensity activities, the concept of accumulating activity throughout the day by means of multiple short (8- to 10-minute) sessions, and the total duration of daily accumulated activity ranging from 30 to 60 minutes or more. However, one can also take the position that the major message—that a physically active lifestyle throughout the lifespan is important to maintain good health—has been consistent across all the guidelines and that the following statements account for the major points in existing physical activity guidelines for Americans.

- For chronic disease prevention, sedentary adults should strive to get 30 minutes or more of moderate-intensity activity on most days—preferably daily—above that required for activities of daily living.
- More studies have been conducted to evaluate the benefits of activity performed in a single long session (≥30 minutes) than to evaluate the benefits of accumulating activity by performing multiple short bouts (6–10 minutes). However, sufficient data exist to support the concept of accumulation (at least, in bouts of 8–10 minutes; very few studies have looked at bouts shorter than this).
- For general health and fitness promotion and disease prevention, greater benefits can be expected with greater amounts of moderate-intensity activity (up to 60 minutes daily) and/or more vigorous-intensity physical activity.
- For younger and older adults who have been active and are free of medical contraindications, vigorous exercise (such as jogging or running) performed for 20 minutes or more approximately every other day will provide significant health and fitness benefits (but at a greater risk of injury; *see* Chapter 14 for additional details).
- School-age youth should participate in 60 minutes/day or more of moderate-to-vigorous physical activity that is developmentally appropriate and enjoyable and involves a variety of activities (CDC, 1997; Strong, 2005).
- When considering physical activity recommendations for the control of body weight, it is absolutely necessary to account for calorie intake. Target activity levels can be set for the prevention of weight gain or re-gain in individuals or populations, but they only apply under conditions of a constant calorie intake. The weight control benefits of physical activity can easily be negated by quite moderate increases in food intake (we can eat more than we can run).

- For prevention of unhealthy weight gain in a sedentary population where "daily required physical activity" results in a PAL of about 1.25, it is likely that more than 30 minutes of moderate-intensity physical activity will be needed by many people (without calorie restriction below a level where good nutrition is jeopardized).
- For adults striving to lose weight, an increase in physical activity can contribute to a negative calorie balance. No target for the amount of activity to achieve weight loss has been set by existing guidelines, but generally more is better, and a target of 30 to 60 minutes/day of moderate-intensity activity is consistent with most recommendations.
- For prevention of weight re-gain in many adults who have lost more than 30 pounds, moderate-intensity activity of 60 to 90 minutes/day is probably necessary. Here again, success depends on energy balance by controlling both intake and expenditure.

Personal Perspective

Development of consensus statements and guidelines is a critical process in the translation of research findings into health policy and practice. When conducted well, the consensus process considers all of the relevant research and distills a complex compilation of data into a concise set of recommendations that can lead to specific actions by health care providers and the public. When data are inadequate to draw definitive conclusions and recommendations, expert opinion needs to determine the best course of action. As the science of physical activity and health advances along with other medical sciences, it should be possible to develop more precise guidelines in areas where detailed information currently is lacking.

Over the past 35 years I have been personally involved in the discussions surrounding and the preparation of physical activity guidelines, recommendations, and consensus statements issued by the ACSM, CDC, NIH, and AHA. Frequently the "panel of experts" convened by these organizations consisted of many of the same people; thus, the various documents were based on the expertise and opinions of a relatively small portion of the investigators involved in the science of physical activity and health. Such a situation can contribute to a biased representation of the data and recommendations not based on all the available science. It seems that this has not been a major problem given the stability of the key recommendations over time and the adoption of modifications as new data have become available. However, it is important that all scientific-based views be considered during the consensus statement process and that this process stimulate research and not constrain it.

References

American Association of Cardiovascular and Pulmonary Rehabilitation. 1995. Guidelines for Cardiac Rehabilitation Programs. Human Kinetics, Champaign, Ill.

American College of Sports Medicine. 1978. The recommended quantity and quality of exercise for developing and maintaining fitness in healthy adults. *Med Sci Sports* 10: vii–x.

American College of Sports Medicine. 1990. The recommended quantity and quality of exercise for developing and maintaining cardiorespiratory and muscular fitness in healthy adults. *Med Sci Sports and Exer* 22: 265–74.

American College of Sports Medicine. 1998. The recommended quantity and quality of exercise for developing and maintaining cardiorespiratory and muscular fitness, and flexibility in healthy adults. *Med Sci Sports Exerc* 31: 975–1008.

American College of Sports Medicine. 2005. ACSM's Guidelines for Exercise Testing and Prescription. Lippincott Williams and Wilkins, Philadelphia, 7th Edition (also editions published in 1975, 1980, 1989, 1991, 1995, 2000).

American Heart Association. 1972. Exercise Testing and Training of Apparently Healthy Individuals: A Handbook for Physicians. Dallas; American Heart Association.

American Heart Association. 1975. *Exercise Testing and Training of Individuals with Heart Disease or at High Risk for its Development*. Dallas: American Heart Association.

Blair SN, Kohl HW, Paffenbarger RS, Clark DG, Cooper KH, Gibbons LW. 1989. Physical fitness and all-cause mortality: a prospective study of healthy men and women. *J Am Med Assoc* 26: 2395–401.

Blair SN, LaMonte MJ, Nichaman MZ. 2004. The evolution of physical activity recommendations: how much is enough? *Am J Clin Nutr* 79: 913S20S.

Bouchard C, Shephard RJ, Stephens T, Sutton JR, McPherson BD (Eds.). 1988. Exercise, Fitness and Health. Human Kinetics Books, Champaign.

Bouchard C, Shephard RJ, Stephens T (Eds.). 1992. Physical Activity, Fitness and Health. Human Kinetics Publishers, Champaign.

Bouchard C. 2001. Physical activity and health: Introduction to the dose-response symposium. *Med Sci Sports Ex* 33: S347–50.

Breslow L, Buel P. 1960. Mortality from coronary heart disease and physical activity of work in California. *J Chron Dis* 11: 428–44.

Brooks GA, Butte N, Rand WM, Flatt J-P, Caballero B. 2004. Chronicle of the Institute of medicine physical activity recommendation: how a physical activity recommendation came to be among dietary recommendations. *Am J Clin Nutr* 79: 921S-30S.

Buchanan F. 1909. The physiological significance of the pulse rate. *Trans. Oxford University Scientific Club* 34: 351–6.

Byford, WH. On the physiology of exercise. 1855. *Am J Med Sci* 30: 32–42.

Centers for Disease Control and Prevention. 1997. Guidelines for School and Community Programs to Promote Lifelong Physical Activity Among Young People. U. S. Department of Health and Human Services. Superintendent of Documents, U.S. Government Printing Office. Washington, DC.

Cooper KH. 1968. Aerobics. M. Evans and Company, New York.

DeBusk RF, Hakansson U, Sheehan M, Haskell WL. 1990. Training effects of long vs. short bouts of exercise. *Am J Cardiol* 65: 1010–3.

Duncan JJ, Gordon NF, Scott CB. 1991. Women walking for health and fitness. How much is enough? *J Am Med Assoc* 266: 3295–9.

Ebisu T. 1985. Splitting the distance of endurance running on cardiovascular endurance and blood lipids. *Jap J Phys Ed* 30: 37–43.

Fletcher GF, Balady G, Froelicher VF, Hartley LH, Haskell WL, Pollock ML. 1990. Exercise Standards: A statement for healthcare professionals from the American Heart Association. *Circulation* 82: 2288–322.

Fletcher GF, Blair SN, Blumenthal J, et al. 1992. Statement on exercise. Benefits and recommendations for physical activity programs for all Americans. A statement for health professionals by the Committee on Exercise and Cardiac Rehabilitation of the Council on Clinical Cardiology, American Heart Association. *Circulation* 86: 340–4.

Fox SM, Skinner J. 1964. Physical activity and cardiovascular health. *Am J Cardiol* 14: 731–746.

Franz SI. 1900. On the methods for estimating the force of voluntary muscular contractions and on fatigue. *Am J Physiol* 4: 348–72.

Gibbs DD. 1969. Sir John Floyer, M. D. (1649–1734). *Br Med J* 25: 242–5.

Gossard D, Haskell, WL, Taylor B, et al. 1986. Effects of low- and high-intensity home-based exercise training on functional capacity in healthy middle-aged men. *Am J Cardiol* 57: 446–9.

Guy WA. 1843. Contributions to a knowledge of the influence of employments on health. *J Royal Stat Soc* 6: 197–211.

Hardman AE. 2001. Issues of fractionization of exercise (short vs long bouts. *Med Sci Sports Exerc* 33: S421-7.

Hartley PHS, Llewellyn GF. 1939. The longevity of oarsmen: a study of those who rowed in the Oxford and Cambridge boat race from 1839–1928. *Br Med J* 1: 657–62.

Haskell WL. 1984. Physical activity and health: The need to define the required stimulus. *Am J Cardiol* 55: 4D–9D.

Haskell WL. 1994. Health consequences of physical activity: understanding and challenges regarding dose-response. *Med Sci Sports Exer* 6: 649–60.

Heberden W. 1772. Some account of a disorder of the breast. *Med Trans (Coll Phys London)* 2: 59–67.

Hill J, Wyatt HR, Reed GW, Peters JC. 2003. Obesity and the environment: Where do we go from here? *Science* 299: 853–5.

Hu FB, Sigal R, Rich-Edwards J, et al. 1999. Walking compared with vigorous physical activity and risks of type 2 diabetes in women: a prospective study. *JAMA* 282: 1433–9.

Hedley OF. 1939. Analysis of 5116 deaths reported due to acute coronary occlusion in Philadelphia 1933–1936. *US Week Pub Health Rep* 54: 972.

Holloszy JO, Skinner JS, Toro G, Cureton TK. 1964. The effects of a six-month program of endurance exercise on serum lipids in middle-aged men. *Am J Cardiol* 14: 753–60.

Institute of Medicine. 2002. Dietary reference intakes: energy, carbohydrates, fiber, fat, fatty acids, cholesterol, protein, and amino acids. Washington, DC. National Academy Press.

Jakicic JM, Wing RR, Butler BA, Robertson RJ. 1995. Prescribing exercise in multiple short bouts versus one continuous bout: effect on adherence, cardirespiratory fitness, and weight loss in overweight women. *Intern J Obes* 19: 893–901.

Kahn HA. 1963. The relationship of reported coronary heart disease mortality to physical activity of work. *Am J Public Health* 53: 1058–67.

Karvonen MJ, Kentala E, Mustala O. 1957. The effects of training on heart rate; a longitudinal study. *Ann Med Exp Biol Fenn* 35(3): 307–15.

Karvonen MJ, Rautaharju PM, Orma E, Punsar S, Takkunen J. 1961. Heart Disease and employment: cardiovascular studies on lumberjacks. *J Occupational Med* 3: 49–53.

Lee I-M, Sesso HD, Paffenbarger RS. 2000. Physical activity and coronary heart disease risk in men: does the duration of exercise episodes predict risk? *Circulation.* 102: 981–6.

Lee, I-M, Rexrode KM, Cook NR, Manson JE, Buring JE. 2001. Physical activity and coronary heart disease in women: Is "no pain, no gain passe? *JAMA* 285: 1447–54.

Leon AS, Connett J, Jacobs DR, Rauramaa R. 1987. Leisure-time physical activity and risk of coronary heart disease and death. *JAMA*. 258: 2388–95.

Mann GV, Garrett HL, Farhi A, Murray H, Billings FT. 1969. Exercise to prevent coronary heart disease: An experimental study of the effects of training on risk factors for coronary heart disease in men. *Am J Med* 46: 12–27.

Manson JE, Greenland P, LaCroix AZ, et al. 2002. Walking compared with vigorous exercise for the prevention of cardiovasculae events in women. *N Engl J Med* 347: 716–25.

Mason JO, Powell KE. 1985. Physical activity, behavioral epidemiology and public health. *Pub Health Rep* 100: 113–5.

Marceau M, Kouame N, Lacourciere Y, Cleroux J. 1993. Effects of different training intensities on 24-hour blood pressure in hypertensive subjects. *Circulation* 88: 2803–11.

McCurdy JH. 1901. The effect of maximum muscular effort on blood pressure. *Am J Physiol* 5: 95–103.

Mercurialis H. 1569. De Arte Gymnastica. 2nd. Paris: Du Puys.

Morgan JE. 1873. University oars being a critical enquiry into the after health of men who rowed in the Oxford and Cambridge Boat Race from the year 1829–1869, based on the personal experience of the rowers themselves. London; Macmillan.

Morris JN, Chave SPW, Adam C, Sirey C, Epstein L, Sheehan DJ. 1973, Vigorous exercise in leisure-time and the incidence of coronary heart disease. *Lancet* 7799: 333–9.

Morris JN, Heady JA, Raffle PAB, Roberts CG, Parks JW. 1953. Coronary heart-disease and physical activity of work. *Lancet* ii: 1053–7; 1111–20.

NIH Consensus Development Panel on Physical Activity and Cardiovascular Health.1996. Physical activity and cardiovascular health. *JAMA* 276: 241–6.

Paffenbaeger RS, Hale WE, Brand RJ, Hyde RT. 1970. Work-energy level, personal characteristics, and fatal heart attack: A birth cohort study. *Am J Epidemiol* 105: 200–13.

Pate RR, Pratt M, Blair SN, et al. 1995. A recommendation from the Centers for Disease Control and Prevention and the American College of Sports Medicine. *JAMA* 273: 402–7.

Pollock ML, Cureton TK, Greninger L. 1969. Effects of Frequency of training on working capacity, cardiovascular function and body composition of adult men. *Med Sci Sports* 1: 70–4.

Pollock ML. 1973. The quantification of endurance training programs. In: JH Wilmore, (Ed.), *Exercise and Sport Sciences Reviews*. New York: Academic Press. Pp. 155–88.

Pollock ML, Broida J, Kendrick Z, Miller HL, Janeway R, Linnerud AC. 1972. Effects of training two days per week at different intensities on middle-aged men. *Med Sci Sports* 4: 192–7.

Powell KE, Paffenbarger RS. 1985. Workshop on epidemiology and public health aspects of physical activity and exercise: a summary. *Public Health Rep* 100: 118–26.

Saltin B, Bloomqvist G, Mitchell JH, Johnson RL, Wildenthal K, Chapman CB. 1968. Response to exercise after bedrest and after training: A longitudinal study of the adaptive changes in oxygen transport and body composition. *Circulation* 37 (Suppl 7): VII,1-VII,78.

Saris WHM, Blair SN, van Bakk MA, et al. 2003. How much physical activity is enough to prevent unhealthy weight gain? Outcome of the IASO 1st Stock conference and consensus statement. *Obes Rev* 4: 101–14.

Schneider EC, Ring GC. 1929. The influence of moderate amounts of physical training on respiratory exchange and breathing during exercise. *Am J Physiol* 91: 103–7.

Shaper AG, Wannamethee G. 1991. Physical activity and ischaemic heart disease in middle-aged British men. *Br Heart J* 66: 384–94.

Silverstern I, Dalstrom AW. 1922. The relation of muscular activity to carcinoma: a preliminary report. *J Cancer Res* 6: 365–78.

Smith E, Milner WR. 1861. Report on the action of prison diet and discipline on the bodily functions of prisoners. Part I. 31st Meeting *Br Assoc Adv Sci* 44–81.

Strong WB, Malina RM, Bumkie CJR, et al. 2005. Evidence based physical activity for school-aged youth. *J Pediatr* 146: 7732–7.

Taylor HL, Klepetar E, Keys A, et al. 1962. Death rates among physically active and sedentary employees of the railroad industry. *Am J Public Health* 52: 1697–707.

Tanasescu M, Leitzmann MF, Rimm EB, Willett WC, Stampfer MJ, Hu FB. 2002. Exercise type and intensity in relation to coronary heart disease in men. *JAMA* 288: 1994–2000.

Thompson PD, Buchner D, Pina IL, et al. 2003. Exercise and physical activity in the prevention and treatment of atherosclerotic cardiovascular disease. *Circulation* 107: 3109–16.

U.S. Department of Agriculture. 2005. Nutrition and Your Health: Dietary Guidelines for Americans. 2005 Dietary Guidelines Advisory Committee Report. U.S. Department of Agriculture, Washington, D.C.

U.S.Department of Health and Human Services. 1996. *Physical Activity and Health: A Report of the Surgeon General*. Atlanta: USDHSS/CDC.

USDA. 2000. Nutrition and Your Health: Dietary Guidelines For Americans. USDA, Washington, DC.

Williams PT. 2005. Nonliner relatiopnships between weekly walking distance and adiposity in 27,596 women. *Med Sci Sports Ex* 37: 1893–901.

World Health Organization/FIMS Committee on Physical Activity for Health. 1995. Exercise for health. *Bull World Health Organ* 73: 135–6.

World Health Organization. 1998. Obesity: Prevention and Managing the Global Epidemic. Division of Noncommunicable Diseases, World Health Organization, Geneva.

Yu S, Yarnell JWG, Sweetnam PM, Murray L. 2003. What level of physical activity protects aganist premature cardiovascular death? The Caerphilly study. *Heart* 89: 502–6.

16

How Can We Increase Physical Activity Levels?

Adrian Bauman and
Philayrath Phongsavan

Approaches to Increasing Physical Activity at the Population Level

Physical inactivity is now regarded as a major global risk factor for non-communicable disease in developed and developing countries (World Health Organization [WHO], 2002). Despite the increasing evidence of the health benefits of physical activity, the majority in most populations remain physically inactive. Trends in physical activity at the population level generally have been stable or have shown slight declines in recent years in many of the countries that have conducted routine population surveillance surveys (Craig et al., 2004).

The challenge is how to address inactivity at the individual and community levels. Acknowledging the need for disease prevention and health promotion strategies, the WHO supports the development of a Global Strategy for Diet and Physical Activity (WHO, 2004). This strategy sets the agenda for a health promotion approach to developing interventions to increase physical activity (Bauman et al., 2005).

In developed countries, many people understand that being physically active confers positive physical and mental health benefits, but levels of physical activity participation remain low. In developing countries, there may be an information gap, and approaches are required to inform and motivate the sedentary in the population (Haase et al., 2004). The gaps between evidence and practice and between individual beliefs and actual behavior represent a substantial challenge for public health practitioners as well as for government and non-government agencies.

Developing interventions to measure the efficacy and effectiveness of programs to increase physical activity provides information that will ensure that limited resources are appropriately channeled to where they are most needed. Identifying effective approaches to increasing physical activity remains a public health challenge. This chapter focuses on the resultant research tasks, specifically the methodological and epidemiological issues in developing and evaluating physical activity programs.

What and Whom Are We Trying to Change?

First, how much physical activity are we trying to promote? Until the publication of the U.S. Centers for Disease Control/American College of Sports Medicine (CDC/ACSM) recommendation on physical activity and health (Pate et al., 1995), health-related recommendations for "exercise" targeted aerobic or fitness enhancing levels of physical activity, with minimal criteria set at 20 minutes, three times per week of vigorous- or high-intensity activity (ACSM, 1990). One of the key messages that emanated from the CDC/ACSM recommendation was that physical activity of moderate intensity could confer health benefits, with the optimal goal for all adults to accumulate at least 30 minutes of physical activity on most days of the week. The notion of "accumulate" further complicated the physical activity concept. These new data suggested broader approaches regarding the quantum and duration of physical activity for health—that is, it could be moderate intensity and accumulated over several bouts during the day. This changed the kind of activity that health promotion experts became interested in—now, we can recommend that people walk to the bus, perform more vigorous domestic chores or yard work, and use the stairs instead of the elevator. The concept of shorter bouts of activity and the different settings or domains of activity provided new ways of thinking about physical activity interventions.

One of the complexities of epidemiological evidence is that not all health outcomes are influenced equally by physical activity. For diabetes prevention or reducing the risk of cardiovascular disease, 30 minutes is sufficient; for breast or colon cancer prevention, more time and greater intensity may be required; for falls prevention, different modes of activity, such as strength training, may be optimal. Finally, for weight loss, at least 1 hour/day or more may be required, at least for some people. These different messages make disseminating health promotion messages slightly more complicated. For example, for whole population interventions, the message "half an hour of moderate activity on most days" suffices; for disease-specific preventive programs, other recommended amounts may be needed.

The second issue is whom we are trying to encourage to become more active. A clinical or high-risk approach targets the most sedentary or those at risk of chronic disease—for example, those who are obese or pre-diabetic. The approach here is that interventions should target these individuals and the proximal causes of inactivity, as their relative risk is greatest for adverse outcomes or disease incidence. Structured and tailored programs can be targeted to these individuals to increase leisure-time physical activity.

A different approach is required to target the whole population, and hence a different set of causes (e.g., distal factors such as changing physical and policy environments) and research issues need to be considered. Whole-population interventions are carried out for some risk factors that demonstrate a dose–response relationship between exposure and outcomes. This model proposes that shifting the entire distribution curve of a risk factor is an optimal public health strategy, as much of the population-attributable risk is in the middle of the distribution curve (Rose, 2001); using this thinking, strategies would be required to shift the whole community and to encourage everyone to expend a little more energy as part of their day.

Frameworks for Promoting Physical Activity: A Typology of Physical Activity Interventions

There are different ways of conceptualizing physical activity programs based on settings, target or population groups, or the type of program being offered. There are also differences in the underpinning theory or proposed mechanism for change and the outcomes that are being changed through the program. Irrespective of the purpose, there has been a dramatic increase in the number of published physical activity interventions in the scientific literature, especially since the 1996 U.S. Surgeon General's report (U.S. Department of Health and Human Services, 1996; *see* Text Box 16.1 and Fig. 16.1). This reflects increased interest in the area but also an increasing diversity of research methods, ranging from smaller scale clinical interventions to broad programs targeting whole communities.

Box 16.1 Is there an increase in published physical activity interventions?

How many more physical activity interventions have been published since the U.S. Surgeon General's report on physical activity and health? A brief bibliometric analysis examined trends in published physical activity interventions since 1960. Before 1996, the term "physical activity" was used infrequently, and the term "exercise program" was a more frequent descriptor. The approach used in Figure 16.1 was non-selective, with all studies included and no stratification by group or target population size. This trend depicts the recent explosion of interventions specifically in "physical activity," increasing from around 12 published interventions annually in the early 1990s to over 175 per year in the period from 2000 onward. Different search terms produce slightly different findings, but the exponential increase is consistently seen. More interventions are conducted and reported, as the issue of inactivity becomes a public health priority and receives more research funding (Healthy People 2010 objectives). This makes the research quality even more important—good designs will produce policy-relevant information for decision makers. Indifferent research methods will not contribute to the evidence base.

Some of the research issues relevant to physical activity program evaluation are evident from a consideration of the examples in Table 16.1. These interventions are described in terms of their setting and target population size, from individual level interventions to macro-level policy and environmental changes. All have the broad objectives of increasing physical activity for those that attend, participate, or access the intervention but reach different sized target groups. Table 16.1 shows some examples of programs in each category of settings as well as some target population, selection, and measurement issues germane to each type of program.

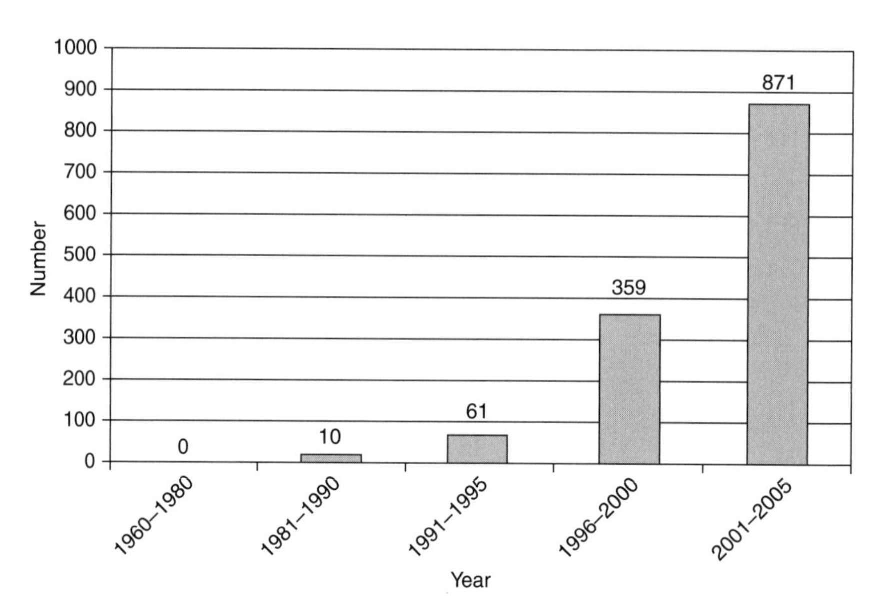

Figure 16.1 Bibliometric analysis—trends in the number of "physical activity" interventions published in the peer-reviewed literature between 1960 and 2005. Medline, PsychINFO, CINAHL, and SPORTDiscus were searched for physical activity interventions; duplicate studies were excluded. Search terms used included keywords "physical activity," and MESH terms included "Program Evaluation or Randomized Controlled Trial(s) or Intervention Studies." A total of 1301 interventions published from 1960 to 2005 were identified.

Until the 1995 CDC/ACSM recommendation on physical activity and health (Pate et al., 1995), most programs addressed physical activity from an individual-change perspective, where people were reached as individuals, or in an organization such as a worksite. Individual information, counseling, or structured group programs were attended by selected groups of individuals who enrolled in the intervention or received resources. In recent years, other types of programs have developed, including broader policy and environmental change

Table 16.1 Interventions to Promote Physical Activity

Settings for intervention	*Examples of intervention*	*Size and attributes of target*	*Examples of published interventions*
Physical activity interventions targeting individuals	Personal trainers	Volunteers; motivated; can afford to pay	Few published intervention studies
	Individualized programs for people with or at risk of chronic disease	High-risk individuals	Motl et al., 2005a; Pinto et al., 2005
	Individual mailed materials/website	Volunteers; motivated to participate; may have larger population reach	Plotnikoff et al., 2005; Rydell et al., 2005
	Physician or professional counseling	Individualized; potential for larger population reach	Little et al., 2004; Marshall et al., 2005; Hillsdon et al., 2002; van Sluijs et al., 2005
Group programs	Group physical activity programs for people with or without chronic conditions; gym- or health center-based group programs; worksite group programs for volunteers	May be high-risk groups; willing to attend the group sessions for the duration of the program	Diabetes Prevention Program (DPP) Research Group, 2002; Stigglebout et al., 2004
Organizational or community level physical activity interventions	School or whole worksite programs	May target whole schools or worksites—nonselective	Luepker et al., 1996; Proper et al., 2003; Yancey et al., 2004
	Local community programs, faith-based programs; special or disadvantaged populations	Community setting for accessing larger groups, including specific disadvantaged or minority populations	Resnicow et al., 2002; Fisher and Li, 2004; Nguyen et al., 2003; Reijneveld et al., 2003
Large-scale, whole community or population-level interventions	Mass media campaigns; national programs/ national guidelines implementation	Reach large populations with information and health promoting physical activity messages	Marshall et al., 2004; Bauman et al., 2001, 2003; Huhman et al., 2005
	Environmental change interventions; policy interventions; collaborative/integrated interagency partnerships	Make changes to physical environment, regulation and policy changes to improve physical activity environments or facilities; outcomes may be measured at individual or supra-individual level	Merom et al., 2003; Evenson et al., 2005; Brownson et al., 2004; Sallis et al., 2003

strategies and partnerships beyond the health sector. Potential partners include government agencies such as parks, sport and recreation, school education, transportation, urban planning, and the private sector. For many public health approaches to physical activity, these agencies have become the effector arm of physical activity initiatives, and the health sector may have a catalytic facilitator role.

There are also differences in the outcome measures for different interventions. Individual level and group programs may seek to influence objective measures of cardiorespiratory fitness, muscle strength, or other metabolic outcomes. Group programs often consist of structured exercise programs, with a fixed duration (such as attendance twice weekly for 12 weeks). Objective measures of physical activity are usual in these individual and group studies. Broader programs attempt to change the behaviors of physical activity and sedentarism, with mass reach programs such as media campaigns changing community awareness and understanding and setting the agenda for behavior change. At the largest scale, national level physical activity programs might comprise influencing inter-agency partnerships, monitoring policy changes, and creating environmental enhancements that support physical activity.

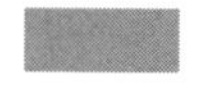

Methodology for Evaluating Physical Activity Interventions

Principles of Program Evaluation Applied to Physical Activity

Evaluation is the process of judging the worth or value of a single intervention or of a whole program of work to address a problem. For physical activity, evaluation of the overall efforts to promote physical activity can be conceptualized in several phases, starting with an initial scene setting to justify the intervention to decision makers, funding bodies, or regional health or other agencies (phase i). Phases ii through iv are the stages of evaluation of an individual program, which is tested under ideal or real-world conditions (efficacy or effectiveness trials). Phase v follows after the results of the individual program are known and relate to the replication, dissemination, and institutionalization of the program.

The stages in a comprehensive program are indicated here (adapted from Nutbeam and Bauman, 2006):

i. Developing the case and rationale for intervention; writing proposals; and seeking support for the program to be developed.
ii. Formative evaluation—assessing the development of the intervention, resources and materials. Is it developed using a theoretical framework? Are the components pilot tested with experts and with people similar to the target group? The development of a logic model is also part of the program-planning phase, to document in advance the anticipated program elements, inputs, and expected outputs for each component. This is important in planning multistrategy interventions, so that each can be monitored for both implementation and impact.
iii. Process evaluation (also known as implementation evaluation) starts when the intervention is launched and is (usually qualitative) monitoring of the program delivery, receipt of the intervention by the target group, monitoring of attendance/ participation in the intervention components, fidelity (intervention delivered as designed), and satisfaction with the program by stakeholders, professionals and the target audience.
iv. Impact and outcome evaluation is scientific appraisal of the achievement of the intervention objectives using reliable and valid outcome measures and using epidemiological criteria for causality. Impact evaluation is usually short term and

includes changes in awareness of the physical activity message, beliefs about physical activity, cognitive measures of intention or self-efficacy, and behavioral physical activity measures. Outcome evaluation is longer term and usually implies changes in health status, such as falls prevented, or incident cases of diabetes averted. Economic evaluation may be conducted here, assessing the costs of interventions relative to each other or the cost savings attributable to a given intervention (Sturm, 2005; Wang et al., 2005).

v. Following the evaluation of the initial intervention, if it has been shown to be effective, can the effects be replicated in other populations? Can the intervention be generalized to the wider community? If it is widely adopted, can it become institutionalized without the need for investigators to continue to advocate for it? (Glasgow et al., 2003).

For example, the Child and Adolescent Trial for Cardiovascular Health (CATCH) program, a comprehensive physical activity and nutrition intervention, was developed using best practice principles for elementary schoolchildren (Zucker et al., 1995; Perry et al., 1997) and was then tested in 96 schools across the United States (Luepker et al., 1996). It was shown to be effective in increasing moderate-to-vigorous physical activity among participants at 2 years follow-up and was then disseminated to hundreds of schools across the Texas school system (Hoelscher et al., 2001). Aspects of the CATCH program were found to be institutionalized 5 years after the main research trial, although the implementation of the whole program was less than desirable (Hoelscher et al., 2004). A next step would be if its delivery were to become part of ongoing educational policy across the region.

Several approaches have been made to summarize effective physical activity interventions. The most comprehensive and systematic reviews were conducted by the CDC within a larger prevention review, known as the Community Guide to Preventive Services (Kahn et al., 2002). This series of systematic reviews concluded that point of decision prompts (such as stair promotion signs), community-wide interventions, school-based curriculum programs, social support interventions, and individual behavior change programs were strongly recommended (Kahn et al., 2002). New areas of environmental interventions were considered promising but were based on changing environments and policies in small-scale ways in worksites and regulated settings—with minimal perspective on external validity. The overall field of environments and physical activity is of great interest at present, but the evidence can be summarized as ecological associations within cross-sectional datasets, with very few intervention studies. Further evidence of the impact of building trails, redesigning urban space, and encouraging active commuting remains to be demonstrable as effective population-wide approaches (Bauman, 2005). A critique of the overall evidence is beyond the scope of this chapter, but maintaining a critical appraisal perspective is important for physical activity intervention research to ensure that realistic policy decisions are made on affordable, achievable, and generalizable interventions.

As an alternate conceptual framework, an adaptation of a CDC-developed logic model is shown in Text Box 16.2. This model describes the first four stages of the aforementioned evaluation framework, using a logic model approach; here, the process and impact outcomes are described in a slightly different way. These are developed before the program starts, as a roadmap for assessing the implementation and effects of an intervention.

Optimizing Research Designs

Evaluation is essential for determining program effects and providing the evidence base for policy. A key element of whether the intervention caused the observed outcomes is the quality of the study design. Experimental evidence, from randomized controlled trials,

Box 16.2 Logic model. Steps for evaluating physical activity programs. (Adapted from: Physical Activity Evaluation Handbook. CDC, 2002. http://www.cdc.gov/nccdphp/dnpa/physical/handbook [Accessed March 2008])

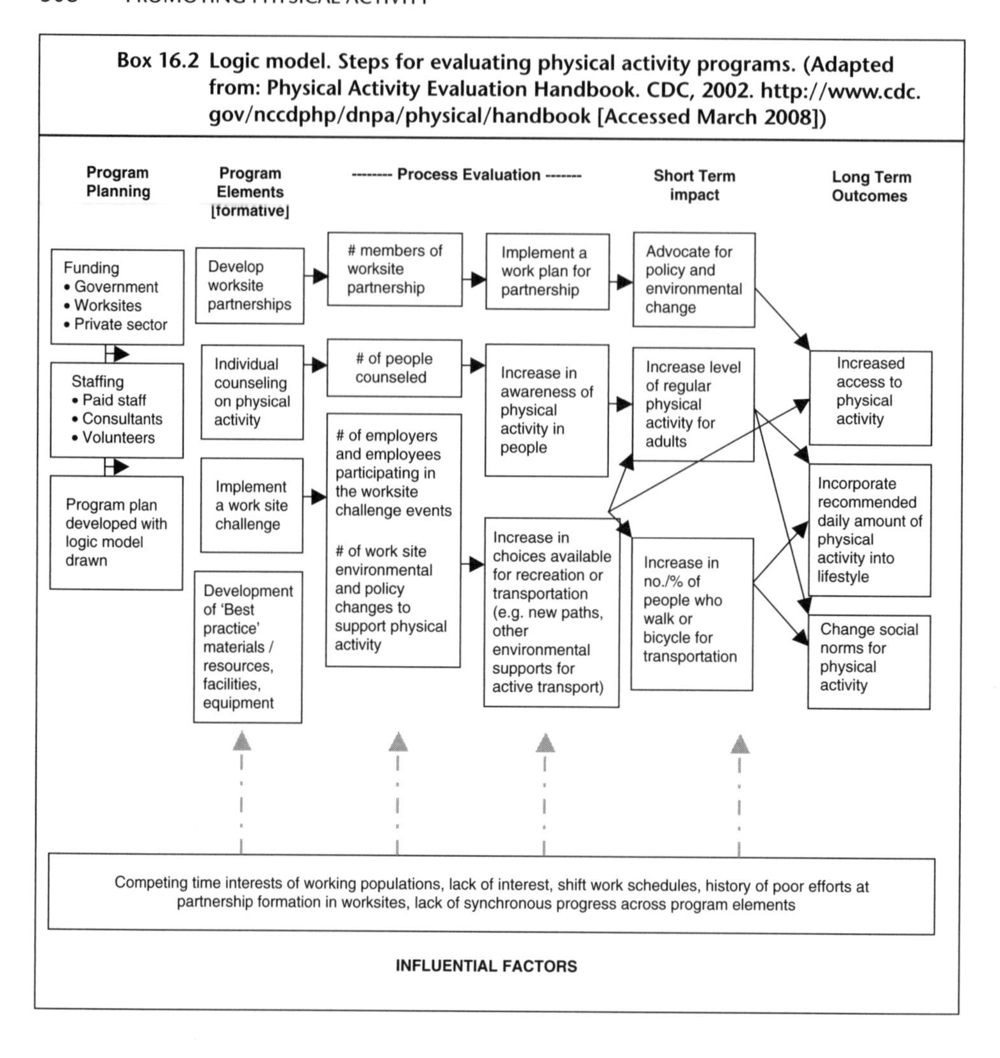

provides the strongest evidence of efficacy. This design is possible in settings that can be tightly controlled, such as clinical settings or other individual-level interventions, where people can be randomly allocated to intervention or control groups. An extension of this design is the cluster or group randomized controlled trials, where communities or organizational units such as worksites, schools, or medical practices can be randomly allocated; this design allocates at the group level, so special analytic techniques are required to adjust for the within-group correlation of outcomes (Bauman and Koepsall, 2005). If exposures and outcomes are comparable across studies, the pooled effects can be estimated through meta-analysis; this increases the statistical power over that within an individual study. However, given the varied nature of physical activity outcome measurements, it is often difficult to formally pool studies. Sometimes this has been attempted, and one example has provided evidence for the lack of clear effects on physical activity following worksite interventions (Dishman et al., 1998).

Evaluation designs other than randomized trials are often required in health promotion because of practical limitations preventing randomization. For example, it may not be possible to randomize in evaluating a national or large-scale regional intervention. The complex and multicomponent parts of an a priori-planned, community-wide intervention or mass media campaign may preclude randomization, or even if comparison communities

Experimental designs

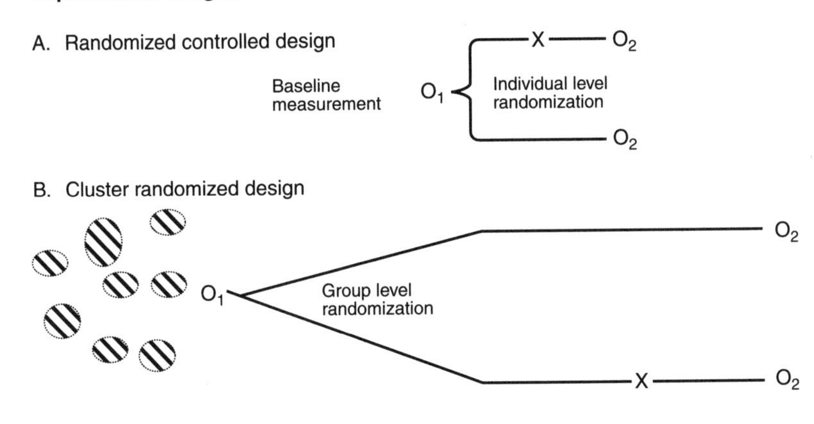

C. Meta analyses
Pooled data from multiple studies (for intervention meta analyses, usually pooling of randomized controlled trials)

Pre-experimental and quasi-experimental designs

D. Before–After with no control group [pre experimental] — O_1------X------O_2

E. Before–After with control group — O_1------X------O_2 Intervention
O_1--------------O_2 Control

F. Time series design — O_1---O_2---O_3---X---O_4---O_5---O_6

G. Time series design with control group — O_1---O_2---O_3---X---O_4---O_5---O_6
O_1---O_2---O_3-------O_4---O_5---O_6

Figure 16.2 Research designs for physical activity programs.
O_n is the nth measurement (observation) of individuals or groups, such as a physical activity questionnaire or interview or more objective measure of fitness or other outcome.
X = intervention

are chosen, there may be too few units to randomize. Community interventions may take years to produce the complex set of changes required to influence whole populations, and randomization cannot be maintained for that length of time. In these situations, quasi-experimental designs are used, whereby individuals or groups are non-randomly allocated to intervention or control (Fig. 16.2). The most limited evidence comes from pre-experimental designs, such as before–after studies, but for national campaigns this may be all that is possible (e.g., Hillsdon et al., 2001), although regional controls are possible (Bauman et al., 2001; Reger-Nash et al., 2005). The key issues are to match control communities to be as similar as possible to intervention communities, so that unknown or known confounders are unlikely to be a problem in assessing intervention effects. The addition of multiple pre-intervention measurement points, called a time series design, is a methodological strength, and study design can be further enhanced by adding time series measures in a control site as well.

For interventions promoting physical activity, quasi-experimental designs are used to evaluate whole-community programs as well as primary care-, worksite-, and school-based interventions (e.g., Smith et al., 2000; Kronenfeld et al., 1987; Baxter et al., 1997). The latter three examples could be assessed using randomized controlled trials or cluster randomized controlled trials if resources are available and the investigators can influence the design (Proper et al., 2003; Luepker et al., 1996; Elley et al., 2003).

The notion of "causality" is central—did the intervention cause the changes to physical activity to occur? Although experimental design studies are best, there are other causal criteria that, in concert with a well-designed quasi-experiment, do suggest that the effects result from the intervention. Matching of control groups is important, because it reduces confounding that might contribute to the observed differences. Theoretically well-designed programs, based on good formative evaluation, provide "causal evidence" analogous to biologic plausibility. As in all science, the effect size is important—how much better did the intervention do compared to controls? Is the difference of both statistical and practical significance? Replication of similar effects across studies also supports the intervention—this is phase v of the evaluation steps, where the program is tested in different settings to see if it still works prior to widespread dissemination.

Finally, understanding the processes of what happened, how the program was implemented, and who attended and participated is an important contributor to assessing outcomes. If few of the intervention group attended or read the resources, then a non-significant result is expected. Other types of research methods are starting to explore the factors leading to positive outcomes; this is the analysis of intervening causal variables or mediators. For example, did those who changed their physical activity level do so via a change in confidence that they could be active? The approaches to mediator analysis are increasingly using new psychometric statistical techniques to explore the strength and direction of mediator effects (Bauman et al., 2002; Motl et al., 2005b).

Other Epidemiological Issues in Assessing Physical Activity Programs

Physical Activity Measurement Principles for Interventions

The same measurement principles apply to the measurement of physical activity interventions as in other studies, such as in longitudinal epidemiological studies or in surveillance (*see also* Chapters 2–4 and 7 for additional discussion). Measures should be repeatable, should show good test–retest agreement, and should show criterion or construct validity.

It is essential to ensure that physical activity measures capture the intervention target behavior as specifically as possible; for example, a generic total physical activity measure is less likely to demonstrate change if the intervention specifically targeted walking. Similarly, a measure of leisure-time physical activity may not be influenced in a program encouraging active transport, where the domain of the targeted behaviors (walking or cycling as part of routine travel) may be outside the scope of the leisure-time physical activity measure. Measures should be reliable, valid, and responsive, the latter being the capacity of the measure to respond acutely to change. Note that criterion validity may be reduced when domains of incidental physical activity are concerned, as there are no objective criteria against which to compare; the intensity and duration of "increased walking in everyday tasks" may be insufficient to change "gold standard" or objective criteria, such as fitness levels or percentage of body fat. However, the use of accelerometers or pedometers that measure the behavior more accurately may be a preferable alternative for validation, as well as being objective outcome measures themselves (see also Chapter 3 for additional discussion).

Self-reported measures, such as beliefs or other cognitive measures, are regularly used in physical activity program evaluation. These may require psychometric statistical techniques to assess their internal consistency, factor structure, or construct validation, because they usually measure phenomena that are not directly observable. Other outcome measures may be beyond the level of assessments at the individual level. For example, measures of policy, organizational outcomes, or measures of the physical environment may be relevant to physical activity interventions. Some of this is qualitative (such as policy measurement—it is typically categorized as present/ absent policy—and, perhaps, the degree of implementation or uptake). Measures of the physical environment can be self-reported perceptions of the environment or objective measures—for example, using Geographic Information Systems, which provide accurate spatial data. For interventions, objective measurements of trail usage or of other facilities could be carried out using Global Position System and accelerometer measurement at the individual level or by external infrared or other trail monitoring devices. Indirect measures such as stair usage, bikeway traffic, or facility or park users is useful only at the aggregate level, because it may reflect increased use by those who are already active, rather than new users in the population.

Some self-reported physical activity measurements have the potential for measurement error. The first is social desirability, where people will report what they want the investigators to hear. Second, is pretest sensitization, where asking the same sets of questions multiple times has a training effect, such that responses may become more accurate or fatigue may set in, but subsequent answers result partly from the previous completion of the same instrument. Other sources of error, such as the Hawthorne effect and the potential for regression to the mean, are true of many health promotion measures. Therefore, many interventions attempt to have some degree of objective assessment or to have more than one self-reported measure to be able to *triangulate* the results from different measures of similar outcomes.

Physical activity may change over several years through natural development, maturation, and changes in socioeconomic positions—for example, increases in strength or fitness through adolescence and these trends being reversed in older age. Thus, multiyear interventions would need to adjust for these, and other secular effects, such as national strategies contaminating control regions. These secular effects may reduce the power of community-wide interventions, but estimating their magnitude in advance is not possible (Bauman and Koepsall, 2005). These are challenges in field studies of physical activity, where there is increasing interest everywhere and where *de novo* interventions may arise in control regions or there is contamination from the media coverage of the intervention communities, and these problems are increasingly difficult to prevent.

The Concept of Population Reach

Epidemiology, as the research discipline underpinning public health, is particularly concerned with research evidence around population level change. Although epidemiologic methods can be applied to clinical interventions, or even to genetic or physiological studies of exercise, the purpose of this chapter is to discuss epidemiologic issues in population-level approaches to increasing physical activity. Given that the magnitude of the program effects in optimally controlled studies are important, it is also important to consider the concept of reach into the population. The number of people in a group who engage with or access the intervention is a measure of its reach (Glasgow et al., 1999).

The notion of whether the program is efficacious for those who participate has also been termed "internal validity." This establishes the best causal evidence possible between program and outcomes (Glasgow et al., 2003). The idea of program reach has been termed "external validity." This is related to the extent to which the results in the study are able to be generalized to the wider population—in other words, was the intervention sample similar enough to the total population that if the intervention were conducted in the wider community, similar effects would be produced? A hypothetical example is shown in Text Box 16.3.

Box 16.3 A hypothetical primary care intervention—assessing population reach

A public health impact is based on reach and effectiveness or effect size. Assume a community has 50000 sedentary adult inhabitants and 100 physicians (i.e., 500 people/physician). For this example, population reach depends on the number of adults who participate but, even more importantly, on the number of physicians who provide physical activity advice.
Assume there are two interventions, a proven intervention (with, say, an effect size of increasing physical activity by 10%) and a less effective "brief counseling" minimal intervention (effect size to increase physical activity by 3%).
Low reach: If only 5% of these physicians counseled their patients about physical activity, the "reach" to the whole community is relatively small. Assume these 5% of physicians delivered the "proven" intervention to all their patients. Here the impact would be small (increasing activity in 10% of the people attending the five interested physicians, and of these 2500 people, only around 250 adults would increase their physical activity levels, or 0.5% of the total population).
By contrast, the minimal intervention (3% improvement) will have a larger population impact if delivered by half of all the physicians in the community—here, if delivered by 50 physicians to 25,000 people; in this scenario, 3%, or 750 adults, would increase their activity level. This is three times as great an effect as the intensive intervention only taken up by five doctors, These ideas of population reach are central to the understanding of population-level impact and highlight key issues in efforts to increase physical activity.

Conclusions

A Conceptual Model of Research, Science, and Evaluation Practice for Physical Activity Promotion

There is an ongoing tension between researcher- and practitioner-related approaches in public health and health promotion, and physical activity interventions are no exception. Practitioners traditionally carry out "program evaluation," which is more focused on accountability, meeting the needs of stakeholders, focusing on quality control of programs, and having limited interest in research design, measurement, and optimal statistical analyses. In contrast, university researchers and academicians place ultimate faith in the experimental design and careful measurement, dealing with selection effects of dropouts and confounders through careful multivariate analyses. Although this is realistic for controlled studies of structured exercise programs, it is unlikely to make a population difference. To deal with the real-world, public health problems of inactivity, one needs to cross these artificial research/practice boundaries and to think like an epidemiologist, but this thinking needs to be applied pragmatically in the context of the real-world situations, environments, and time pressures that people present as barriers to physical activity.

The best compromise is to aspire to the best methodological solutions to the problems posed by multicomponent community interventions, within budgets that may be insufficient for perfect science. Compromise needs to become a new term for field epidemiologists, with slightly more flexibility in research designs, tolerance for some level of study dropouts, and acceptance of self-reported measures in population research. All of these can be tightly controlled in clinical or laboratory interventions. For example, assessing the impact of a walking/biking trail on physical activity levels may be opportunistic research, and not all design issues may be achievable, but the "best possible" research methods will be a large leap forward to generating better evidence from practice (Glasgow et al., 1999).

A summary of the decision-making processes required is shown as a "Rubik's cube" in Figure 16.3. The first step is whether the program is likely to make a public health impact based on its target population size and composition. Is the intervention likely to be effective,

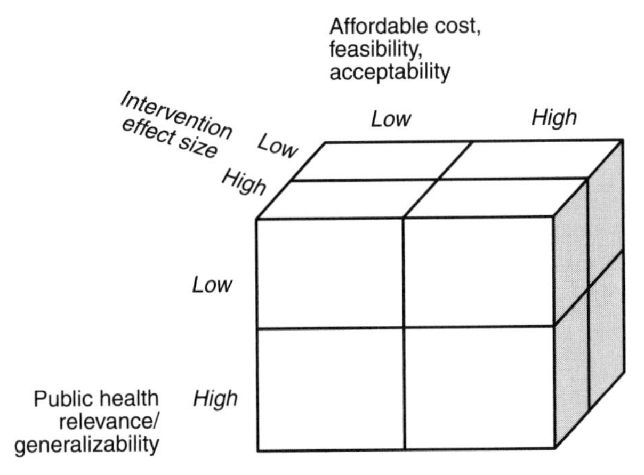

Figure 16.3 The "Rubik cube" model of developing population health-relevant research: integrating research, science, and evaluation practice.

represented by the effect size axis? Finally, is it relatively low-cost and feasible? The best public health approach would have high generalizability, high effectiveness, and high feasibility and affordability. This is a set of judgments, with contributions from both epidemiologist and policymaker. For example, a trail that is being built by a conservation agency might be affordable and feasible, theoretically would have a small-to-moderate effect size acting on the whole population, and would be cost-effective. In this example, the epidemiologist could then utilize a time series research design that included matched control sites, objective and self-reported measures, and sample the whole surrounding population, not just trail users. It is about compromise, with the trade-off between internal and external validity.

Moving Forward

To appraise population-level efforts to promote physical activity, researchers need to focus on innovative methods for the design and measurement of studies with high external validity or studies of program replication or dissemination. The technical aspects to support this include better measurements of physical activity and physical environments using objective measures at the individual and ecologic levels. More efforts should be made to explore process evaluation and to improve understanding of "how programs work"; the epidemiological methods to do this are being developed through increased attention to intervening causal variables and to effect modifiers in physical activity programs (Bauman et al., 2002). New designs should be applied to program assessment, including time series quasi-experiments, with multiple pre-intervention measures. The use of population surveillance measures at the state or national level (such as the Behavioral Risk Factor Surveillance System in the United States) in program evaluation could be developed; here, the community-wide intervention will be monitored through state-level population surveys over several years. Researchers will need to become advocates for funding and publishing studies that attempt public health change; this involves going beyond only accepting research papers based on the "best science" for internally valid studies but assessing components of external validity, such as program reach and uptake (Glasgow et al., 2003), as central to public health effectiveness. Finally, the areas of evidence generation—especially environment and policy interventions—remain unproven (Bauman, 2005), and despite repeated cross-sectional and significant associations, there is limited known intervention effectiveness; the design and conduct of these macro-level studies is the greatest research challenge for the future but is evidence that a plethora of agencies and policymakers most urgently need.

Personal Perspective

The ongoing tension between maximizing scientific rigor and the need for public health-relevant interventions has impeded progress toward the evaluation of programs to increase physical activity levels. Despite consistent epidemiological evidence for the health-enhancing benefits of physical activity, gaps in the evidence base remain for understanding the effects of physical activity interventions and for generalizing that information to wider populations, organizations, and settings. To assess the effects of programs to increase physical activity, all the traditional elements of epidemiology are required, including minimizing selection bias, using good measures, and considering confounders. Research designs should be optimal but cannot always be randomized trials in field settings. Finding the right compromise in conceptual and methodologic approaches between "health promotion" and "disease prevention research" will enhance the translation of evidence into practice. Making the boundaries between "research" and "evaluation" more fuzzy, with funding of the best possible research methods applied to practical settings, may substantively contribute to interventions that increase physical activity at the population level.

References

ACSM. American College of Sports Medicine. 1990. Position stand: the recommended quantity and quality of exercise for developing and maintaining cardiorespiratory and muscular fitness in healthy adults. *Med Sci Sports Exerc* 22: 265–74.

Bauman A, Bellew B, Owen N, Vita P. 2001. Impact of an Australian mass media campaign targeting physical activity in 1998. *Am J Prev Med* 21: 41–7.

Bauman AE, Sallis JF, Dzewaltowski DA, Owen N. 2002. Toward a better understanding of the influences on physical activity: the role of determinants, correlates, causal variables, mediators, moderators, and confounders. *Am J Prev Med* 23(2S): 5–14.

Bauman A, McLean G, Hurdle D, et al. 2003. Evaluation of the national 'Push Play' campaign in New Zealand—creating population awareness of physical activity. *N Zeal Med J* 116: U535.

Bauman A, Craig CL, Cameron C. 2005. Low levels of recall among adult Canadians of the CSEP/Health Canada physical activity guidelines. *Can J Applied Physiol* 30: 246–52.

Bauman A. 2005. The physical environment and physical activity: moving from ecological associations to intervention evidence. *J Epidemiol Commun Health* 59: 535–6.

Bauman A, Koepsall TD. 2005. Epidemiologic Issues in Community Interventions. In RC Brownson, D Petiti (Eds.), *Applied Epidemiology: Theory to Practice*, 2nd Edition 2005, Oxford University Press.

Baxter AP, Milner PC, Hawkins S. et al. 1997. The impact of heart health promotion on coronary heart disease lifestyle risk factors in schoolchildren: lessons learnt from a community-based project. *Public Health* 111: 131–7.

Brownson RC, Baker EA, Boyd RL, et al. 2004. A community-based approach to promoting walking in rural areas. *Am J Prev Med* 27: 28–34.

CDC. Centers for Disease Control and Prevention. US Department of Health and Human Services. *Physical Activity Evaluation Handbook.* Atlanta, GA: US Department of Health and Human Services, 2002. http://www.cdc.gov/nccdphp/dnpa (accessed December 2005).

Craig CL. Russell SJ, Cameron C, Bauman A. 2004. Twenty–Year trends in physical activity among Canadian Adults. *Can J Publ Health* 95(1): 59–63.

Diabetes Prevention Program (DPP) Research Group. 2002. The Diabetes Prevention Program (DPP): description of lifestyle intervention. Diabetes Care 25(12): 2165–2171.

Dishman RK, Oldenburg B, O'Neal H, Shephard RJ. 1998. Worksite Physical Activity Interventions. *Am J Prev Med* 15: 344–61.

Elley CR, Kerse N, Arroll B, Robinson E. 2003. Effectiveness of counselling patients on physical activity in general practice: cluster randomised controlled trial. *Br Med J* 12;326(7393): 793.

Evenson KR, Herring A, Huston S. 2005. Evaluating change in physical activity with the building of a multi-use trail. *Am J Prev Med* 28(2s): 177–85.

Fisher KJ, Li F. 2004. A community-based walking trial to improve neighborhood quality of life in older adults: a multilevel analysis. *Ann Behav Med* 28(3): 186–94.

Glasgow RE, Vogt TM, Boles SM. 1999. Evaluating the public health impact of health promotion interventions: the REAIM framework. *Am J Publ Health* 89(9): 1322–7.

Glasgow RE, Lichtenstein E, Marcus AC. 2003. Why don't we see more translation of health promotion research to practice? Rethinking the efficacy-to-effectiveness transition. *Am J Publ Health* 93(8): 1261–7.

Haase A, Steptoe A, Sallis JF, Wardle J. 2004. Leisure-time physical activity in university students from 23 countries: associations with health beliefs, risk awareness, and national economic development. *Prev Med* 39(1): 182–90.

Hillsdon M, Cavill N, Nanchahal K, et al. 2001. National level promotion of physical activity: results from England's ACTIVE for LIFE campaign. J Epidemiol Commun Health 55: 755–61.

Hillsdon M, Thorogood M, White I, Foster C. 2002. Advising people to take more exercise is ineffective: a randomized controlled trial of physical activity promotion in primary care. *Intern J Epidemiol* 31: 808–15.

Hoelscher DM, Kelder SH, Murray N, et al. 2001. Dissemination and adoption of the Child and Adolescent Trial for Cardiovascular Health (CATCH): a case study in Texas. *J Publ Health Man Prac* 7(2): 90–100.

Hoelscher DM, Feldman HA, Johnson CA, et al. 2004. School-based health education programs can be maintained over time: results from the CATCH Institutionalization study. *Prev Med* 38: 594–606.

Huhman M, Potter LD, Wong FL, et al. 2005. Effects of a mass media campaign to increase physical activity among children: Year 1 results of the VERB campaign. *Pediatrics* 116(2): e277–84.

Kahn E, Ramsey L, Brownson R, et al. 2002. The effectiveness of interventions to increase physical activity. A systematic review. *Am J Prev Med* 22(4s): 73–107.

Kronenfeld JJ, Jackson K, Blair SN, et al. 1987. Evaluating health promotion: a longitudinal quasi-experimental design. *Health Education Quarte*r 14(2): 123–39.

Little P, Dorward M, Gralton S, et al. 2004. A randomised controlled trial of three pragmatic approaches to initiate increased physical activity in sedentary patients with risk factors for cardiovascular disease. *Br J Gen Prac* 54(500): 189–95.

Luepker RV, Perry CL, McKinlay SM, et al. 1996. Outcomes of a field trial to improve children's dietary patterns and physical activity: the Child and Adolescent Trial for Cardiovascular Health (CATCH). *JAMA* 275: 768–776.

Marshall AL, Bauman AE, Owen N, et al. 2004. Reaching out to promote physical activity in Australia: a statewide randomized controlled trial of a stage-targeted intervention. *Am J Health Promot* 18(4): 283–287.

Marshall AL, Booth ML, Bauman AE. 2005. Promoting physical activity in Australian general practices: a randomised trial of health promotion advice versus hypertension management. *Pat Educ Counsel* 56(3): 283–90.

Merom D, Bauman A, Vita P, Close G. 2003. An environmental intervention to promote walking and cycling—the impact of a newly constructed Rail Trail in Western Sydney. *Prev Med* 36(2): 235–42.

Motl RW, Konopack JF, McAuley E, et al. 2005a. Depressive symptoms among older adults: long-term reduction after a physical activity intervention. *J Behav Med* 28: 385–94.

Motl RW, Dishman RK, Ward DS, et al. 2005b. Perceived physical environment and physical activity across one year among adolescent girls: self-efficacy as a possible mediator? *J Adolesc Health* 37: 403–8.

Nguyen MN, Gauvin L, Martineau I, Grignon R. 2003. Sustainability of the impact of a public health intervention: lessons learned from the Laval walking clubs experience. *Health Promot Prac* 6(1): 44–52.

Nutbeam D, Bauman A. 2006. *Evaluation in a Nutshell.* McGraw-Hill Sydney 2006.

Pate RR, Pratt M, Blair SN, Haskell WL, et al. 1995. Physical activity and public health. A recommendation from the Centers for Disease Control and Prevention and the American College of Sports Medicine. *JAMA* 273: 402–7.

Perry CL, Sellers DE, Johnson E, et al. 1997. The Child and Adolescent Trial for Cardiovascular Health (CATCH): intervention, implementation, and feasibility for elementary schools in the United States. *Health Educ Behav* 24: 716–35.

Pinto BM, Frierson GM, Rabin C, et al. 2005. Home-based physical activity intervention for breast cancer patients. J Clin Oncol 23(15): 3577–87.

Plotnikoff RC, McCargar LJ, Wilson PM, Loucaides CA. 2005. Efficacy of an E-mail intervention for the promotion of physical activity and nutrition behavior in the workplace context. *Am J Health Prom* 19(6): 422–9.

Proper KI, Hildebrandt VH, Van der Beek AJ, et al. 2003. Effect of individual counseling on physical activity fitness and health: a randomized controlled trial in a workplace setting. *Am J Prev Med* 24(3): 218–26.

Reger-Nash B, Bauman A, Butterfield-Booth S, et al. 2005. Wheeling Walks—long term evaluation. *Family Commun Health* 28(1): 64–78.

Reijneveld SA, Westhoff MH, Hopman-Rock M. 2003. Promotion of health and physical activity improves the mental health of elderly immigrants: results of a group randomised controlled trial among Turkish immigrants in the Netherlands aged 45 and over. *J Epidemiol Commun Health* 57(6): 405–11.

Resnicow K, Jackson A, Braithwaite R, et al. 2002. Healthy Body/Healthy Spirit: a church-based nutrition and physical activity intervention. *Health Educ Res* 17(5): 562–73.

Rose G. 2001. Sick individuals and sick populations. *Int J Epidemiol* 30: 427–32.

Rydell SA, French SA, Fulkerson JA, et al. 2005. Use of a web-based component of a nutrition and physical activity behavioral intervention with girl scouts. *J Am Diet Assoc* 105(9): 1447–50.

Sallis JF, McKenzie TL, Conway TL, et al. 2003. Environmental interventions for eating and physical activity: a randomized controlled trial in middle schools. *Am J Prev Med* 24(3): 209–17.

Smith BJ, Bauman AE, Bull F, et al. 2000. Promoting physical activity in general practice: a controlled trial of written advice and information materials. *Br J Sports Med* 34: 262–7.

Stiggelbout M, Popkema DY, Hopman-Rock M, et al. 2004. Once a week is not enough: effects of a widely implemented group based exercise programme for older adults; a randomised controlled trial. *J Epidemiol Commun Health* 58(2): 83–8.

Sturm R 2005. Economics and physical activity. *Am J Prev Med* 28(2S2): 141–9.

USDHHS. United States Department of Health and Human Services. 1996. *Physical activity and health: a report of the Surgeon General.* Atlanta, GA: U.S. Department of Health and Human Services, Centers for Disease Control and Prevention, National Center for Chronic Disease Prevention and Health Promotion.

van Sluijs EM, van Poppel MN, Twisk J, et al. 2005. Effect of a tailored physical activity intervention delivered in general practice settings: results of a randomized controlled trial. *Am J Publ Health* 95(10): 1825–31.

Wang G, Macera C, Scudder-Soucie B, et al. 2005. A cost-benefit analysis of physical activity using bike/pedestrian trails. *Health Prom Prac* 6(2): 174–9.

WHO. World Health Organization. 2002. *The World Health Report 2002—Reducing Risks, Promoting Healthy Life.* Geneva, Switzerland: World Health Organization.

WHO. World Health Organization. 2004. *Global Strategy on Diet, Physical Activity and Health.* 22 May 2004. WHA57.17. Geneva, Switzerland: World Health Organization.

Yancey AK, McCarthy WJ, Taylor WC, et al. 2004. The Los Angeles Lift Off: a sociocultural environmental change intervention to integrate physical activity into the workplace. *Preventive Med.* 38(6): 848–56.

Zucker DM, Lakatos E, Webber LS, et al. 1995. Statistical design of the Child and Adolescent Trial for Cardiovascular Health (CATCH): implications of cluster randomization. *Control Clin Trial* 16: 96–118.

Index